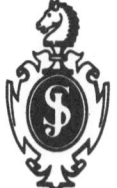

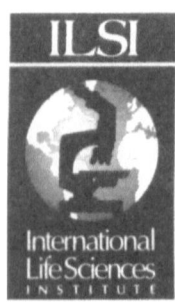

ILSI Human Nutrition Reviews

Series Editor: Ian Macdonald

Already published:

Sweetness
Edited by John Dobbing

Calcium in Human Biology
Edited by B.E.C. Nordin

Sucrose: Nutritional and Safety Aspects
Edited by Gaston Vettorazzi and Ian Macdonald

Zinc in Human Biology
Edited by C.F. Mills

Dietary Starches and Sugars in Man: A Comparison
Edited by John Dobbing

Diet and Behavior
Edited by G. Harvey Anderson, Norman A. Krasnegor,
Gregory D. Miller and Artemis P. Simopoulos

**Modern Lifestyles, Lower Energy Intake and
Micronutrient Status**
Edited by K. Pietrzik

Thirst: Physiological and Psychological Aspects
Edited by D.J. Ramsay and D.A. Booth

Dietary Fibre –
A Component of Food
Nutritional Function
in Health and Disease

Edited by Thomas F. Schweizer and
Christine A. Edwards

With 28 Figures

Springer-Verlag London Ltd.

Dr. Thomas F. Schweizer
Nestlé Research Centre, Nestec Ltd,
Vers-chez-les-Blanc, PO Box 44, CH-1000 Lausanne 26, Switzerland

Dr. Christine A. Edwards
Department of Human Nutrition, University of Glasgow,
Yorkhill Hospital, Glasgow G3 8SJ, UK

Series Editor
Ian MacDonald MD, DSc, PhD, FIBiol
Emeritus Professor of Applied Physiology
University of London, UK

ISBN 978-1-4471-1930-2   ISBN 978-1-4471-1928-9 (eBook)
DOI 10.1007/978-1-4471-1928-9

British Library Cataloguing in Publication Data
Dietary fibre – a component of food: nutritional function in health and disease
    (ILSI human nutrition)
I. Schweizer, Thomas F.   II. Edwards, Christine A.   III. Series
613.28

Library of Congress Cataloging-in-Publication Data
Dietary fibre: a component of food: nutritional function in health and disease/edited by Thomas F.
Schweizer, Christine A. Edwards.
    p. cm. – (ILSI human nutrition reviews)
Includes index.

1. Fiber in human nutrition.   I. Schweizer, Thomas F.   II. Edwards, Christine A. (Christine
Ann), 1959–.   III. Series
[DNLM: 1. Dietary Fiber–analysis.   2. Dietary Fiber–therapeutic use. WB 427 D5648]
QP143.D54 1992
612.3'96–dc20
DNLM/DLC   91–5132
for Library of Congress   CIP

© Springer-Verlag London 1992
    Originally published by Springer-Verlag London Ltd. 1992
Softcover reprint of the hardcover 1st edition 1992

Typeset by Genesis Typesetting, Laser Quay, Rochester, Kent, UK
28/3830–543210 Printed on acid-free paper

Foreword

Fibre, a non-nutrient component of the diet of man since time began, has over the last two decades come to assume an important role in the prevention of disease. There is no clinical condition that is associated with acute fibre deficiency, as with, say, protein, but as a component of the diet that plays a role in the prevention of disease, fibre is probably of considerable consequence.

To assess the current situation about the role of fibre in health and disease, the European branch of the International Life Sciences Institute (ILSI) convened a panel of distinguished scientists at an April 1991 workshop in Brussels. Well before the workshop, the panellists prepared chapters on a comprehensive range of subjects relating to fibre. Each participant was given the opportunity to read and comment on the other chapters, with the objective of producing a comprehensive, accurate, and up-to-date volume on the subject of fibre in health and disease.

This volume is one of a series concerned with topics of growing interest to those who want to increase their understanding of human nutrition. Written for workers in the nutritional and allied sciences rather than for the specialist, these volumes aim to fill the gap between the textbook on the one hand and the many publications addressed to the expert on the other. The target readership spans medicine, nutrition, and the biological sciences generally and includes those in the food, chemical, and allied industries who need to take account of advances in those fields relevant to their products.

ILSI, is a non-profit, world-wide scientific foundation with branches in each continent, established in 1978 to advance the understanding of scientific issues relating to nutrition, food safety, toxicology, and the environment. By bringing together scientists from academia, government, and industry, ILSI promotes a balanced approach to solving problems with broad implications for the well-being of the world community. Headquartered in Washington, D.C., ILSI has branches in Agentina, Brazil, Europe, Japan, Mexico, and North America.

London
April 1992

Ian Macdonald
Series Editor

Preface

This book is the result of a three day ILSI workshop on dietary fibre held in Brussels in spring 1991. Distinguished experts from all over Europe were invited by a Scientific Planning Committee (Chairman Professor Jean Mauron) to participate. Drafts of the individual chapters were written before the workshop and circulated to all participants for critical review. During the meeting these chapters were further discussed and edited. This often gave rise to substantial modifications and improvements of the original manuscripts and to written commentaries and sometimes authors' replies printed at the end of a chapter. In this way a unique collection of peer reviewed "state of the art" papers on dietary fibre has been obtained.

The General Discussion is a slightly shortened and edited account of the final workshop discussion which included practical issues such as definition, analysis, physico-chemical properties and energy values of dietary fibre. At a time when European legislation, directives and guidelines are being prepared, it seemed worthwhile to make this discussion available to the reader.

We wish to thank all the authors for contributing to such a demanding project. In several chapters, leading European scientists from different institutes and countries have successfully co-operated to present a balanced and objective assessment of their topic. Thanks to the indefatigable efforts of Professor Nils-Georg Asp, this was also possible for the most controversial subject of dietary fibre analysis which is co-authored by main representatives of analytical techniques presently in use.

We would also like to thank Dr. David Kritchevsky who chaired the whole workshop in a stimulating and sovereign way which was essential to the workshop's success.

Finally, we extend our thanks to ILSI Europe and its head office in Brussels, especially Professor Michel Fondu and Dr. Uta Priebe who were both excellent organisers and hosts of this conference. The publisher and series editor have kindly agreed to publish the product of all these efforts.

Lausanne and Glasgow
November 1991

Thomas Schweizer
Christine Edwards

Contents

List of Contributors xvii

SECTION I.   Background Papers

1. The Dietary Fibre Hypothesis: A Historical Perspective
D.A.T. Southgate 3
Introduction 3
Developments in the Chemistry and Analysis of Food
     Carbohydrates: Early Studies on the Chemistry of Foods   4
Concerns about the Energy Value of Foods 4
Studies on the Chemistry of Plant Cell Walls 5
Nutritional Studies on Food Carbohydrates 5
The Impact of New Techniques on the Study of Carbohydrates   7
The Energy Values of Carbohydrates in the Human Diet 8
Studies on the Analysis of Fibre 8
Dietary Fibre as a Protective Component of the Diet 9
The Dietary Fibre Hypothesis Emerges 10
Initial Responses to the Hypothesis 11
Major Themes in the Initial Development of the Dietary Fibre
     Hypothesis 13
    Definition and Analysis 13
    Studies with Isolated Polysaccharides 14
    Dietary Fibre as a Source of Energy 14
    Mechanism of Faecal Bulking 15
The Status of the Dietary Fibre Hypothesis 16
Commentary 19

2. Physico-chemical Properties of Food Plant Cell Walls
J.-F. Thibault, M. Lahaye and F. Guillon 21
Introduction 21
Ion-Exchange Properties 21
    The Ionic Groups Associated with Fibres 22
    Methods of Cation-Exchange Capacity Determination 23
    The Cation-Exchange Capacity Values 23
    Determination of pK 25

Hydration Properties 26
    Hydration Properties of Polysaccharides 26
    Methods for the Determination of Hydration Characteristics ... 27
    Variations of the Hydration Value 29
    Examples of Hydration Value 31
Adsorption of Organic Molecules 32
Effect of Processing 33
    Grinding 33
    Chemical Treatments 33
    Heat Treatment 34
Conclusions 34

3. Physico-chemical Properties of Food Polysaccharides
E.R. Morris 41
Introduction 41
Structure and Shape of Polysaccharide Chains 41
Order and Disorder 42
Inter-residue Linkage Patterns and Ordered Packing 43
Hydrated Networks 45
Polysaccharide "Weak Gels" 47
Hydrodynamic Volume of Disordered Polysaccharide Chains 47
Coil Overlap and Entanglement 48
Shear-Rate Dependence of Viscosity 50
Implications for Digesta Viscosity 51
Transport and Release of Nutrients 53
Susceptibility to Digestive Enzymes and Colonic Fermentation ... 54
Conclusions 54
Commentary 55

4. Dietary Fibre Analysis
N.-G. Asp, T.F. Schweizer, D.A.T. Southgate and O. Theander   57
Classification of Carbohydrates in Foods as Related to Dietary
        Fibre Analysis 57
    Principal Criteria for Classification 58
    Degree of Polymerisation 58
    Classification of the Polysaccharides 58
    Recommendations for Nomenclature for use in the
        Classification of Carbohydrates in Nutritional Studies ... 61
The Definition of Dietary Fibre: A Determinant of Analytical
        Strategy 62
    Main Features of Analytical Strategies 63
    Implications for the Choice of Analytical Methods for the
        Carbohydrates in Foods 64
    Criteria for the Choice of Method: The Conflict Between the
        Requirements of Research and Regulation 65
Development of Crude Fibre, Detergent Fibre and Enzymatic
        Methods 65
    Crude Fibre 66
    Detergent Fibre Methods 67

Enzymatic Methods 67
The Method of Asp et al. 69
The AOAC Method 69
The Various Steps in Enzymatic Gravimetric Methods 70
Comparison of Methods 72
Other Current Gravimetric Methods 72
The Southgate Method for Unavailable Carbohydrates 73
Principles 74
Performance 74
Limitations 75
Analysis of Individual Components of Dietary Fibre 75
Determination and Chemical Characterisation of Total
    Dietary Fibre by the Uppsala Methodology 77
Analysis and Characterisation of Soluble and Insoluble
    Dietary Fibre 79
Main Features of the Method of Englyst et al. 79
Alternatives for the Determination of Dietary Fibre
    Constituents 82
Collaborative Studies 85
Studies under Review and Performance Criteria 85
Total Dietary Fibre with Gravimetric Methods 89
Non-starch Polysaccharides with the Englyst Procedures 90
Separate Measurement of Insoluble and Soluble Dietary
    Fibre 91
Inter-method Comparisons 91
Summary and Conclusions 93
Note Added in Proof 99
The MAFF IV Study 99
The AOAC Method 100
Commentary 100

5. Gastro-intestinal Physiology and Function
N.W. Read and M.A. Eastwood 103
Introduction 103
How Do Non-starch Polysaccharides Reduce Absorption of
    Nutrients in the Small Intestine? 103
How Does Increasing the Viscosity of Gastro-intestinal
    Contents Delay Absorption? 103
Unresolved Issues 107
Can Non-starch Polysaccharides Reduce Absorption by
    Mechanisms Other than Increasing the Viscosity of
    Gastro-intestinal Contents? 109
Effects on the Colon 112
Increased Stool Output 112
Transit Time 113
Laxative Action of Sequestered Bile Acids and Fatty Acids   113
Direct Irritant Effect of Particles 113
Gas Formation 114
How does the Colon Adapt to Fibre? 115

6. Bacterial Fermentation in the Colon and Its Measurement
C.A. Edwards and I.R. Rowland 119
Introduction 119
Fermentation 119
Colonic Bacteria 119
Carbohydrate Fermentation by Gut Bacteria 120
    Dietary Fibre 120
    Oligosaccharides 122
    Resistant Starch 122
    Mucins and Mucopolysaccharide 122
    Enzymes Involved in Polysaccharide Degradation 123
Fermentation Products 123
    Short Chain Fatty Acids 123
    Products of Protein and Amino Acid Degradation 124
    Gaseous Products 125
Measurement of Colonic Fermentation In Vivo 125
    Human Models 125
    Patients with Colostomies 127
    Faecal Analysis 127
    Animal Models 127
Measurement of Colonic Fermentation In Vitro 128
    Static In Vitro Systems 129
    Continuous and Semi-continuous Culture Systems 130
    Studies of Carbohydrate Fermentation 131
Conclusions 132
Commentary 136

**7. Metabolism and Utilisation of Short Chain Fatty Acids
Produced by Colonic Fermentation**
C. Rémésy, C. Demigné and C. Morand 137
Background 137
Metabolism of SCFA by the Digestive Tract 137
Comparison of SCFA and Glucose Absorption 139
Hepatic Metabolism of SCFA 139
    Acetate Metabolism 141
    Propionate Metabolism 142
    Butyrate Metabolism 144
Extrasplanchnic Metabolism of Acetate 145
SCFA and Lipid Metabolism 145
Energy Aspects 146
Conclusion 147
Commentary 150

SECTION II. Physiological Effects

**8. The Influence of Dietary Fibre on Protein Digestion and
Utilisation**
B. O. Eggum 153
Introduction 153

Experiments with Rats 154
    Conclusion from Experiments with Rats 157
Experiments with Pigs 157
    Conclusion from Experiments with Pigs 159
Experiments with Humans 159
    Conclusion from Experiments with Humans 161
General Conclusion 161

9. The Influence of Dietary Fibre on Lipid Digestion and Absorption

I. T. Johnson 167
Introduction 167
Digestion and Absorption of Dietary Fat 167
Inhibition of Lipolytic Activity 169
Formation and Composition of Micelles 171
Effects of Fibre on Intraluminal Lipid Transport 172
The Cellular Phase: Adaptation to Prolonged Fibre Intake 174
Conclusions 176
Commentary 179

10. The Influence of Dietary Fibre on Carbohydrate Digestion and Absorption

B. Flourié 181
Introduction 181
Acute Effects of Dietary Fibre on Factors Affecting Digestion
    and Absorption of Carbohydrates 182
    Influence of Dietary Fibres on Gastric Emptying 182
    Influence of Dietary Fibres on Small Intestinal Digestion and
        Absorption 185
Chronic Effects of Dietary Fibre on Factors Affecting Digestion
    and Absorption of Carbohydrates 190
Conclusion 192
Commentary 196

11. The Influence of Dietary Fibre on Mineral Absorption and Utilisation

L. Rossander, A.-S. Sandberg and B. Sandström 197
Introduction 197
Methodological Considerations in Studies on Mineral
    Absorption in Humans 197
Effects of Fibre and Fibre-Associated Compounds on Mineral
    Absorption in Humans 198
    Effect of Non-starch Polysaccharides and Lignin 198
    Effect of Fibre-Associated Compounds 199
    Mineral Absorption from Fibre-Rich Diets 204
    Interactions Between Dietary Components 205
    The Significance of the Phytate Content in the Diet 206
The Influence of Food Processing on Mineral Absorption 207
    Extrusion Cooking 207

Soaking and Malting 207
Fermentation 208
The Possibility of Predicting Absorption Using In Vitro and
    Animal Models 208
In Vitro Studies 208
Animal Models 210
Conclusions 210
    Points of Consensus 210
    Implementation of Present Knowledge by the Food Industry
        and Legislative Bodies 211
    Areas for Future Research 211
Commentary 216

12. Dietary Fibre and Bile Acid Metabolism
F.M. Nagengast 217
Introduction 217
Bile Acid Metabolism 217
Colonic Carcinogenesis 218
    Fibre 218
    Fat 219
Dietary Fibre and Bile Acid Metabolism 219
    Fibre and Biliary Bile Acids 220
    Fibre and Faecal Bile Acids 223
Conclusions 228

13. Faecal Bulking and Energy Value of Dietary Fibre
E. Wisker and W. Feldheim 233
Introduction 233
Faecal Bulking Effect of Dietary Fibre 233
    Physico-chemical Properties 234
    Personality Factors 235
    Mechanisms of Action 235
    Conclusions 236
Energy Value of Dietary Fibre 236
    Estimation of the Digestible and Metabolisable Energy of
        Dietary Fibres 237
    Calculation of the Metabolisable Energy of Fibre-Rich Diets   241
Commentary 246

SECTION III. Prevention and Treatment of Disease

**14. Dietary Fibre in the Prevention and Treatment of
Gastro-intestinal Disorders**
K. W. Heaton 249
Introduction 249
Sliding Hiatus Hernia 249
Duodenal Ulcer 250
Gallstones 250
Crohn's Disease 252

Appendicitis 252
Constipation 253
Irritable Bowel Syndrome 255
Diverticular Disease of the Colon 256
Cancer of the Large Bowel 257
Conclusions 259
Commentary 263

15. Dietary Fibre in the Prevention and Treatment of Obesity
S. Rössner 265
Introduction 265
Fibre Trial Design Problems in Obesity 265
Indicators of Success of Obesity Treatment 267
Dietary Fibre in Obesity 268
Dietary Fibre and Energy Intake 269
Effects of Dietary Fibre on Hunger, Appetite, Satiation and
    Satiety 270
Effects of Dietary Fibre on Weight Loss 271
Dietary Fibre in the Prevention of Obesity 273
Dietary Fibre, Obesity and Hypertension 273
Conclusions 274
Commentary 276

16. Dietary Fibre in the Prevention and Treatment of Diabetes Mellitus
M. Berger and A. Venhaus 279
Introduction 279
Different Glycaemic Responses of Foods 279
Metabolic Effects of Fibre 280
    Studies with Soluble Fibre 281
    Insoluble Fibre and High-Carbohydrate, High-Fibre Studies 281
    Acceptability of High-Carbohydrate, High-Fibre Diets 283
No Direct Effects of Fibre in Diabetes Treatment? 283
Evidence Suggesting Starch as the Responsible Factor for
        Different Glycaemic Responses 284
    Effects of Thermal Processing and Starch Characteristics 284
    Mechanical Processing and "Antinutrients" 285
    Studies Including Fibre and the Effect of Processing 286
Conclusions and Areas for Future Research 287
Commentary 292

17. Dietary Fibre and Plasma Lipids: Potential for Prevention and Treatment of Hyperlipidaemias
A.S. Truswell and A.C. Beynen 295
Introduction 295
Wheat Fibre 296
Pectin 298
Guar 303
Oat Fibre 309
Cellulose 316

Lignin 317
Other Types of Dietary Fibre 317
Legumes 318
Whole Foods 322
Discussion 323
Conclusion 324
Commentary 332

General Discussion 333

Subject Index 349

Contributors

Authors

Prof. N.-G. Asp
Department of Applied Nutrition and Food Chemistry, Chemical
Centre, University of Lund, PO Box 124, S-221 00 Lund, Sweden

Prof. M. Berger
Medizinische Klinik der Universität Düsseldorf, Abteilung
Stoffwechsel und Ernährung, Moorenstrasse 5, D-4000 Düsseldorf 1,
Germany

Prof. A. C. Beynen[1]
Department of Lab. Animal Science, Veterinary Faculty, University
of Utrecht, PO Box 80166, NL-3508 TD Utrecht, The Netherlands

Dr. C. Demigné
I. N. R. A., Laboratoire des Maladies Métaboliques, Centre de
Clermont Ferrand-Theix, F-63122 Ceyrat, France

Dr. M.A. Eastwood[1]
Gastrointestinal Unit, Western General Hospital, University of
Edinburgh, Edinburgh EH4 2XU, UK

Dr. C.A. Edwards
Department of Human Nutrition, University of Glasgow, Yorkhill
Hospital, Glasgow G3 8SJ, UK

Prof. B.O. Eggum
National Institute of Animal Science, Animal Physiology and
Biochemistry, Foulum, PO Box 39, DK-8830 Tjele, Denmark

Prof. W. Feldheim
Institut für Humanernährung und Lebensmittelkunde, Christian-
Albrechts-Universität, Düsternbrooker-Weg 17-19, D-2300 Kiel,
Germany

Dr. B. Flourié
Service de Gastroentérologie, Hôpital Saint-Lazare, Rue du
Faubourg Saint-Denis 107, F-75475 Paris Cédex 10, France

Dr. F. Guillon[1]
I. N. R. A., Laboratoire de Biochimie et Technologie des Glucides,
Boîte postale 527, F-44026 Nantes Cédex 03, France

Dr. K.W. Heaton
Department of Medicine, Bristol Royal Infirmary, Bristol BS2 8HW,
UK

Dr. I.T. Johnson
AFRC Institute of Food Research, Norwich Laboratory, Colney
Lane, Norwich NR4 7UA, UK

Dr. M. Lahaye[1]
I. N. R. A., Laboratoire de Biochimie et Technologie des Glucides,
Boîte postale 527, F-44026 Nantes Cédex 03, France

Dr. C. Morand[1]
I. N. R. A., Laboratoire des Maladies Métaboliques, Centre de
Clermont Ferrand-Theix, F-63122 Ceyrat, France

Prof. E.R. Morris
Cranfield Institute of Technology, Silsoe College, Bedford MK45
4DT, UK

Dr. F.M. Nagengast
Department of Medicine, Division of Gastroenterology, Academic
Hospital Nijmegen, PO Box 9101, NL-6500 HB Nijmegen, The
Netherlands

Prof. N.W. Read
Centre for Human Nutrition, University of Sheffield, Northern
General Hospital, Sheffield S5 7AU, UK

Dr. C. Rémésy[1]
I. N. R. A., Laboratoire des Maladies Métaboliques, Centre de
Clermont Ferrand-Theix, F-63122 Ceyrat, France

Dr. L. Rossander
Department of Medicine II, Sahlgrenska Hospital,
S-413 45 Göteborg, Sweden

Prof. S. Rössner
Obesity Unit, Karolinska Hospital, S-104 01 Stockholm, Sweden

Dr. I.R. Rowland
British Industrial Biological Research Association, Woodmansterne
Road, Carshalton, Surrey SM5 4DS, UK

Dr. A.-S. Sandberg
Department of Food Science, Chalmers University of Technology,
c/o SIK – The Swedish Institute for Food Research, Box 5401,
S-402 29 Göteborg, Sweden

Dr. B. Sandström
Institute of Human Nutrition, Rolighedsvej 25, DK-1958
Fredriksberg C, Denmark

Dr. T.F. Schweizer
Nestlé Research Centre, Nestec Ltd, Vers-chez-les-Blanc,
PO Box 44, CH-1000 Lausanne 26, Switzerland

Prof. D.A.T. Southgate
AFRC Institute of Food Research, Norwich Laboratory, Colney
Lane, Norwich NR4 7UA, UK

Prof. O. Theander[1]
Department of Chemistry, Swedish University of Agricultural
Sciences, Box 7015, S-740 07 Uppsala, Sweden

Dr. J.-F. Thibault
I. N. R. A., Laboratoire de Biochimie et Technologie des Glucides,
Boîte postale 527, F-44026 Nantes Cédex 03, France

Prof. A.S. Truswell[2]
Human Nutrition Unit, University of Sydney, New South Wales
2006, Australia

Dr. A. Venhaus[1]
Medizinische Klinik der Universität Düsseldorf, Abteilung
Stoffwechsel und Ernährung, Moorenstrasse 5, D-4000 Düsseldorf 1,
Germany

Dr. E. Wisker[1]
Institut für Humanernährung und Lebensmittelkunde, Christian-
Albrechts-Universität, Düsternbrooker-Weg 17-19, D-2300 Kiel,
Germany

Invited Discussants

Dr. J.H. Cummings[3]
Dunn Clinical Nutrition Centre, 100 Tennis Court Road, Cambridge
CB2 1QL, UK

Dr. H.N. Englyst[3]
Dunn Clinical Nutrition Centre, 100 Tennis Court Road, Cambridge
CB2 1QL, UK

Scientific Planning Group

Prof. J. Mauron (Chairman)
Av. de Blonay 2, 1800 Vevey, Switzerland

Prof. N.-G. Asp (Coordinator for Chapter 4)
Department of Applied Nutrition & Food Chemistry, Chemical
Centre, University of Lund, PO Box 124, S-221 00 Lund, Sweden

Dr. M.A. Eastwood
Gastrointestinal Unit, Western General Hospital, University of
Edinburgh, Edinburgh EH4 2XU, UK

Prof. M. Fondu
ILSI Europe, Avenue E. Mounier 83, Bte 6, B-1200 Bruxelles,
Belgium

Dr. T.F. Schweizer
Nestlé Research Centre, Nestec Ltd, Vers-chez-les-Blanc,
PO Box 44, CH-1000 Lausanne 26, Switzerland

Workshop Chairman

Dr. D. Kritchevsky
The Wistar Institute of Anatomy and Biology, 3601 Spruce Street,
Philadelphia, Pennsylvania 19104, U. S. A.

[1] Did not participate in the workshop.
[2] On sabbatical leave at Department of Human Nutrition,
   Wageningen Agricultural University.
[3] Were invited to contribute chapters but participated in the
   workshop only and did not want to be associated with a chapter.

Section I
Background Papers

Chapter 1

The Dietary Fibre Hypothesis: A Historical Perspective

D.A.T. Southgate

Introduction

Most major scientific advances have not developed in a vacuum but have had their foundations in the body of scientific knowledge derived from previous work. This is particularly true of the dietary fibre hypothesis (Walker, 1974; Burkitt, 1983; Burkitt and Trowell, 1975) whose foundations were laid in three major strands of scientific endeavour. A historical account of the dietary fibre hypothesis must, therefore, start with an account of the research that provided the base from which the hypothesis emerged in the early 1970s.

A number of conditions need to be satisfied for a new hypothesis to attract sufficient interest: first, that the hypothesis provides a paradigm that is in accord with current scientific thinking when the hypothesis is first proposed (Carpenter, 1986); second, that technical developments in the field are such that the hypothesis can be tested; and third, it should, ideally, offer the possibility of understanding relationships that could not be understood by the application of existing concepts (Trowell, 1985). In discussing the development of scientific or other concepts there is the danger that hindsight may delineate paths that were not at all evident to those working at the time. Nevertheless the dietary fibre hypothesis, like all integrative scientific concepts, depended on research findings in several different fields (Southgate, 1975a).

The three major strands of research that provided the foundation for the hypothesis are closely interdependent and I have endeavoured to present them as an interwoven account. First of these three strands is the developing understanding of the chemistry of the carbohydrates in general, but of the plant cell wall carbohydrates in particular. The parallel developments in analysis are inseparable from this strand and the chapter on the analysis of dietary fibre should be read in conjunction with this element of the present account.

The second strand relates to developments in the understanding of the physiological role of the carbohydrates in foods. The third strand concerns the relationships between diet and the incidence of chronic diseases, in particular the role of the polysaccharides in the diet. The dietary fibre hypothesis arose amongst researchers working in this field (Trowell, 1985) but its subsequent development has depended on bringing these three strands of research to focus on the issue of the relationship between diet and health and the incidence of disease.

Developments in the Chemistry and Analysis of Food Carbohydrates: Early Studies on the Chemistry of Foods

Simple sugars had been isolated from fruits, milk and blood and it was known that starch could be hydrolysed to sugars by acid and by malt diastase by the middle of the nineteenth century, but these early studies were not linked to any nutritional role (McCollum, 1957). This was primarily due to the difficulties of analysis and the lack of any conceptual framework for nutrition. In the elemental systems for analysing foods, carbohydrates were merely hydrates of carbon. As the proximate system developed, in the absence of specific analytical techniques, it was reasonable to measure the water, the nitrogenous material, the lipid-solvent soluble material and the mineral matter and consider the remainder carbohydrate (Henneberg and Stohmann, 1860).

As the proximate system for analysis began to be used in studies of ruminant nutrition at the Weende Experimental Station in Germany it became clear that the digestion of the carbohydrates showed that two fractions could be distinguished, an insoluble fibrous fraction and the soluble fraction that was digested during the course of ruminant digestion; this observation led to the development of the classical crude fibre method (AOAC, 1980), using successive acid and alkaline digestion simulating the digestive processes (*sic*). The soluble fraction was given the rather strange designation "nitrogen free extractives" a term that remained in use until the 1960s.

Concerns about the Energy Value of Foods

At the forefront of nutritional questions in the late nineteenth and early twentieth centuries was the issue of whether the laws of thermodynamics applied to animals (Atwater, 1900). The interest was both practically based, because of the economics of animal production, and theoretical. In these studies both Rubner and Atwater applied the proximate system of analysis to the diets of their experimental animals and human subjects. The detailed calorimetric studies of Atwater (1900) in particular, showed that carbohydrate "by difference" gave a very good prediction of the digestible energy of the human diet. Atwater, however, realised that foods that contained significant amounts of crude fibre increased faecal energy losses and he evolved a series of specific energy conversion factors that corrected for the effects of indigestible fibre on the energy value of foods (Merrill and Watt, 1955). These factors adjusted the protein and fat conversion factors to correct for the effects on the apparent digestibility of the indigestible components. Atwater's studies suggested that crude fibre did not contribute metabolisable energy to the body.

Rubner and his colleagues took up this topic again during the First World War when food shortages in Germany necessitated a search for alternative sources of energy for both animals and humans (Rubner, 1917a). Analytical chemistry had advanced considerably since the proximate system had been proposed and Rubner was able to carry out some detailed analyses of the components of the plant cell wall, using hydrolysis and reducing sugar methods and distillation for the measurement of pentosans with gravimetric measurements of residual Klason lignin (Rubner, 1917b).

Studies on the Chemistry of Plant Cell Walls

The chemical studies on the carbohydrates continued to develop following the war as new techniques for elucidating the structures of the polysaccharides were developed and the structures of the monosaccharides were better understood. Fractionation studies of the cell wall polysaccharides particularly of woody tissues established nomenclature for the water-soluble, alkali-soluble, cellulosic and lignin fractions (O'Dwyer, 1926; Norman, 1937).

Nutritional Studies on Food Carbohydrates

As these chemical studies were developing, another stimulus to the study of the nutritional role of carbohydrates in man became very strong; this stimulus was diabetes mellitus which, until the availability of insulin, could only be managed by dietary means. For this the values for food carbohydrate "by difference" in the proximate system were very unreliable because foods that contained plant cell wall were incorrectly excluded. McCance and Lawrence (1929) carried out a very thorough and perceptive review of the information that was emerging about the chemistry of the carbohydrates and proposed that the carbohydrates in foods should be considered in two categories depending on whether or not they were digested in the small intestine and were absorbed as carbohydrate. Those that were digested made up the "Available Carbohydrates" that were glucogenic in man and therefore needed to be controlled in the diabetic diet. The indigestible, structural carbohydrates from the plant cell walls in foods made up the second category: the "Unavailable Carbohydrates" or roughage. It was well established at that time that these cell wall components were fermented in the large intestine to short chain fatty acids and McCance and Lawrence debated whether these fatty acids would provide energy to the body. Their use of the word "unavailable" applied to the capacity of these components to provide carbohydrate for absorption not energy. In any case they argued that the amounts of energy provided would be relatively small in relation to total intake.

In the context of the nutrition of the ruminant and non-ruminant herbivore, the fermentation of plant cell walls and the provision of energy from this source was, however, of much greater importance and there was a large body of research on the digestion of fibre which was reviewed by Mangold (1934). This review came to the conclusion that there was no evidence for the existence of small intestinal enzymes that could hydrolyse the polysaccharides present in the plant cell wall and that the losses observed in the course of transit through the gut were due to the activities of the microflora. The review also commented on the variability in the values for apparent digestibility of fibre which at that time was ascribed to differences in cell wall composition, although it was recognised that analytical techniques were unsatisfactory.

The report of McCance and Lawrence (1929), while commenting on the unsatisfactory features of the proximate system for carbohydrates, recommended that, for human nutritional purposes, the carbohydrates in foods and in the diet should be measured directly as the techniques were available, which was not the case when the proximate system of analysis was developed 60 years previously. This recommendation led Widdowson and McCance (1935) to develop methods for measuring the available carbohydrates separately as free reducing sugars, sucrose and starch. By using a series of different reductiometric methods they showed that it was possible to measure glucose, fructose and sucrose separately in foods. Starch was measured after enzymatic hydrolysis with takadiastase, again using a combination of reducing methods to measure the glucose and maltose produced by the enzyme. This work laid the foundations for the UK practice of measuring and recording the carbohydrates directly in food composition tables and nutritional databases (McCance and Widdowson, 1940; Paul and Southgate, 1978). Alongside the development of methods for measuring available carbohydrates, techniques for measuring the unavailable components were developed for fruits, nuts and vegetables (McCance et al., 1936). The application of the method produced a value for the non-starch polysaccharides plus lignin which was called "Unavailable Carbohydrate" or roughage although the latter term was dropped in the first edition of *The chemical composition of foods* (McCance and Widdowson, 1940).

In the United States parallel developments for the measurement of available carbohydrates were made by Williams et al. (1940). These authors also turned their attention to the limitations of the crude fibre procedure; a procedure which had remained virtually unchanged in principle since it was first proposed. Williams and Olmsted were concerned, however, with the so-called simulation of digestion and developed a more physiological approach in a biochemical method for indigestible material. Their method (Williams and Olmsted, 1935) involved a preliminary proteolytic digestion using pepsin in dilute acid followed by a amylolytic hydrolysis using pancreatin in alkaline buffer. The residue was hydrolysed in dilute acid and the reducing sugars measured to give a measure of hemicelluloses and the cellulosic fraction was solubilised in strong 72% w/w sulphuric acid. The residual insoluble "lignin" was measured gravimetrically. Both soluble and insoluble hemicellulose fractions could be measured by variations in the procedures.

At about this time there was growing interest in clinical research on the significance of laxation for health and the studies of the chemistry and nutritional role of the carbohydrates start to interact with the strand that links the consumption of carbohydrates with health.

The Ancient Greek physicians were well aware of the effects of high extraction cereal foods on faecal performance and had strong views on the desirability of avoiding constipation (British Nutrition Foundation, 1990). Their views show some inconsistencies in that the Pythagoreans regarded beans as being undesirable components of the diet because of the flatulence they caused. It is possible to identify a consistent belief since that time that constipation was undesirable and some extreme views were held about the significance for health of fermentation in the large bowel. The activities of Graham, Kellogg and Allinson (Heaton, 1991) in promoting the value of high extraction cereal products because of their beneficial effects on laxation were all seminal to this growing interest in the effects of diet on large bowel function. Cowgill and Anderson (1932) had suggested that a minimum intake of crude fibre was essential for normal laxation.

Williams and Olmsted used their technique for the analysis of the indigestible residue to try to establish the mechanism of laxation by feeding residues from different plants (with different proportions of cellulose, hemicellulose and lignin). They were able to show that the faecal bulk was more influenced by the hemicelluloses than the cellulose or lignin, the two components of crude fibre, and that the concentrations of short chain fatty acids in the stools did not seem to be related to laxation rates (Williams and Olmsted, 1936). The methods were also used by Macy and her colleagues in their study of the nutrition of children (Macy, 1942; Macy et al., 1943).

The Impact of New Techniques on the Study of Carbohydrates

In the years following the Second World War a number of significant developments occurred in the study of the chemistry of the carbohydrates. These included the development of colorimetric analytical procedures that permitted the measurement of small amounts of carbohydrates (Dische, 1955); the use of nuclear magnetic resonance (NMR) as a powerful tool for investigating the structure and configuration of carbohydrates and most significantly the introduction of chromatographic methods for separating the component monosaccharides (Jermyn and Isherwood, 1956). These led to an upsurge in the studies of the polysaccharides in plant tissues and research programmes on the biosynthesis of the plant cell wall. Paper chromatography combined with the new colorimetric procedures opened up the study of the fractions of the plant cell wall obtained by the classical procedures developed earlier (Thornber and Northcote, 1961). Ion exchange chromatography of carbohydrates proved more difficult and the application of gas chromatographic methods had to await the development of volatile derivatives (Bishop, 1964).

These new techniques were applied vigorously in the study of digestion in the ruminant where the plant cell wall materials in forages provided the major source of energy for growth and production. The studies were assisted by the fact that volatile fatty acids could be studied directly by the new chromato-graphic methods and that the methyl esters of the longer chain fatty acids were also suitable for analysis by gas chromatography. These studies were accompanied by complementary researches on the interaction between the rumen microflora and the polysaccharides so that understanding of the anaerobic fermentation of the carbohydrates developed rapidly (Hungate, 1966). The research on the structure of polysaccharides was accompanied by research on the physical properties of isolated materials, especially the gums whose physical properties had been found empirically to be useful as food additives (Glicksman, 1969).

The Energy Values of Carbohydrates in the Human Diet

The problems of feeding Europe after the war reawakened an interest in the energy value of carbohydrates in the diet. The initial difficulties stemmed from the continued use of carbohydrate "by difference" values in the USA for the composition of foods and the use of direct values for the available carbohydrates in the UK. The use of the two systems resulted in the projected energy values of cereal supplies changing as they crossed the Atlantic and a controversy developed over the validity of using the Atwater energy conversion factors, derived for use with carbohydrate by difference values, for available carbohydrate (Maynard, 1944).

In order to resolve the issue the Medical Research Council supported an experimental re-evaluation of the energy conversion factors (Durnin, 1961; Southgate and Durnin, 1970). As part of this research it was clearly necessary to develop procedures for measuring the unavailable carbohydrates directly. In starting this work a number of different approaches were examined following the McCance and Widdowson principle that direct measurement of the carbohydrates was desirable. The Southgate procedure (Southgate, 1969a, b; Southgate, 1981) was the outcome of these studies. The procedure was developed so that a complete carbohydrate analysis of sugars, starches, non-cellulosic polysaccharides, cellulose and lignin could be carried out sequentially on the same sample. The methods could be applied to foods and faeces and we were able to measure the intake and excretion of the complex carbohydrates in 54 subjects on two levels of intake of unavailable carbohydrates and 10 subjects on three levels (Southgate and Durnin, 1970). The studies confirmed the fact that both the non-cellulosic and cellulosic polysaccharides were degraded during intestinal transit. The studies also showed that when intakes of wholemeal bread were increased there was a very substantial increase in the pentosan content of the faeces. The increased faecal losses of energy when the intakes of unavailable carbohydrates were increased were consistent with the view that for practical dietetic purposes the unavailable carbohydrates could be discounted in calculations of energy intake. At the same time the more detailed analysis of the conceptual basis of energy conversion factors showed that it was theoretically unsound and that an empirical system based on measurements of gross energy content (heat of combustion) and dietary analysis for protein, fat, available and unavailable carbohydrates would not have these theoretical limitations (Southgate and Durnin, 1970; Southgate, 1975b).

Studies on the Analysis of Fibre

Over the same period in the USA Peter Van Soest was engaged in detailed studies of the analysis of fibre in forages. The crude fibre method had been the subject of much criticism within the animal nutritional community; in fact the criticism is evident in unpublished material in the reports of the Weende Experimental Station at the time the method was published (Van Soest and McQueen, 1973). The criticisms were mainly technical because the empirical nature of the method required very strict attention to the prescribed protocol if consistent and repeatable results were to be obtained. The value of the method of predicting the indigestible fraction in forages was also questioned and Van Soest was given the task of assessing the procedure and improving it. One of the problems related to the variable nitrogen content of the residue. Walker (1959) showed that inclusion of a detergent in the acid stage of the procedure resulted in low nitrogen residues and that the modified Normal Acid Fibre method was a more repeatable and reliable method. Van Soest further developed the use of detergents in fibre analysis and produced a series of methods (Van Soest, 1966). The Acid Detergent Fibre (ADF) method (Van Soest, 1963) gave a good measure of cellulose and lignin; Neutral Detergent Fibre (NDF) (Van Soest and Wine, 1967) gave a good estimate of the insoluble cell wall material. In addition procedures for lignin, cutin and silica were also developed (Van Soest and Wine, 1968). These procedures were all gravimetric.

The application of the new techniques for the analysis of plant cell wall material in foodstuffs was very much focused on cereal foods especially wheat and bread. Fraser and his colleagues at the Laboratory of the Government Chemist in the UK combined the new techniques with some well established carbohydrate methods in detailed analyses of wheat flours (Fraser et al., 1956). Thomas in Berlin developed a series of studies on the cell wall material in wheat flours and bran, and also carried out some physiological studies on the effects of "Ballastoffe" (Thomas, 1964).

Dietary Fibre as a Protective Component of the Diet

There was at this time little clinical interest in the complex carbohydrates in foods apart from the link with constipation. However, in 1953 a paper appeared in the British Medical Journal (Hipsley, 1953) which reported the results of an epidemiological study of toxaemia in pregnancy and made the claim that the results showed that the plant cell walls in the diet, the "dietary fibre" intake, appeared to be protective. The paper seemed to attract little interest at the time.

There were a number of significant pieces of research conducted during this period that are relevant to the subsequent development of the dietary fibre hypothesis. These concerned firstly a growing interest in the relation between diet and disease incidence, in particular that of atherosclerosis and coronary heart disease (CHD). These studies focused very strongly on the relation between the intake of fat in different communities and the relation between fat intake, cholesterol levels in the blood and the incidence of CHD. Here the work of Ancel Keys and his colleagues was very influential in the development of views about the relation between diet and disease incidence (Keys, 1970). Although the work at that time was focused on saturated fat intakes some other findings emerged for example there was evidence that a diet rich in fruits and vegetables had cholesterol-reducing properties (Keys et al., 1961). Studies on bile salt metabolism also showed that some plant materials had profound bile salt binding effects (Kritchevsky and Story, 1974). In vitro studies of bile salt binding also showed that lignin preparations had strong binding properties (Eastwood and Girdwood, 1968).

This was the period when Hugh Trowell, working in East Africa, was developing his ideas on non-infective diseases in Africa which showed a very different pattern to that seen in the affluent Western world (Trowell, 1960). Walker, working in Southern Africa, had also noticed the difference in the patterns of disease incidence (Walker, 1956) and had been intrigued by it, as had Burkitt on the basis of his surgical experience. Burkitt and Trowell, as a result of their observations, became convinced that an environmental factor was involved and focused on diet as being the most likely reason for the differences in disease patterns. Burkitt was influenced by the book by Surgeon Captain Cleave and his colleagues *Diabetes, coronary thrombosis and the saccharine disease* (1969) which attributed the diseases of Western civilisation to the excessive consumption of refined sugars and starches. However, Burkitt began to realise that it was more probable that the removal of fibre from the plant foods during the refining process was the key to the problem.

The Dietary Fibre Hypothesis Emerges

In 1971 a paper appeared that I regard as marking the start of the dietary fibre hypothesis; the paper by Painter and Burkitt (1971) which postulated that diverticular disease was a deficiency disease of Western civilisation caused by a lack of fibre in the diet. Painter's experimental work on measuring pressures developing in the large intestine, the pathological features of the condition, and his experience in treating the condition with cereal bran all provided a range of evidence that supported the hypothesis. In the same year two papers by Burkitt proposed that appendicitis (Burkitt, 1971a) and colorectal cancer (Burkitt, 1971b) were also related to a low consumption of fibre. The data on consumption of fibre were calculated from values for crude fibre in foods.

Trowell at this time had retired from medicine and was collecting a substantial volume of literature that linked other diseases to fibre intake. These included obesity, diabetes and coronary heart disease (Trowell, 1972a, b). This linked back to his work on non-infective diseases and the differences in their incidence in rural Africa and Western countries. In his reading he became convinced that it was the presence of plant cell wall material in the foods that was the important component, not just crude fibre, and he resuscitated the term "Dietary Fibre" used by Hipsley (1953) as a shorthand for the components of the plant cell wall that resisted digestion. He published the results of his work on the literature in 1972.

At this time, I think that it is fair to say that neither Burkitt nor Trowell was familiar either with the body of knowledge on the chemistry or physiology of the food carbohydrates, or with the problems the analysis of these substances posed. Trowell visited me in Cambridge while his 1972 papers were in proof and we spent a day on what became a seminar on the "unavailable carbohydrates", the plant cell wall and their analysis. I tried very hard to persuade him to abandon the term fibre because I was convinced that it would lead to confusion amongst the food chemists and the clinical nutritionists using food composition tables.

In 1968, Alison Paul and I had started work on the fourth edition of *The composition of foods* and as part of the preparations for the revision we had conducted a questionnaire amongst dietitians on the nutrients that they considered desirable in the tables to support their clinical work (Paul and Southgate, 1970). Unavailable carbohydrates were considered dispensable in 1969, but by 1972 there was a growing call for fibre values as a result of the interest generated by the early papers of Burkitt and Trowell. These papers together formed a unifying hypothesis regarding the relation between dietary intake and the incidence of a range of hitherto unrelated conditions comprising metabolic diseases such as obesity, diabetes and cardiovascular disease (Trowell, 1973), and the diseases that Burkitt proposed which were a result of straining at stool (as a consequence of constipation) and included appendicitis, hiatus hernia, diverticular disease and haemorrhoids on low fibre diets, and colorectal cancer where a protective effect was proposed. Burkitt suggested that the mechanism of protection was that the bulky stools of a high fibre diet diluted the concentrations of environmental carcinogens in the contents of the tract derived either from the diet or formed by bacterial metabolism from unabsorbed dietary components such as bile acids (Burkitt, 1973). The more rapid transit produced by the high fibre diet would reduce the time that the mucosa would be exposed to the putative carcinogens. A low fibre intake on the other hand would permit extensive bacterial modification, and maximise the concentrations of carcinogens and the time that the mucosa was in contact with the active substances.

Thus the dietary fibre hypothesis, drawn from observations on populations consuming different types of diets, could be extended into a series of subsidiary hypotheses regarding mechanism (Southgate and Penson, 1983).

Initial Responses to the Hypothesis

The initial reactions to the hypothesis that diets rich in foods that contain plant cell wall material are protective against a range of diseases prevalent in Western affluent societies, and that a low intake of these foods may, for certain diseases, be causative, varied considerably depending in large part on both the current views about the relationships between diet and health and past prejudices. Both Burkitt and Trowell were very persuasive evangelists of their ideas because they saw the unifying attractiveness of the hypothesis. Furthermore, as Burkitt said, it was up to the critics to either refute the hypothesis or come up with a better one.

There was considerable interest in the general public, due in part to the effective presentation of the concepts and because the mechanisms were plausible. One group that responded very positively to the ideas were those whose systems of beliefs led them to the view that processed and refined foods were undesirable and that natural wholefoods had special properties. These included some food "cranks" but also groups whose views were based on more scientific principles, often stemming from the view that organic food production systems were preferable and that the nutrient losses associated with some forms of processing could be avoided if unprocessed natural foods formed the major part of the diet. In many ways the dietary fibre hypothesis was very much in accord with the emergent "green" environmental movement.

The food industry, however, saw the hypothesis in a different light because of the criticisms of processing that the ideas implied. Burkitt, in particular, identified the introduction of roller milling as the starting point when fibre intakes started to fall because roller milling permitted more effective separation of the bran from the germ and endosperm of wheat than sieving (Burkitt, 1973). Trowell also carried out an analysis of the deaths from diabetes from before the start of the Second World War and argued that the introduction of national high extraction bread flours in the UK corresponded with the time that deaths started to decline (Trowell, 1973). The flour milling and baking industries were thus identified as a major cause of low fibre intake and by implication the increased incidence of disease. Accordingly a very detailed critique of the dietary fibre hypothesis was prepared (Eastwood et al., 1974). This dealt primarily with the specific effects of cereal foods and bread in particular, and challenged the view that significant changes in the intake of fibre from cereals had occurred. The paper was problematic for several reasons: firstly, it argued much of its case using data on crude fibre although the authors were aware that dietary fibre was different from crude fibre; secondly, it managed to equate wheat bran with dietary fibre; finally, and more significantly, it raised a barrier to exploring the scientific issues. The conclusions, however, contain an important recognition that the dietary fibre hypothesis derived from observations on diets that differed in many attributes.

In the nutritional research community the hypothesis raised many questions; my initial view was that although the ideas were plausible it was difficult to believe that the intake of one component, fibre, could be linked to these diverse conditions, clearly crude fibre was not at all likely to be the dietary component but the range of materials present in the plant cell wall had a range of chemical and physical properties that could produce diverse physiological effects. My reaction as a researcher was that this was an important hypothesis that deserved experimental study, if only to refute it and prevent the dissemination of the dietary advice that was already beginning to be published in popular articles (Southgate, 1973).

Several other workers had a similar view – Martin Eastwood had written an essay that debated the issue (Eastwood, 1972) and also on the basis of his previous researches on the effects on bile acid metabolism argued that more detailed study of the physico-chemical properties of cell wall constituents was required. Ken Heaton, whose interests included bile acid metabolism and gallstones, argued the case for gallstones being caused by fibre-depleted diets (Heaton, 1973a) and also, in relation to obesity, drew attention to the ability of intact plant cell wall material to diminish energy intake and absorption, a major factor in this being the solid chewy texture of unprocessed plant foods (Heaton, 1973b).

John Cummings, from the viewpoint of a gastroenterologist, also saw that the dietary fibre hypothesis raised issues of profound importance in relation to understanding gastro-intestinal function and disease (Cummings, 1973). Bo Drasar and Mike Hill, with interests in the bacterial ecology of the large bowel, saw important questions that needed to be answered (Drasar and Hill, 1972). The epidemiological evidence relating disease to dietary intake did not support the hypothesis that crude fibre intakes were linked with colorectal cancer; the dietary factor that dominated both cancer and CHD was fat intake with animal protein close behind for the former (Draser and Irving, 1973).

The body of analytical information on crude fibre and the more limited studies on unavailable carbohydrates and plant cell wall material in foods was such at that time to indicate that there was no direct quantitative relationship between crude fibre and dietary fibre and therefore the definitive epidemiological studies depended on obtaining comprehensive data on dietary intakes through extending the information on the dietary fibre in foods (Southgate, 1975a). Proposals to include these analyses in the work on the composition of foods were rejected because of the doubts raised about the scientific soundness of the hypothesis while the welcome given to the hypothesis by the health food lobby was viewed with grave doubts. Nevertheless the research need was there and the analytical work was developed with postgraduate students (Southgate et al., 1976). At this time an extensive review of food and nutrition research was being undertaken in the UK and this recognised that if the dietary fibre hypothesis was to be tested more detailed work on the chemistry and physical properties of dietary fibre and its components was needed (Medical Research Council and Agricultural Research Council, 1974).

Major Themes in the Initial Development of the Dietary Fibre Hypothesis

The scientific evidence for the physiological role of dietary fibre and the links between these effects and the aetiology of diseases will form the major themes to be discussed in later chapters and in concluding this "historical" account I would like to focus on four major topics that formed the early concerns in the development of the hypothesis: definition and analysis; studies with isolated polysaccharides; dietary fibre as a source of energy; and the mechanism of faecal bulking. Some of these topics form the specific subject matter of later chapters and I will only try to summarise the initial stages.

Definition and Analysis

The debate over the definition of dietary fibre began before Trowell's papers in 1972 (Trowell, 1972a, b) had appeared and the concept of "the skeletal remains of the plant cell wall that were indigestible" was immediately viewed as too imprecise to develop quantitative studies that were essential for testing the epidemiological elements of the hypothesis. Several authors used crude fibre data which was all that was available in databases outside the UK. The issue of definition cannot be separated from the identification of analytical methods because the chosen definition determines the analytical strategy to be adopted. The debate over the definition continues at the present time and is developed elsewhere (Chapter 4).

Studies with Isolated Polysaccharides

The researchers who contemplated experimental studies to establish the possible mechanisms whereby dietary fibre exerted its effects were faced with two major dilemmas. The first of these was the complexity of the plant cell walls in foods (Southgate, 1976) and the fact that the cell wall material was present in relatively low concentrations so that increasing the intake of dietary fibre resulted in a range of other changes in dietary intake which served to confound the interpretation of the results. The second was that if one contemplated human studies there was an ethical obligation to be sure that the materials fed were safe; this constrained the use of those concentrated preparations that were available such as citrus waste, apple pomace and various cereal hull preparations. Wheat bran was seized upon by many workers who initially failed to appreciate that it was a complex mixture which invariably contained starch, polyunsaturated fats and plant sterols. Furthermore the concentrations of dietary fibre could vary over a two-fold range (James and Southgate, 1975).

This led many groups to turn their attention to isolated polysaccharides, especially those that were already established and approved for use in foods. Pectin was an immediate candidate followed by the galactomannan gums used as food additives, guar and locust bean gum (Jenkins et al., 1976; Cummings et al., 1978); isolated cellulose preparations were also studied as was the arabinoxylan mucilage from *Plantago ovata* (Prynne and Southgate, 1979). The studies with pectin and guar gum produced some very interesting findings: first they reduce fat apparent digestibility and they lowered serum cholesterol levels; in addition they reduced the postprandial glucose levels in diabetic subjects and appeared to be of value in the management of non-insulin dependent diabetics (Jenkins et al., 1976).

Trowell was disturbed by the studies on isolated polysaccharides because this moved away from the dietary fibre concept of the plant cell wall in foods; however, he was persuaded that the use of isolated polysaccharides provided a powerful experimental tool for studying the mode of action of dietary fibre. Nevertheless he suggested the term "dietary fibre" should be reserved for cell wall materials and proposed that "edible fibre" be used for other sources (Trowell et al., 1978).

This debate still continues and there is strong evidence that the physiological effects of isolated polysaccharides are not identical to those when they are consumed as part of intact cell wall structures; the architecture of the wall confers other properties.

Dietary Fibre as a Source of Energy

This topic, as I have shown above, has been a central feature of the interest in the nutritional role of plant cell wall material. The large body of evidence from studies of the nutrition of the ruminant and the more limited human studies show that the plant cell wall polysaccharides are extensively degraded by the microflora of both the rumen and the large bowel. The conditions in the contents of both organs are very similar and are anaerobic so that the products of digestion are principally short chain fatty acids and the stoichiometry of rumen anaerobic fermentation is such that approximately 75% of the gross energy is released in these fatty acids (Southgate, 1989). McCance and Lawrence (1929) debated whether the fatty acids would be absorbed and came to the conclusion that if so their contribution to energy intake would be small. This view led McCance and Widdowson (1940) to adopt a convention of discounting the unavailable carbohydrates in calculations of the energy value of foods; this was based on the reasoning that unavailable carbohydrates increased the faecal losses of fat and protein and that this loss of energy counterbalanced the small amounts of energy gained from short chain fatty acids. The studies of Southgate and Durnin (1970) confirmed that at modest levels of unavailable carbohydrate intake this was true for practical dietetic purposes but at higher levels of intake might not apply.

In the early 1970s there was considerable debate about whether the short chain fatty acids were absorbed from the large bowel, a discussion that seemed at the time to ignore the evidence from the studies of non-ruminant herbivores such as the horse, elephant and rhinoceros which obtained most of their energy from fermenting forages in their large bowel. Fortunately the studies of McNeil (McNeil et al., 1978) resolved the issue by showing that short chain fatty acids were absorbed rapidly from the human colon.

Studies of the energy value of plant cell wall materials and isolated polysaccharides remain of considerable interest especially to the food industry in relation to energy claims and nutritional labelling (Livesey, 1990). In most Western diets the energy derived from dietary fibre is small but where intakes of dietary fibre are high and total energy limiting, may have wider nutritional significance.

In the context of energy metabolism Trowell's original writings included the proposition that obesity was rare in communities that habitually consumed high-fibre diets and that there was a protective effect. Initially the experimental evidence was drawn from studies that showed an increased faecal loss of energy on increased intakes of dietary fibre but the magnitude of the effects was small. Heaton suggested that dietary fibre in the form of intact cell wall materials in unrefined, fibre-replete foods acted as a barrier to excessive food consumption and was thus of value in the prevention of obesity (Heaton, 1973b). Some interesting experimental observations have demonstrated effects of foods with their cell walls intact (Haber et al., 1977) but the debate on whether high-fibre intakes assist in regulation of appetite remains to be established.

Mechanism of Faecal Bulking

When the hypothesis was first proposed there was substantial evidence that increased intakes of dietary fibre resulted in increased faecal bulk both on a wet and dry basis. Initially there was some surprise that relatively small changes in crude fibre intakes produced such dramatic effects but the substitution of unavailable carbohydrate values into these studies resolved the issue. The early studies of Williams and Olmsted (1936) which had shown that different sources of plant cell wall material had different bulking effects were not appreciated by many workers who expected all fibre sources to have equal effects and some comparisons of sources were made where intakes were not quantitatively identical. Hellendoorn argued that the effects on faecal bulking were due to the osmotic effects of the fermentation products analogous to the effects of lactulose and the sugar alcohols (Hellendoorn, 1969, 1973, 1978). Studies with highly fermentable sources showed very low effects on faecal bulking and this hypothesis was rejected (Jenkins et al., 1976). Studies with concentrated preparations with different proportions and types of polysaccharides and lignin showed that faecal bulking of the different sources, fed at the same intakes, was very different and that the preparations that were least fermented had the most pronounced effects and the completely fermented materials had low bulking effects (Cummings et al., 1978). This led to the recognition that faecal bulking was due to the combined effects of residual material that resisted fermentation together with the bacterial mass produced from the fermentation (Stephen and Cummings, 1980). At the same time it was clear that other factors influenced both transit rate and faecal bulking. These studies have focused attention on the effects of the dietary fibre components on the environment of the large bowel and particularly the interaction with the microflora, which may provide the link to the effects on large bowel disease.

The Status of the Dietary Fibre Hypothesis

The dietary fibre hypothesis has been compared with the vitamin hypothesis that dominated nutritional research in the 1930s and 1940s and if one judges the hypothesis by the research that it has stimulated it can already been seen as successful because it has brought contact between researchers on carbohydrates, cell wall chemistry and architecture, gastro-intestinal physiology and clinical nutrition, and thus has promoted studies at the interfaces between these disciplines which, until Burkitt and Trowell proposed their hypothesis, had been unaware of the relevance of each others' work. Thus the hypothesis has the characteristics of many major scientific advances. One could argue that the original mechanisms have not been substantiated but there have been new understandings of the physiology of the intestinal tract and new findings in the way diet influences metabolism. The hypothesis has transformed nutritional views on the role of the carbohydrates in foods. As part of the wider debate on the relation between dietary intake and health/disease it has profoundly influenced nutritional guidance to the consumer and through them has influenced the range of foods available.

References

Association of Official Analytical Chemists (1980) Official methods of analysis, 11th edn, Horwitz W (ed) AOAC, Washington DC, p 129

Atwater WO (1900) Discussion of the terms digestibility, availability and fuel value. Twelfth Annual Report of the Storrs Agricultural Experimental Station, p 69

Bishop CT (1964) Gas-liquid chromatography of carbohydrate derivatives. Adv Carb Chem 19:95–147

British Nutrition Foundation (1990) Complex carbohydrates in foods. Chapman and Hall, London

Burkitt DP (1971a) The aetiology of appendicitis. Br J Surg 58:695–699

Burkitt DP (1971b) Epidemiology of cancer of colon and rectum. Cancer 28:3–13

Burkitt DP (1973) The role of refined carbohydrate in large bowel behaviour and disease. Plant Foods for Man 1:5–9

Burkitt DP (1983) The development of the fibre hypothesis. In: Birch GG, Parker KJ (eds) Dietary fibre. Applied Science Publishers, London, pp 21–27

Burkitt DP, Trowell HC (eds) (1975) Refined carbohydrate foods and disease; some implications of dietary fibre. Academic Press, London

Carpenter KJ (1986) The history of scurvy and vitamin C. Cambridge University Press, Cambridge

Cleave TL, Cambell GD, Painter NS (1969) Diabetes, coronary thrombosis and the saccharine disease, 2nd edn. Wright, Bristol

Cowgill GR, Anderson WE (1932) Laxative effects of wheat bran and washed bran in healthy men. A comparative study. JAMA 98:1866–1875

Cummings JH (1973) Dietary fibre. Progress report. Gut 14:69–81

Cummings JH, Southgate DAT, Branch W, Houston H, Jenkins DJA, James WPT (1978) Colonic response to dietary fibre from carrot, cabbage, apple, bran and gaur gum. Lancet i:5–9

Cummings JH, Southgate DAT, Branch W et al. (1979) The digestion of pectin in the human gut and its effect on calcium absorption and large bowel function. Br J Nutr 41:477–485

Dische Z (1955) New color reactions for determination of sugars in polysaccharides. In: Glick D (ed) Methods of biochemical analysis, vol II. Interscience, New York, pp 313–358

Drasar BS, Hill MW (1972) Intestinal bacteria and cancer. Am J Clin Nutr 25:1399–1404

Drasar BS, Irving D (1973) Environmental factors and cancer of the colon and breast. Br J Cancer 27:167–172

Durnin JVGA (1961) The availability of nutrients in diets containing differing quantities of unavailable carbohydrate: a study on young and elderly men and women. I. General description and proportionate loss of calories. Proc Nutr Soc 20:ii

Eastwood MA (1972) Vegetable dietary fibre – fad or farago? Van de Berghs and Jorgens Nutrition Award

Eastwood MA, Girdwood RH (1968) Lignin: a bile salt sequestering agent. Lancet ii:1170–1172

Eastwood MA, Fisher N, Greenwood CT, Hutchinson JB (1974) Perspectives on the bran hypothesis. Lancet i:1029–1033

Fraser JR, Brendon-Bravo M, Holmes DC (1956) The proximate analysis of wheat flour carbohydrates. I. Methods and scheme of analysis. J Sci Food Agric 7:577–589

Glicksman M (1969) Gum technology in the food industry. Academic Press, New York

Haber GB, Heaton KW, Murphy D, Burroughs IF (1977) Depletion and disruption of dietary fibre, effects on satiety, plasma glucose and serum insulin. Lancet ii:679–682

Heaton KW (1973a) Gallstones and dietary carbohydrates. Plant Foods for Man 1:33–44

Heaton KW (1973b) Food fibre as an obstacle to energy intake. Lancet ii:1418–1421

Heaton KW (1991) Concepts of dietary fibre. In: Southgate DAT et al. (eds) Dietary fibre: Chemical and biological aspects. Royal Society of Chemistry, Cambridge

Hellendoorn EW (1969) Intestinal effects following ingestion of beans. Food Technol 23:87–92

Hellendoorn EW (1973) Physiological importance of indigestible carbohydrates in human nutrition. Voeding 34:618–635

Hellendoorn EW (1978) Some critical observations in relation to 'dietary fibre', the methods for its determination and the current hypotheses for the explanation of its physiological action. Voeding 39:230–235

Henneberg W, Stohmann F (1860) Beiträge zur Begründung einer rationellen Fütterung der Wiederkäuer, I. Braunschweig

Hipsley EH (1953) Dietary "fibre" and pregnancy toxaemia. Br Med J ii:420–422

Hungate RE (1966) The rumen and its microbes. Academic Press, New York

James WPT, Southgate DAT (1975) Bran and blood lipids. Lancet i:800

Jenkins DJA, Goff DV, Leeds AR et al. (1976) Unabsorbable carbohydrates and diabetes: decreased postprandial hyperglycaemia. Lancet ii:172–174

Jermyn MA, Isherwood FA (1956) Changes in the cell wall of the pear during ripening. Biochem J 64:123–132

Keys A (1970) Coronary heart disease in seven countries. Circulation [Suppl] 41:1

Keys A, Grande F, Anderson JT (1961) Fiber and pectin in the diet and serum cholesterol concentration in man. Proc Soc Exp Biol Med 106:555–558

Kritchevsky D, Story WA (1974) Binding of bile salts in vitro by non-nutritive fiber. J Nutr 104:458–462

Livesey G (1990) The energy values of unavailable carbohydrates and diets: an enquiry and analysis. Am J Clin Nutr 51:617–637

Macy IG (1942) Nutrition and chemical growth in childhood, vol. I, Evaluation. C. C. Thomas, Springfield, Illinois

Macy IG, Hummel FC, Shepherd ML (1943) Value of complex carbohydrates in diets of normal children. Am J Dis Child 65:195–206

Mangold DE (1934) The digestion and utilisation of crude fibre. Nutr Abstr Rev 3:647–656

Maynard LA (1944) The Atwater system of calculating the caloric value of diets. J Nutr 28:443–452

McCance RA, Lawrence RD (1929) The carbohydrate content of foods. HMSO, London (special report series of the Medical Research Council, no. 135)

McCance RA, Widdowson EM (1940) The chemical composition of foods. HMSO, London (special report series of the Medical Research Council, no. 235)

McCance RA, Widdowson EM, Shackleton LRB (1936) The nutritive value of fruits, vegetables and nuts. HMSO, London (special report series of the Medical Research Council, no. 213)

McCollum EV (1957) A history of nutrition. Houghton Mifflin, Boston, Mass

McNeil NI, Cummings JH, James WPT (1978) Short chain fatty acid absorption by the human large intestine. Gut 19:819–822

Medical Research Council and Agricultural Research Council (1974) Food and nutrition research. Report of the Neuberger committee. HMSO, London

Merrill AL, Watt BK (1955) Energy value of foods basis and derivation. US Dept. Agric., Washington (US Department of Agriculture, Handbook no. 74)

Norman AG (1937) The biochemistry of cellulose, the polyuronides [etc]. Oxford University Press, Oxford

O'Dwyer MH (1926) The hemicelluloses of beech wood. Biochem J 20:656–664

Painter NS, Burkitt DP (1971) Diverticular disease of the colon: A deficiency disease of Western civilisation. Br Med J ii:450–454

Paul AA, Southgate DAT (1970) Revision of "The composition of foods", some views of dietitians. Nutrition 24:21–24

Paul AA, Southgate DAT (1978) McCance and Widdowsons' The composition of foods, 4th edn. HMSO, London

Prynne CJ, Southgate DAT (1979) The effects of a supplement of dietary fibre on faecal excretion by human subjects. Br J Nutr 31:495–503

Rubner M (1917a) Die Verwertung aufgeschlossenen Strohes für die Ernährung des Menschen. Arch Anat Physiol 74

Rubner M (1917b) Untersuchungen über Vollkornbrot. Arch Anat Physiol 74:245–372

Southgate DAT (1969a) Determination of carbohydrates in foods. I. Available carbohydrates. J Sci Food Agric 20:326–330

Southgate DAT (1969b) Determination of carbohydrates in foods. II. Unavailable carbohydrates. J Sci Food Agric 20:331–335

Southgate DAT (1973) Dietary fibre. Plant Foods for Man 1:45–47

Southgate DAT (1975a) Fibre in nutrition. Bibl Nutr Dieta 22:109–124

Southgate DAT (1975b) Fiber and other unavailable carbohydrates and energy effects in the diet. In: White PL, Selvey N (eds) Proceedings of Western Hemisphere nutrition congress IV. Publishing Sciences Group, Acton, Mass, pp 51–55

Southgate DAT (1976) The chemistry of dietary fiber. In: Spiller GA, Amen RJ (eds) Fiber in human nutrition. Plenum Press, New York, pp 31–72

Southgate DAT (1981) Use of the Southgate method for unavailable carbohydrates in the measurement of dietary fiber. In: James WPT, Theander O (eds) The analysis of dietary fiber. Dekker, New York, pp 1–19

Southgate DAT (1989) The role of the gut flora in the digestion of starches and sugars: with special reference to their role in the metabolism of the host, including energy and vitamin metabolism. In: Dobbing J (ed) Dietary starches and sugars in man: a comparison. Springer, London, pp 67–83

Southgate DAT, Durnin JVGA (1970) Calorie conversion factors. An experimental re-assessment of the factors used in the calculation of the energy value of human diets. Br J Nutr 24:517–535

Southgate DAT, Penson JM (1983) Testing the dietary fibre hypothesis. In: Birch CG, Parker KJ (eds) Dietary fibre. Applied Science Publishers, London, pp 1–19

Southgate DAT, Bailey B, Collinson E, Walker AF (1976) A guide to calculating intakes of dietary fibre. J Hum Nutr 30:303–313

Stephen AM, Cummings JH (1980) Mechanism of action of dietary fibre in the human colon. Nature 284: 283–284

Thomas M (1964) Die Nähr und Ballastoffe der Getreidemehle in ihrer Bedeutung für die Brotnahrung. Wissenschaftliche Verlagsgesellschaft, Stuttgart

Thornber JP, Northcote DH (1961) Changes in the chemical composition of a cambial cell during its differentiation into xylem and phloem tissues in trees. Major Components. Biochem J 81:449–454

Trowell HC (1960) Non-infective disease in Africa. Edward Arnold, London

Trowell HC (1972a) Ischemic heart disease and dietary fibre. Am J Clin Nutr 25:926–932

Trowell HC (1972b) Dietary fibre and coronary heart disease. Rev Eur Etud Clin Biol 17:345–349

Trowell HC (1973) Dietary fibre, coronary heart disease and diabetes mellitus. Plant Foods for Man 1:11–16

Trowell HC (1985) Dietary fibre: a paradigm. In: Trowell H et al. (eds) Dietary fibre, fibre-depleted foods and disease. Academic Press, London, pp 1–20

Trowell H, Godding E, Spiller G, Briggs G (1978) Fiber bibliographies and terminology. Am J Clin Nutr 31:1489–1490

Van Soest PJ (1963) Use of detergents in the analysis of fibrous feeds. II. A rapid method for the determination of fiber and lignin. J Assoc Off Analyt Chem 46:829–835

Van Soest PJ (1966) Non-nutritive residues: A system of analysis for the replacement of crude fiber. J Assoc Off Analyt Chem 49:546–551

Van Soest PJ, McQueen RW (1973) The chemistry and estimation of fibre. Proc Nutr Soc 32:123–130

Van Soest PJ, Wine RH (1967) Use of detergents in the analysis of fibrous feeds. IV. Determination of plant cell-wall constituents. J Assoc Off Analyt Chem 50:50–55

Van Soest PJ, Wine RH (1968) Determination of lignin and cellulose in acid-detergent fiber with permanganate. J Assoc Off Analyt Chem 52:780–785

Walker ARP (1956) Some aspects of nutritional research in South Africa. Nutr Rev 14:321–324

Walker ARP (1974) Dietary fibre and the patterns of disease. Ann Intern Med 80:663–664

Walker DM (1959) A note on the composition of normal-acid fibre. J Sci Food Agric 10:415–418

Widdowson EM, McCance RA (1935) The available carbohydrates of fruits. Determination of glucose, fructose, sucrose and starch. Biochem J 29:151–156

Williams RD, Olmsted WH (1935) A biochemical method for determining indigestible residue (crude fiber) in faeces: lignin, cellulose and non-water soluble hemicelluloses. J Biol Chem 108:653–666

Williams RD, Olmsted WH (1936) The effect of cellulose, hemicellulose and lignin on the stool: a contribution to the study of laxation in man. J Nutr 11:433–449

Williams RD, Wicks L, Bierman HR, Olmsted WH (1940) Carbohydrate values of fruits and vegetables. J Nutr 19:593–604

Commentary

Schweizer: Trowell's various definitions always comprised three criteria of dietary fibre, namely a *physiological*, a *botanical* and a *chemical* one. Of these, only the first remained unchanged throughout the years, i.e. the resistance of dietary fibre against human digestive enzymes. The botanical description changed from "skeletal remains of plant cells" (Trowell 1972a) to "remnants of plant *cells*" (Trowell 1974) and only later to "remnants of the plant cell *wall*" (Trowell 1975) or to "structural polymers of the plant cell *wall*" (Trowell 1976). Trowell's chemical descriptions of dietary fibre were not very precise and changed repeatedly. However, indigestible non-wall polysaccharides were not excluded from dietary fibre by Trowell et al. (1978).

Thus, Trowell's definitions – including the working definition of Trowell et al. (1976) – give no ground for preferring any particular analytical strategy. Also, no analytical strategy is able to meet any of these definitions fully. Therefore, the statement that dietary fibre is effectively being defined by the method used applies to all methods, whether they attempt to measure indigestible residues, cell walls, or unavailable carbohydrate.

References

Trowell HC (1974) Definitions of fibre. Lancet i:503
Trowell HC (1975) Refined carbohydrate foods and fibre. In: Burkitt DP, Trowell H (eds) Refined carbohydrate foods and disease. Academic Press, London, pp 23–41
Trowell H (1976) Definition of dietary fiber and hypotheses that it is a protective factor in certain diseases. Am J Clin Nutr 29:417–427
Trowell H, Southgate DAT, Wolever TMS, Leeds AR, Gassull MA, Jenkins DJA (1976) Dietary fibre redefined. Lancet i:967
(Other references given in chapter)

Author's reply: Non-wall polysaccharides were indeed included in the definition of dietary fibre because they were frequently used as model substances in dietary fibre studies and because they cannot be distinguished in analytical practice from cell wall polysaccharides.

Heaton: This chapter is very well written and accurately reflects a food analyst's perspective. However, the originators of the "fibre hypothesis" were practising doctors and amateur epidemiologists. In my opinion, an account like this should acknowledge that the whole motivation for the work of Cleave, Burkitt and Trowell was the striking variation in disease prevalence with place and time. In addition, it should be recognised that the rapid acceptance of the hypothesis in the early 1970s was aided by clinical studies on the effects of wheat bran on faecal weight and composition, transit time, colonic pressures and bile composition.

Chapter 2

Physico-chemical Properties of Food Plant Cell Walls

J.-F. Thibault, M. Lahaye and F. Guillon

Introduction

The benefits of dietary fibre intake are now established and the physiological as well as technological aspects of fibre or of fibre-enriched products are well documented. The chemical structure and their physico-chemical properties are both thought to determine their nutritional effects and/or their functional properties.

Plant cell walls are constituted by a tridimensional and heterogeneous network with amorphous and crystalline zones, hydrophilic and hydrophobic areas. The cohesion of the network is realised by both chemical and physical links of different strengths; furthermore negatively charged groups are always present. The ion-exchange properties, the hydration properties and the organic compound absorptive properties are therefore the main physico-chemical properties of the plant cell walls. They play an important role in the digestion flow, nutrient availability, viscosity, and mixing and determine their incorporation into food. The physico-chemical properties depend on various parameters, including processing which will be discussed in this chapter. Each property will be considered individually but it is clear that the nutritional or functional effects of fibres result from complex combinations of all these properties.

Ion-Exchange Properties

Dietary fibres have been shown to bind nutritionally important minerals in vitro and therefore they may influence electrolyte and mineral absorption and heavy metal toxicity (cf. Chap. 5). Calcium ions in particular may bind through carboxyl groups to pectins and to some dietary anions involved in cholesterol metabolism (see "Adsorption of Organic Molecules"). However, fibres are more or less degraded in the digestive tract by colonic bacteria and thus their ion-exchange capacity in these dynamic conditions is perhaps far from that determined in vitro.

The Ionic Groups Associated with Fibres

Fibres from vegetable or fruit appear to be weak monofunctional ion-exchange resins because of the presence of uronic acids (galacturonic acid, glucuronic acid, 4-O-methyl glucuronic acid) (Fig. 2.1). In contrast, fibres from cereals behave as polyfunctional exchangers indicating the presence of different ionogenic groups and probably phytates (Fig. 2.1). Fibres from algal cell walls contain carboxylic and sulphate groups.

Galacturonic acid is the basic constituent of pectins which can amount to 25%–30% of some fibres (Voragen et al., 1983; Brillouet et al., 1988). However, all these acids are not available for ion-exchange because they are partly esterified by methanol, the degree of methylation being generally in the range 50%–70% (Voragen et al., 1983). Very good agreements have been obtained between experimental cation-exchange capacities and values calculated from the amount of unmethylated galacturonic acid residues (Bertin et al., 1988).

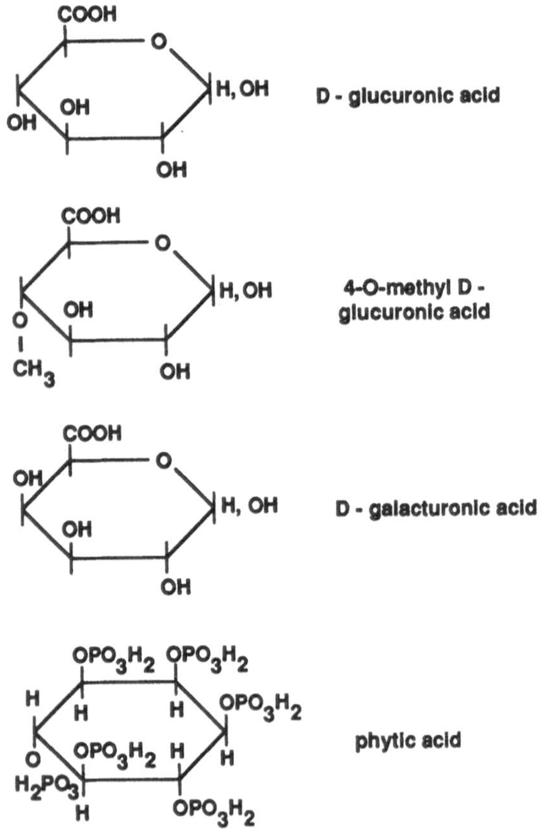

Fig. 2.1. Structure of the main ionic moieties of fibres.

Glucuronic acid and its 4-O-methyl derivative are found in secondary plant cell walls where they form sidechains attached to the C-2 of the major hemicelluloses, namely xylans. They are not esterified and their content in brans from cereals is about 5% (Selvendran et al., 1987).

Phytic acid (myo-inositol hexaphosphoric acid) is associated with cereal brans. It can amount to about 1% of the oat bran (Frölich and Nyman, 1988), or to 3.7% in wheat bran (Schweizer et al., 1984).

Methods of Cation-Exchange Capacity Determination

Cation-exchange capacity (CEC) can be measured on fibres "as received" but exchange into a known ionic state is sometimes preferable, as fibres contain charges bearing possibly different counterions. The acidic form can be obtained by suspending the fibres in an acidic medium followed by extensive washings in order to eliminate the excess of acid. Salt forms can be obtained by exact neutralisation of the acid form or directly from the native fibres by immersion in a concentrated salt solution and then by extensive washings in order to eliminate the excess salt. These treatments may partially solubilise or degrade fibres and optimal conditions (normality, concentration, time, solid to liquid ratio) for complete conversion of the ionic groups should keep losses to a minimum (Bertin et al., 1988). Indeed the yield of material on which the CEC is performed must be stated, particularly for vegetable fibres since pectins are particularly sensitive to these treatments (Bertin et al., 1988; Ralet et al., 1990).

The method most often used for determination of CEC is pHmetry. Conductimetry is sometimes used (Bertin et al., 1988) since this method allows the determination of the CEC of fibres whatever their ionic form (H^+, Na^+, K^+ ...).

Exchange with monovalent, divalent, or even trivalent ions was also used to determine the CEC after washing out the original counterion, generally in acidic medium, and subsequent determination of the liberated counterions using various ion indicators (Van Soest and Robertson, 1976; MacBurney et al., 1983; Allen et al., 1985).

The Cation-Exchange Capacity Values

The CEC of vegetable, fruit and cereal fibres ranges between 0.2 to 3.1 meq/g (Tables 2.1 and 2.2). Lower values are generally observed for cereal fibres.

The nature of the counterion is unlikely to determine CEC because the porosity of fibres is always larger than the size of the counterions, and all the charges in fibres are accessible for ion exchange. The only limitation (not yet studied) may arise from high proportions of lignin which can impregnate some secondary walls in bran fractions and thus hinder charges.

Table 2.1. Cation-exchange capacity (CEC) of some vegetable and fruit fibres

Fibre	CEC (meq/g)	Ionic form of the fibre	Fibre content (%)	Reference[a]
Pea	0.80	H^+	23.7	1
Apple	1.90	H^+	64.0	1
Sugar beet	0.57	Pr^{3+}, Nd^{3+}	51.0	2
	0.70	Cu^{2+}	51.0	3
	0.60	H^+	56.0	4
	0.47	H^+	75.3	5
Carrot	0.82	H^+	nd	6
	2.40	H^+	57.0	1
Lettuce	0.94	H^+	nd	6
	3.10	H^+	52.2	1
Potato	0.62	Ca^{2+}	4.7	7
	0.30	H^+	4.1	1
	0.77	H^+	nd	6

[a] 1, MacConnell et al., 1974; 2, Allen et al., 1985; 3, MacBurney et al., 1983; 4, Michel et al., 1988; 5, Bertin et al., 1988; 6, Yoshida and Kuwano, 1989; 7, Van Soest and Robertson, 1976.

Table 2.2. Cation-exchange capacity (CEC) of some cereal brans

Bran	CEC (meq/g)	Ionic form of the fibre	Fibre content (%)	Reference[a]
Corn	0.20	H^+	71.9	1
	0.38	Ca^{2+}	nd	2
	0.41	Pr^{3+}, Nd^{3+}	93.7	3
	0.04	H^+	nd	4
Wheat	0.22	Ca^{2+}	38.4	2
	0.41	Pr^{3+}, Nd^{3+}	43.2	3
	0.07	H^+	nd	4
	0.87	Cu^{2+}	44.1	5
	1.6	H^+	50.4	6
	0.7–1.2	H^+	19.2	7
Rice	0.49	Pr^{3+}, Nd^{3+}	30.7	3

[a] 1, Schimberni et al., 1982; 2, Van Soest and Robertson, 1976; 3, Allen et al., 1985; 4, Moorman et al., 1983; 5, Van Soest et al., 1983; 6, Ralet et al., 1990; 7, Kirwan et al., 1974.

In contrast, CEC depends on the physiological state or on the stage of development of plant fibres because chemical or structural changes concerning the ionic groups, especially in pectins, can occur. More unmethylated galacturonic residues can be formed after the action of pectinmethylesterase as the plant ages. The CEC of carrot fibres (Robertson et al., 1980a) was constant between varieties but increased within each variety with aging.

Binding of ions to fibres depends on the CEC value but also on the pH, the ionic strength, and the nature of ions (Thompson and Weber, 1979; Garcia-Lopez and Lee, 1985). Generally, a high ionic strength and a low pH is unfavourable for strong binding because fewer charges are available. Interesting developments on ion-binding properties of fibres have been made by Laszlo (1987) using equations involving Donnan potential, chemical equilibrium, and conservation of electrical neutrality. Applied to soy hull, these equations were used to predict the extent of cation binding. Uronic acid-containing fibres are able to bind calcium very strongly because of interaction with contiguous residues (Grant et al., 1973; Thibault and Rinaudo, 1986). Cereal fibres are able to bind calcium essentially due to the presence of phytates which form insoluble salts.

Determination of pK

The neutralisation curves may be used to determine the pK value of the charged groups. Tentative approaches were carried out on pectin-rich fibres. The range of pK values reported for carrot fibres is between 4.4 and 5.3 (Robertson et al., 1980a). However, these values must be considered only as apparent pK at one degree of dissociation and at a given ionic strength. Indeed, the neutralisation curves give the pH of the surrounding solution and not that of the insoluble

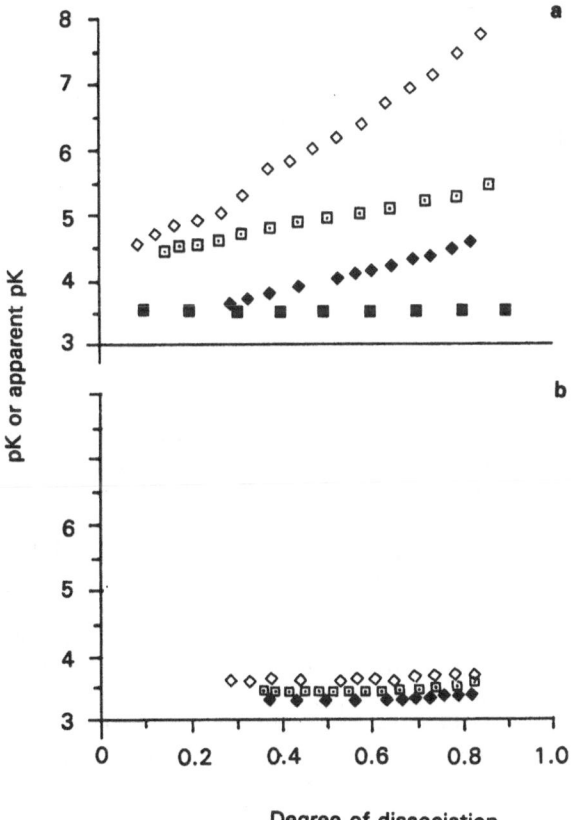

Fig. 2.2. Determination of pK and apparent pK (pK$_a$). **a** In absence of added salt. **b** In presence of 0.1 M NaCl of: *filled squares*, galacturonic acid; *filled diamonds*, beet pectins; *open squares*, crosslinked beet pectins; and *open diamonds*, beet fibres.

fibres. Furthermore, only apparent pK (pK_a) is thus obtained as it depends especially on the degree of dissociation, on the ionic strength of the surrounding solution, and on the degree of swelling of the fibres. For the determination of pH and therefore of pK of fibre, both polyelectrolyte and Donnan effects must also be taken into account (Thibault, 1986). The pK of galacturonic acid is independent of the degree of dissociation and is around 3.5 (Fig. 2.2). The curve for pure pectin demonstrates the polyelectrolyte effect and an intrinsic pK (pK_0) of 3.2 can be obtained on extrapolation to a degree of dissociation of zero. The curves for fibre show the additional effect of the Donnan phenomenon which tends to increase the external pH and therefore the pK_a. All these effects can be suppressed with a high salt concentration and then the pH measured is roughly that of the fibres, and the pK_0 can be estimated at around 3.2.

Hydration Properties

Water plays an important role in the plasticity and in the physiology of the cell wall; for example, it regulates the hydrolase activities involved in the loosening of cell wall fibres during cell elongation and/or division. Often, treatments such as drying, cooking, grinding, freezing, and fermentation are applied to the plant. These treatments affect the chemical composition and the physical structure of fibre (see "Effects of Processing") and precise correlations between treatments and hydration of fibres need to be established.

Hydration Properties of Polysaccharides

Hydration properties of fibres are better described for isolated fractions. The methods of isolation will condition the hydration characteristics of the fibres. Furthermore, these isolates can be mixtures of different polymers (pectin, cellulose, lignin, etc.) with different properties that will probably not be the same as those of the original fibres in the entire food plant cell wall. Basically, four different hydration parameters are measured: swelling, solubility, water-holding and water-binding capacities.

Swelling and solubility are closely related. Indeed, the first event in solubilisation of polymers is swelling. Water coming into the solid spreads the macromolecules (swelling) until they are fully extended and dispersed. They are then solubilised as random coils. However, this dispersion is not possible in the case of polysaccharides that adopt regular, ordered structures such as cellulose for example, and for which only swelling can occur. There, the maintenance of these strong associations in excess water depends on several factors (Whistler, 1973).

The regularity of the linear chemical structure increases the strength of the non-covalent bonds and thus stabilises the ordered conformation. If irregularities in the backbone or branching occur, these bonds will be weaker and the ordered structure will dissociate more easily. Furthermore, the type of linkages between sugar residues, such as $1 \longrightarrow 6$ linkages, induce a chain flexibility and the more flexible, the more soluble is the polysaccharide.

Another important factor influencing solubility is the charge. When dissociated, uronic acid, sulphate or pyruvate groups, for example, will tend to repel polysaccharides from each other and thus will favour solubilisation of the polymers. However, solubilisation is governed by pH, the ionic form of the charge, and by the presence of other solutes such as salts or sugars. Thus, pectic acids will not be soluble at acid pH, nor pectate at neutral pH in presence of calcium, for example.

Temperature increases the solubility of polysaccharides by breaking the weak bonds and thus by melting the ordered structure. Agar in the cell wall of marine algae, for example, will be soluble in water at about 80–100 °C and not at 37 °C. The properties of soluble polysaccharides such as viscosity, gel formation, etc. will be discussed later (see Chap. 3) but it is important to stress that there is no saturation limit for soluble polysaccharides. Thus published values of swelling, water-holding and water-binding capacity for soluble polysaccharides have to be treated with caution.

Methods for the Determination of Hydration Characteristics

Water-binding capacity and water-holding capacity (or water absorption) are two parameters used to describe hydration characteristics. The terms water-holding and water-binding capacities may be used interchangeably but, in common with Rey and Labuza (1981), we will use the term water binding for water content measured after an external force has been applied and water holding for water content measured without stress. The amount of water associated with insoluble fibres is dependent upon the chemical structure, molecular associations, particle size, and porosity of the sample, in addition to the solvent and temperature effects.

Swelling

Swelling is the volume of a given weight of dry fibre after equilibrium has been achieved in excess solvent (Kuniak and Marchessault, 1972). Swelling depends on several factors (amount of material tested, density, porosity, etc.) some of which can not be measured at the present time.

Water-Binding Capacity (WBC)

When measuring WBC, an external force is applied to the fibre equilibrated in solvent. The most widely used method is centrifugation. A fibre sample is equilibrated in solvent and then centrifuged at a set g value [2000 g for 10 minutes (AACC, 1978), 14 000 g for 1 hour (MacConnell et al., 1974), or 6000 g for 15 minutes (Robertson and Eastwood, 1981a)]. The supernatant liquid is drained off and the moisture content of the pellet is determined. It is necessary to specify to which dry weight the moisture content relates, i.e. the starting dry weight or the dry weight calculated after centrifugation. Centrifugal forces are primarily used to expel capillary water from the fibres. MacConnell et al. (1974) observed that WBC of celery fibre decreases with increasing centrifugal force and further noted that depending upon the plant source, centrifugation can lead to separation of the matrix in a layer located between water and the fibrous material. It is not clear whether sample deformation (collapse, separation) or the change in fibre capillary suction pressure is predominant in determining water losses by centrifugation. Furthermore, it is not known how the elasticity of fibre in the pellet can modify WBC through re-swelling once the centrifugal force has stopped.

Stephen and Cummings (1979) designed a method to model physiological conditions, involving an osmotic pressure created across a dialysis membrane. A dry or swollen fibre sample is placed in a dialysis tubing and immersed in a solution of known water activity. This solution is prepared using compounds, usually polyethylene glycol, with high molecular weight to prevent them from passing across the dialysis membrane. The difference in water potential across the dialysis membrane drives water in or out of the tubing depending upon the moisture content of the sample. After equilibrium has been reached, the dialysis bag is weighed and the weight of the solid content inside is determined. The size of the tubing should be chosen so that it can withstand the water volume increase without leakages or bursting; the ionic strength has to be controlled because it will affect the expansion of the fibre by the Donnan phenomenon. Robertson and Eastwood (1981b) reported that the WBC of fibres decreases with increasing suction pressure. This method also allows the determination of a type of WBC for water-soluble polysaccharides. However, the meaning of this value is unclear (Table 2.3).

Simple filtration using suction has also been used to determine WBC of fibres (Robertson et al., 1980a; Robertson and Eastwood, 1981a, b). The drawback of this method is that for it to be reproducible, at least the suction pressure applied

Table 2.3. Hydration characteristics (g of water/g of product) of different soluble fibres measured by different methods

Fibre	Method					
	Isotherms ($a_w = 0.98$)	Freezing-point depression ($a_w = 0.995$)	Baumann	Dialysis (280 mOsm)	Swelling capacity	Water absorbed during swelling
Mixed carrageenan	1.01[a]	8.83[a]	32.9[a]			
ι Carrageenan			138.6[b]		1.9[b]	16.7[b]
κλ Carrageenan			34.0[b]		2.1[b]	32.2[b]
κ Carrageenan			12.3[b]	46.6[c]	1.9[b]	40.3[b]
Agar	0.51[a]	0.92[a]	4.8[a]			
HM pectin[d]	0.81[a]	5.38[a]	4.0[a]		1.5[b]	14.0[b]
LM pectin[e]	1.27[a]	15.84[a]	3.7[a]		1.4[b]	11.6[b]

[a] Wallingford and Labuza, 1983; [b] Weber, 1987; [c] Stephen and Cummings, 1979; [d] high methoxyl pectin; [e] low methoxyl pectin.

and the duration should be standardised. Compression methods (0.5 to 1.0 ton pressure applied for 2 to 60 minutes) were used to determine the WBC of "hard-to-cook beans" (Garcia-Vela and Stanley, 1989; Plhak et al., 1989).

Water-Holding Capacity (WHC)

WHC relates to the amount of water in fibres equilibrated in an environment of known water potential, absorbed through capillarity, or measured by colligative methods.

Drawbacks of the moisture sorption isotherm method are that the equilibrium can take as long as 6 weeks to be reached, that the useful part of the curve near a water activity of one is highly imprecise, and that at certain water chemical potential growth of microorganism on the fibres can occur. This method has been used by Wallingford and Labuza (1983), Chen et al. (1984) and Cadden (1988).

Determination of WHC is also done based on liquid diffusion into a capillary swelling system such as with the Enslin (Enslin, 1933) or the Baumann (Baumann, 1967) apparatus. This method which has been automated (Arrigoni et al., 1987) is the only one allowing the observation of absorption kinetics. A small amount of sample (10–150 mg) is sprinkled on a fritted glass and water uptake is measured on a calibrated capillary as a function of time until equilibrium is reached.

Freezing-point depression has been used by Wallingford and Labuza (1983) and Chen et al. (1984). The osmolality of fibre suspensions at different concentrations is determined with a cryoscopic osmometer. The values obtained are plotted as a function of sample weight and the curve obtained is extrapolated to 280 mOsm corresponding to a water activity of 0.995, and the moisture content at that point is determined.

Variations of the Hydration Value

Variations Associated with the Method Used

All the methods used yield different results because some artefacts may be created and because the amounts measured relate to water associated differently with fibre. This variability is well illustrated by the work of Robertson and Eastwood (1981c) and of Chen at al. (1984) (Table 2.4).

Variations Associated with Experimental Conditions Used

Temperature has been shown to increase WBC of celery fibres (MacConnell et al., 1974) although the increase observed from 20 to 37 °C is not very important and may depend on other solvent conditions such as the presence of particular salts as seen with algal fibres (Fleury and Lahaye, 1991). Swelling of several fibres has been shown to increase with temperature (Parrott and Thrall, 1978;

Table 2.4. Effect of different methods on the water-binding and water-holding capacities (g of water/g of dry fibre) of different fibres

Fibre	Method						
	Centrifugation	Filtration	Dialysis pressure: 1 atm	Dialysis pressure: 10 atm	Baumann	Isotherm $(a_w = 0.98)$	Freezing-point depression
Potato[a]	23.8	16.5	3.3	1.7			
Bran[a]	3.7	3.0	1.4	1.0			
Apple[b]	2.3				2.4	1.4	10.5
Citrus[b]	5.7				1.8	5.7	2.3
Rice bran[b]	1.0				1.3	1.0	4.3
Wheat bran[b]	2.6				1.1	1.1	4.1
Soybean bran[b]	2.4				0.8	0.6	2.3
Oat bran[b]	1.4				0.7	0.4	1.1
Corn bran[b]	2.5				0.3	0.5	0.8

[a] Robertson and Eastwood, 1981c; [b] Chen et al., 1984.

Fleury and Lahaye, 1991). The ionic form of sugar beet fibre fractions was shown to affect WBC and swelling (Bertin et al., 1988). High ionic strength in the solvent was shown to decrease WBC of several fibres (Parrott and Thrall 1978; Bertin et al., 1988); the nature of ions present also affects WBC and swelling of algal fibres (Fleury and Lahaye, 1991), although such variation is fibre dependent as for those observed with different pH (Parrott and Thrall, 1978; Michel et al., 1988). In fact, it is not possible to draw conclusions since effects of solvent conditions are due to the chemical and physical properties of the fibres. Thus, for nutritional purposes, it may be more meaningful to determine these parameters in conditions (temperature, ionic strength, type of ions, pH, etc.) close to those prevailing in the gastro-intestinal tract.

Variations Associated with the Method of Fibre Preparation

Particle size was shown to modify the hydration characteristics of fibres (Mongeau and Brassard, 1982; Cadden, 1986, 1988; Michel et al., 1988; Fleury and Lahaye, 1991), but again, the variations are fibre dependent and may be related in some cases with chemical partitioning (Michel et al., 1988) (see "Effects of Processing"). Rasper (1979) showed that methods of preparation of cereal brans affected their hydration characteristics. They were generally higher with enzyme-prepared fibres than with acetone dried powders. Drying methods, temperature of drying, cooking methods (boiling, steaming, autoclaving, roasting) and extrusion-cooking affect fibre hydration (Rasper, 1979; Robertson and Eastwood, 1981a; Arrigoni et al., 1986; Caprez et al., 1986; Weber, 1987; Ralet et al., 1990).

Examples of Hydration Value

Rasper (1979) found an important correlation between the cellulose content of cereal fibres and hydration properties, while for other fibres the chemical factors controlling these properties were more complex. Holloway and Greig (1984)

Table 2.5. Hydration characteristics of some food plant cell walls

Reference and method	WBC[a] 1[c]	2[c]	3[c]	4[c]	4[d]	WHC[b] 4[e], 5[e]	Swelling 5[f]	4[g]	4[h]
Carrot	33		46.0		3.4	1.2		1.19	13.3
Onion	14	21.7	27.0		4.6	4.0		1.16	20.8
Tomato		14.0	40.7		2.8	7.5		1.26	9.6
Beans		20.8			3.4	1.6			10.9
Cabbage		35.8			3.7	5.9		1.07	29.6
Lettuce	36	25.3			3.1	2.6		1.08	37.0
Pumpkin		13.2							
Cauliflower	28				3.4	3.0		1.13	17.9
Acorn squash					3.3	8.4		1.01	18.9
Cucumber					2.8	4.4		1.06	26.7
Zucchini					3.1	3.8		1.06	12.9
Rutabaga					3.3	2.6		1.09	16.4
Celery					2.6	2.2		1.10	36.4
Broccoli					3.4	1.8		1.15	8.9
Potato	22								
New potato					1.4	0.3		1.46	4.2
Russet potato					2.8	0.2		1.53	2.8
Corn					3.1	1.8		1.22	8.6
Pear		16.4			3.3	3.7		0.86	12.1
Peach		11.5			3.1	8.1		0.86	31.5
Orange	20				3.5	4.2		1.12	17.0
Apple	17				3.2	7.9		1.17	17.8
Prune					3.4	5.6		0.90	19.4
Banana					2.5	0.1		1.04	7.0
Watermelon					3.6	3.1		0.98	43.6
Cantaloupe					3.1	3.6		1.02	41.2
Wheat bran	2.9	5.2			2.4	1.1		1.50	3.9
Hard wheat bran				4.8		4.3	320		
Soft wheat bran				4.2		3.5	250		
Rice bran				4.3		3.8	220		
Oat bran				2.6	2.3	0.7 (ref. 4) 2.8 (ref. 5)	220	1.29	3.2
Rye middlings				3.7		3.4	360		
Corn bran				3.8	2.2	0.3 (ref. 4) 3.7 (ref. 5)	160	1.16	3.6

[a] water-binding capacity (g H_2O/g dry weight); [b] water-holding capacity (g H_2O/g dry weight); [c] method of centrifugation (MacConnell et al., 1974); [d] method of dialysis starting from dry fibres (Weber, 1987); [e] Baumann apparatus; [f] % volume increase after 24 hours in de-ionized water at 25 °C (Rasper, 1979); [g] ratio of hydrated to dry fibre volume (Weber, 1987); [h] g water absorbed per g dry fibre during swelling (Weber, 1987).
References: 1, Heller and Hackler (1977) WHC of raw product; 2, Holloway and Greig (1984) WHC of freeze-dried food; 3, Longe (1984) WHC of raw product; 4, Rasper (1979) acetone dry powder; 5, Weber (1987).

found that lignin contributed to WBC of plant food cell wall and that arabinose and xylose (hemicellulose fraction) were correlated with WBC. It is hard to draw conclusions from the data of Table 2.5 although fruit and vegetable fibres tend to bind more water than cereal fibres. However, WBC is not always calculated in the same manner and results may be different if all the product, acetone dry powder or freeze-dried, or the fibre content is taken into account (Heller and Hackler, 1977). In the case of WHC and swelling values, there are great variations between vegetables, fruits, and cereals so that no generalisation is possible.

Adsorption of Organic Molecules

Lipid-binding capacity of fibre is measured by methods similar to those used for determining water-binding capacity. Fibre is stirred in an excess of oil (peanut oil, for example) in standard conditions of temperature and time, recovered by centrifugation or filtration and weighed. Oil-binding capacity refers to the weight increase of the sample and is expressed as gram of oil per gram of dry sample. Values for vegetables and fruit fibres are low ($<2\,g/g$) but are slightly higher for cereal fibres ($2–4\,g/g$) (Porzio and Blake, 1982; Solsulski and Cadden, 1982; Arrigoni et al., 1986; Caprez et al., 1986; Fleury and Lahaye, 1991). The mechanism of oil binding is unknown but the presence of lignin, particularly in cereal fibres, may have some role in such adsorption.

Investigation of the adsorption capacity of other organic molecules by fibres has been mainly concerned with bile acids (Vahouny, 1982; Eastwood, 1983; Vahouny and Cassidy, 1985; Selvendran et al., 1987; Kritchevsky, 1988; Edwards and Read, 1990) and there have been repeated demonstrations of adsorption of bile acids to various (isolated or not) fibres (Eastwood and Hamilton, 1968; Kritchevsky and Story, 1974; Eastwood et al. 1976; Story and Kritchevsky, 1976; Vahouny et al., 1980, 1981; Selvendran et al., 1987). Adsorption depends on the experimental conditions (duration of exposure, pH, . . .), on the physical and chemical forms of fibres and on the nature of bile acids (Eastwood and Hamilton, 1968; Kritchevsky and Story, 1974; Eastwood and Mowbray, 1976; Vahouny, 1982; Lairon et al., 1985). Certain fibres appear to exhibit preferential adsorption for unconjugated bile acids rather than the taurine or glycine conjugates and may show a degree of specificity for di- or trihydroxylated bile acids (Eastwood and Mowbray, 1976). Among fibres, pectins and lignins seem to have the greatest ability to adsorb bile acids. Hydrophobic interactions were suggested as a mechanism of adsorption of bile acids to lignins (Eastwood and Hamilton, 1968; Story and Kritchevsky, 1976) whereas ionic interactions involving Ca^{2+} or Al^{3+} bridges were proposed for pectins and other acidic polysaccharides (Nagyvary and Bradbury, 1977; Falk and Nagyvary, 1982; Hoagland, 1989). However, other authors also suggested hydrophobic interactions or hydrogen bonding between bile acids and pectins since they observed greater binding when acidic groups were non-ionized (Vahouny and Cassidy, 1985; Selvendran et al., 1987). Mechanisms of bile acids' adsorption to fibres are not fully understood and discrepancies in adsorption behaviour may arise from the method used to determine them and from the ways fibres were prepared. Adsorption is often taken as equivalent to retention but both adsorption and entrapment in the cell wall matrix could be responsible for binding (Eastwood, 1983). The preparation of fibres is important since some components associated with fibres such as lectins, saponins, silicate could be involved in bile acids and steroids adsorption. In fact, the efficiency of lignin as an adsorbent is still an open question since its high bile acid adsorption capacity was deduced from work on Klason lignin (Eastwood and Hamilton, 1986) which is obtained after harsh chemical treatments of cell walls that may expose or create sites for bile acids adsorption that otherwise would not be available or even exist. Variations in bile acids adsorption capacity has been also related to the developmental stage of fibre sources (Robertson et al., 1980b).

The in vivo bile acid-binding capacity of fibres has been indirectly demonstrated by the increase of faecal bile acids and sterols (Anderson and Chen, 1979; Gallaher and Schneeman, 1986). However, the effect of fibres on bile acids metabolism may represent a small part of the overall mechanism related to hyperlipidaemia (Eastwood, 1983; Judd and Truswell, 1985; Kritchevsky, 1988; Adiotomre et al., 1990).

Effect of Processing

Much of the cell wall material we consume is processed, thus modifying the content, the composition, the physico-chemical, functional and nutritional properties of fibres.

Grinding

Most fibres are ground for better acceptance of the final food products. Partitioning may be done but fractions can have different chemical compositions. Wheat bran, which contains different tissue, is especially affected. Milled bran has a lower level of insoluble dietary fibre than coarse bran (Heller et al., 1977; Caprez et al., 1986). In contrast, no marked differences were observed between fractions of sugarbeet fibres, except an enrichment in ash for the fraction with low particle size (Michel et al., 1988).

Grinding may affect hydration characteristics (see "Hydration Properties" above) and possibly CEC (Kirwan et al., 1974). These effects are related to changes in physical structure and chemical partitioning.

Chemical Treatments

Chemical treatments can solubilise some of the constituents such as pectins and lignin. For example, treatment of wheat straw, corn stalk, cereal brans or vegetable or fruit pulp with an alkaline solution of hydrogen peroxide removes part of the lignin and increases water absorption of the resulting fibres (Gould et al., 1989). Treatment of sugar beet fibres successively with acid and alkaline solutions enriches the resulting fibres in hemicellulose and cellulose at the expense of pectins and arabinans and leads to fibres having different CEC and hydration properties (Bertin et al., 1988; Table 2.6).

Table 2.6. Influence of some extractions on the physico-chemical properties of beet fibre (from Bertin et al., 1988)

Treatment	Swelling (ml/g) (in H_2O)	WBC[a] (g/g)		CEC[b] (meq/g)
		in H_2O	in 1 M MaCl	
None	11.5	26.5	20.6	0.47
Extraction by oxalate	25.2	32.0	21.1	0.46
Extraction by acid	16.7	27.5	19.1	0.37
Extraction by alkali	50.8	35.4	14.8	0.51

[a] Water-binding capacity.
[b] Cation-exchange capacity.

Heat Treatment

Heat treatment may alter the fibre content of food as some insoluble compounds such as products of Maillard reactions and resistant starch can be formed and measured as part of cell wall fibres. For example, Björk et al., (1984) showed that the fibre content of wheat products increased with the severity of extrusion-cooking (temperature, screw speed). The additional fibre fraction was attributed to amylose–lipid complexes since they disappeared when a heat stable α-amylase was used in the fibre content determination. On the other hand, heating can also lower fibre content or modify the fibre distribution between water-soluble and insoluble fractions by degrading components into smaller compounds (Anderson and Clydesdale, 1980; Varo et al., 1984; Arrigoni et al., 1986; Asp et al., 1986; Caprez et al., 1986; Ralet et al., 1990, 1991). In particular, extrusion-cooking can increase the amount of water-soluble pectin (Ralet et al., 1991). Wet heat treatment, particularly of vegetable and fruit fibres, increases the amount of soluble fibre by partially degrading pectic polysaccharides. The severity of the different heat treatments determines the physico-chemical properties of fibres (Tables 2.7 and 2.8) (Anderson and Clydesdale, 1980; Varo et al., 1984; Arrigoni et al., 1986; Caprez et al., 1986; Ralet et al., 1990, 1991).

Conclusions

When studying physico-chemical properties of fibre, it is necessary to define their origin, their methods of preparation, and, if possible, their chemical and physical structure. The first crucial step is the preparation of the sample. For

Table 2.7. Influence of some treatments on water-binding capacity (WBC) and fibre content of some fibres (from Arrigoni et al., 1986)

Fibre	Treatment	Fibre content (% dry matter)			WBC (g/g)
		Insoluble	Soluble	Total	
Yellow pea hulls	None	85.3	5.3	90.6	3.3
	Boiled 60 min	82.9	9.8	92.7	5.0
	Autoclaved 15 min	85.3	9.0	94.3	4.0
	Autoclaved 30 min	81.7	9.7	91.3	3.7
	Autoclaved 60 min	80.8	12.5	93.3	3.7
	Extruded	81.1	6.7	87.8	3.3
Apple pomace	None	55.5	10.5	65.9	5.1
	Boiled 15 min	48.5	12.0	60.5	6.2
	Boiled 60 min	45.9	18.4	64.3	6.2
	Autoclaved 30 min	50.2	18.0	68.2	4.5
	Autoclaved 60 min	43.7	19.2	62.9	4.2
De-pectinised apple pomace	None	78.0	14.0	92.0	2.3
	Boiled 15 min	72.0	10.9	82.8	2.5
	Autoclaved 15 min	72.3	10.7	83.0	2.1
	Autoclaved 60 min	69.7	11.0	80.7	2.0
	Extruded	82.0	8.9	90.9	3.0

Table 2.8. Influence of extrusion-cooking on the fibre content and properties of wheat bran (from Ralet et al., 1990)

	Fibre content (% dry matter)			Water-binding capacity (g/g)	Water-holding capacity (g/g)
	Insoluble	Soluble	Total		
Not treated	42.3	8.1	50.4	6.4	2.7
Extruded[a]	41.4	10.8	52.2	6.0	3.8
Extruded[b]	38.3	12.9	51.2	6.0	3.0
Extruded[c]	37.5	13.9	51.4	5.8	3.3
Extruded[d]	30.7	16.0	46.7	6.8	2.2

Conditions of extrusion:
Temperature, 100 °C;
Screw speed (rev/min), 250[a, b], 240[c, d];
Water added (% of dry matter), 17.5[a], 8.7[b], 11.3[c], 6.1[d];
Feed rate (kg/h), 32[a, b, c], 20[d].

material rich in starch and protein and poor in pectins, classical methods for the analysis of cell walls can be used (cf. Chap. 4); however, the soluble fraction has to be taken into account, especially for plant materials such as vegetable or fruit fibre, which are rich in pectins susceptible to solubilisation mainly by β-elimination (Massiot et al., 1988). During this step, artefacts arising from the drying process or grinding may also be produced.

When considering the hydration properties, it is clear that further work is needed to understand:

1. What we measure with all the different methods
2. How water precisely interacts and how we can distinguish between all the types of interactions (physical, chemical)

3. What is the physical structure of fibres, i.e. area, density, shape of fibres, diameter, length and population repartition of capillaries in fibres
4. How treatments affect the physical and chemical characteristics of fibres
5. How all these parameters affect hydration properties of fibres
6. How these parameters can be correlated with physiological response.

Thus, it is important that methods and conditions of measurements be clearly given when reporting hydration properties of fibres. It is also necessary to develop methods leading to the characterisation of the physical structure of insoluble fibre.

The other very important physico-chemical property of dietary fibre is its solubility. In cell walls some polysaccharides may be soluble (β-glucans, pectins, some hemicelluloses, etc.); this soluble fraction is more important in vegetable or fruit cell walls than in cereal cell walls because of the presence of pectic substances. Much more is known about the properties (viscosity, gelling behaviour, etc.) of soluble polysaccharides than those of insoluble fibre, because appropriate methods exist. As most of the fibre found in food may be considered as insoluble aggregates embedded in a more or less viscous surrounding solution, the characterisation of the "texture" of these "suspensions" has to be extensively studied; this is not yet the case because appropriate methods must be developed.

References

AACC methods manual (1978) Water hydration capacity of protein materials method 88-04. American Association of Cereal Chemists, St Paul, MN, USA

Adiotomre J, Eastwood MA, Edwards CA, Brydon WC (1990) Dietary fiber: in vitro methods that anticipate nutrition and metabolic activities in human. Am J Clin Nutr S2:128–134

Allen MS, MacBurney MI, Van Soest PJ (1985) Cation-exchange capacity of plant cell walls at neutral pH. J Sci Food Agric 36: 1065–1072

Anderson JW, Chen WJ (1979) Plant fiber: carbohydrate and lipid metabolism. Am J Clin Nutr 32:346–363

Anderson NE, Clydesdale FM (1980) Effects of processing on the dietary fiber content of wheat bran, puréed green beans and carrots. J Food Sci 45:1533–1537

Arrigoni E, Caprez A, Amadò R, Neukom H (1986) Chemical composition and physical properties of modified dietary fibre sources. Food Hydrocolloids 1:57–64

Arrigoni E, Caprez A, Neukom H, Amadò R (1987) Determination of water uptake by an automated method. Lebens Wiss Technol 20:263–264

Asp NG, Björck I, Nyman M (1986) Effects of processing on dietary fibre. In: Amadò R, Schweizer TF (eds) Nahrungsfasern dietary fibres. Academic Press, London, pp 177–189

Baumann H (1967) Apparatur nach Baumann zer Bestimmung der Flussigkeitsaufnahme von pulvigren Substanzen. Glastechnik und Intrumententechnik – Fachzeitschrift für das Laboratorium 11:540–542

Bertin C, Rouau X, Thibault JF (1988) Structure and properties of sugar beet fibres. J Sci Food Agric 44:15–29

Björck I, Nyman M, Asp NG (1984) Extrusion-cooking and dietary fiber. I. Effects on dietary fiber content and on degradation in the rat intestinal tract. Cereal Chem 61:174–179

Brillouet JM, Rouau X, Hoebler C, Barry JL, Carré B, Lorta E (1988) A new method for determination of insoluble cell walls and soluble non starchy polysaccharides from plant materials. J Agric Food Chem 36:969–979

Cadden AM (1986) Comparative effects of particle size reduction on physical structure and water binding properties of several plant fibers. J Food Sci 52:1595–1599

Cadden AM (1988) Moisture sorption characteristics of several plant fibers. J Food Sci 53:1150–1155

Caprez A, Arrigoni E, Amadò R, Neukom H (1986) Influence of different type of thermal treatment on the chemical composition and physical properties of wheat bran. J Cereal Sci 4:233–239

Chen JY, Pina M, Labuza TP (1984) Evaluation of water binding capacity (WBC) of food fiber sources. J Food Sci 49:59–63

Eastwood MA (1983) Physical properties of fiber towards bile acids, water and minerals. In: Birch GG, Parker KJ (eds), Dietary fibre. Applied Science Publishers, London, pp 149–163

Eastwood MA, Hamilton D (1968) Studies on the adsorption of bile salts to non-absorbed components of the diet. Biochim Biophys Acta 152:165–173

Eastwood MA, Mowbray L (1976) The binding of components of mixed micelles to dietary fibers. Am J Clin Nutr 29:1461–1467

Eastwood MA, Anderson R, Mitchell WD, Robertson J, Pocock S (1976) A method to measure adsorption of bile salts to vegetable fibre of differing water holding capacity. J Nutr 106:1429–1432

Edwards CA, Read NW (1990) Fibre and small intestine function. In: Leeds AR (ed) Dietary fibre perspectives – review and bibliography. John Libbey, London, pp 52–75

Enslin O (1933) Ueber einen Apparat zur Messung der Flussigkeitsaufnahme von quellbaren und porosen Stoffen und zur Charakterisierung der Benetzbarkeit. Die Chemische Fabrik 13:147–148

Falk JD, Nagyvary JJ (1982) Exploratory studies of lipid–pectin interactions. J Nutr 112:182–188

Fleury N, Lahaye M (1991) Chemical and physico-chemical characteristics of fibres from *Laminaria digitata* (kombu breton). J Sci Food Agric 55:389–400

Frölich W, Nyman M (1988) Minerals, phytate and dietary fibre in different fractions of oat grain. J Cereal Sci 7:73–82

Gallaher D, Schneeman BO (1986) Intestinal interaction of bile acids, phospholipids, dietary fibres and cholestyramine. Am J Physiol 250:G420–426

Garcia-Lopez J, Lee K (1985) Iron binding by fiber is influenced by competing minerals. J Food Sci 50:424–425–428

Garcia-Vela LA, Stanley DW (1989) Water-holding capacity in hard-to-cook beans (*Phaseolus vulgaris*): effect of pH and ionic strength. J Food Sci 54:1080–1081

Gould JM, Jasberg BK, Dexter LB, Hsu JT, Lewis SM, Fahey GC (1989) High fiber, non-caloric flour substitute for baked food properties of alkaline peroxide-treated lignocellulose. Cereal Chem 66:201–205

Grant GT, Morris ER, Rees DA, Smith PJC, Thom D (1973) Biological interactions between polysaccharides and divalent cations: the egg-box model. FEBS Lett 32:195–198

Heller SN, Hackler LR (1977) Water-holding capacity of various sources of plant fiber. J Food Sci 42:1137–1139

Heller SN, Rivers JM, Hackler LR (1977) Dietary fiber: the effect of particle size and pH on its measurement. J Food Sci 42:436–439

Hoagland PD (1989) Binding of dietary anions to vegetable fiber. J Agric Food Chem 37:1343–1347

Holloway WD, Greig RI (1984) Water-holding capacity of hemicelluloses from fruits, vegetables and wheat bran. J Food Sci 49:1632–1633

Judd PA, Truswell AS (1985) Dietary fibre and blood lipids in man. In: Leeds AR (ed) Fibre perspectives – review and bibliography. John Libbey, London, pp 52–75

Kirwan WO, Smith AN, MacConnell AA, Mitchell WD, Eastwood MA (1974) Action of different bran preparations on colonic function. Br Med J iv:187–189

Kritchevsky D (1988) Dietary fiber. Ann Rev Nutr 8:301–328

Kritchevsky D, Story JA (1974) Binding of bile salts in vitro by non-nutritive fiber. J Nutr 104:458–462

Kuniak L, Marchessault RH (1972) Study of crosslinking reaction between epichlorhydrin and starch. Starke 4:110–116

Lairon D, Lafont H, Vigne JL, Nalbone G, Léonardi J, Hauton JC (1985) Effects of dietary fibers and cholestyramine on the activity of pancreatic lipase in vitro. Am J Clin Nutr 42:629–638

Laszlo JA (1987) Mineral binding properties of soy hull modeling mineral interactions with an insoluble dietary fiber source. J Agric Food Chem 35:593–600

Longe OG (1984) Water-holding capacity of some African vegetables, fruits and tubers measured in vitro. J Food Sci 49:762–764

MacBurney MI, Van Soest PJ, Chase LE (1983) Cation-exchange capacity and buffering capacity of neutral detergent fibres. J Sci Food Agric 34:910–916

MacConnell AA, Eastwood MA, Mitchell WD (1974) Physical characteristics of vegetable foodstuffs that could influence bowel function. J Sci Food Agric 25:1457–1464

Massiot P, Rouau X, Thibault JF (1988) Structural study of cell wall of carrot (*Daucus carota* L). 1. Isolation and characterisation of cell wall fibres. Carbohydr Res 172:217–227

Michel F, Thibault JF, Barry JL, De Baynast R (1988) Preparation and characterisation of dietary fibre from sugar beet pulp. J Sci Food Agric 42:77–85

Mongeau R, Brassard R (1982) Insoluble dietary fiber from breakfast cereals and brans; bile salt binding and water-holding capacity in relation to particle size. Cereal Chem 59: 413–417

Moorman WFB, Moon NJ, Worthington RE (1983) Physical properties of dietary fiber and binding of mutagens. J Food Sci 48:1010–1011

Nagyvary J, Bradbury EL (1977) Hypocholesterolemic effects of Al^{3+} complexes. Biochim Biophys Res Comm 77:592–598

Parrott ME, Thrall BE (1978) Functional properties of various fibers: physical properties. J Food Sci 43:759–763

Plhak LC, Cadswell KB, Stanley DW (1989) Comparison of methods to characterize water imbibition in hard-to-cook beans. J Food Sci 54:326–336

Porzio MA, Blake JR (1982) Washed orange pulp: characterization and properties. In: Furda I (ed) Unconventional sources of dietary fiber. American Chemical Society, Washington, pp 135–141 (ACS symposium series, no. 214)

Ralet MC, Thibault JF, Della Valle G (1990) Influence of extrusion-cooking on the structure and properties of wheat bran. J Cereal Sci 11:249–259

Ralet MC, Thibault JF, Della Valle G (1991) Solubilisation of sugar beet cell wall polysaccharides by extrusion-cooking. Lebensm Wiss Technol 24:107–112

Rasper VF (1979) Chemical and physical characteristics of dietary cereal fiber. In: Inglett GE, Falkehag SI (eds) Dietary fibers: chemistry and nutrition. Academic Press, New York, pp 93–115

Rey DK, Labuza TP (1981) Characterization of the effect of solutes on the water-binding and gel strength properties of carrageenan. J Food Sci 46:786–789

Robertson JA, Eastwood MA (1981a) An examination of factors which may affect the water-holding capacity of dietary fibre. Br J Nutr 45:83–88

Robertson JA, Eastwood MA (1981b) A method to measure the water-holding properties of dietary fibre using suction pressure. Br J Nutr 46:247–255

Robertson JA, Eastwood MA (1981c) An investigation of the experimental conditions which could affect water-holding capacity of dietary fibre. J Sci Food Agric 32:819–825

Robertson JA, Eastwood MA, Yeoman MM (1980a) An investigation into the physical properties of fibre prepared from several carrot varieties at different stages of development. J Sci Food Agric 31:633–638

Robertson JA, Eastwood MA, Yeoman MM (1980b) Bile salt adsorption ability of dietary fibre from named variety of carrot at different developmental ages. J Nutr 110:1130–1137

Schimberni M, Cardinali F, Sodini G, Canella M (1982) Chemical and functional characterization of corn bran, oat hull flour and barley hull flour. Lebens Wiss Technol 15:337–339

Schweizer TF, Frölich W, Del Vedovo S, Besson R (1984) Minerals and phytate analysis of dietary fiber from cereals. J Cereal Chem 61:116–119

Selvendran RR, Stevens BJH, Du Pont MS (1987) Dietary fiber: chemistry, analysis and properties. Adv Food Res 31:117–209

Solsulski FW, Cadden AM (1982) Composition and physiological properties of several sources of dietary fiber. J Food Sci 47:1472–1477

Stephen AM, Cummings JH (1979) Water-holding by dietary fibre in vitro and its relationship to faecal output in man. Gut 20:722–729

Story JA, Kritchevsky D (1976) Comparison of the binding of various bile acids and bile salts in vitro to several types of fiber. J Nutr 106:1292–1294

Thibault JF (1986) Some physical properties of sugar beet pectins modified by oxidative crosslinking. Carbohydr Res 155:183–191

Thibault JF, Rinaudo M (1986) Chain association of pectic molecules during calcium-induced gelation. Biopolymers 25:455–468

Thompson SA, Weber CW (1979) Influence of pH on the binding of copper, zinc and iron in six fiber sources. J Food Sci 44:752–754

Vahouny GV (1982) Dietary fibres and intestinal absorption of lipids. In: Vahouny GV, Kritchevsky D (eds) Dietary fibre in health and disease. Plenum Press, New York, pp 203–228

Vahouny GV, Cassidy M (1985) Dietary fibres and absorption of nutrients. Proc Soc Exp Biol Med 180:432–446

Vahouny GV, Tombes R, Cassidy M, Kritchevsky D, Gallo LL (1980) Binding of bile salts, phospholipids and cholesterol from mixed micelles by bile acid sequestrants and dietary fibers. Lipids 15:1012–1018

Vahouny GV, Tombes R, Cassidy M, Kritchevsky D, Gallo LL (1981) Dietary fibres. VI. Binding of fatty acids and monoolein from mixed micelles containing bile salts and lecithin. Proc Soc Exp Biol Med 166:12–16

Van Soest PJ, Robertson JB (1976) Chemical and physical properties of dietary fibre. In: Proceedings of the Miles symposium presented by the Nutrition Society of Canada, June 14, Dalhousie University, Halifax, Nova Scotia, pp 13–25

Van Soest PJ, Horvath P, MacBurney M, Jeraci J, Allen M (1983) Some in vitro and in vivo properties of dietary fibers from non-cereal sources. In: Furda I (ed) Unconventional sources of dietary fiber. American Chemical Society, Washington, pp 135–141 (ACS symposium series, no. 214)

Varo P, Veijalainen K, Koivistoinen P (1984) Effect of heat treatment on the dietary fibre contents of potato and tomato. J Food Technol 19:485–492

Voragen FGJ, Timmers JPT, Linssen JPH, Schols HA, Pilnik W (1983) Methods of analysis for cell wall polysaccharides of fruit and vegetables. Z Lebensm Unters Forsch 177:251–256

Wallingford L, Labuza TP (1983) Evaluation of the water-binding properties of food hydrocolloids by physical/chemical methods and in a low fat meat emulsion. J Food Sci 48:1–5

Weber JL (1987) The water-binding capacity of fruit and vegetable fibers. PhD dissertation, University of Minnesota, MN, USA

Whistler RL (1973) Solubility of polysaccharides and their behavior in solution. Carbohydrates in Solution. American Chemical Society, Washington, pp 242–255 (ACS symposium series, no. 117)

Yoshida T, Kuwano K (1989) Methods used in the investigation of insoluble dietary fiber. In: Linskens HF, Jackson JF (eds) Plant fibers. Springer, Berlin, Heidelberg, New York, pp 260–277 (Modern methods of plant analysis, new series 10)

Chapter 3

Physico-chemical Properties of Food Polysaccharides

E.R. Morris

Introduction

Polysaccharides, which are the principal constituents of dietary fibre, show a wide spectrum of physical properties, reflecting the nature and extent of intermolecular association. At one extreme, the polymer chains may be packed together into ordered assemblies, such as cellulose fibrils, which are almost totally resistant to hydration and swelling. At the other extreme, polysaccharide chains can exist in solution as fluctuating, disordered coils, interacting with one another only by physical entanglement. Between these extremes lie the hydrated, swollen networks typical of plant tissue and of many manufactured foods.

The aim of this chapter is to relate the physical properties of food polysaccharides to (1) possible modes of physiological action as dietary fibre, and (2) their composition (primary structure), drawing on the understanding of structure–function relationships that has developed from the use of isolated and purified polysaccharides for control of texture in the food industry.

Certain industrial polysaccharides (notably pectin) also occur as significant constituents of unprocessed foods. Some, such as methylcellulose and carboxymethylcellulose (CMC), are chemically modified forms of natural dietary fibres. Others come from sources that do not form part of the traditional Western diet (from seaweeds, plant exudates, and bacterial fermentation), but would fall within the "non-starch polysaccharide" definition of dietary fibre.

For the benefit of readers unfamiliar with carbohydrate chemistry, a brief introduction to polysaccharide composition and shape (conformation) is given below.

Structure and Shape of Polysaccharide Chains

The basic building block in all industrial polysaccharides is a six-membered (pyranose) sugar ring (Fig. 3.1), composed of five carbon atoms and one oxygen. In the projections shown in Fig. 3.1, carbon atoms are numbered clockwise from the ring oxygen, with C-6 lying outside the ring. The stable conformations of the pyranose ring (see, for example, Stoddart, 1971) are chair forms ($^4C_1$ and $^1C_4$) in

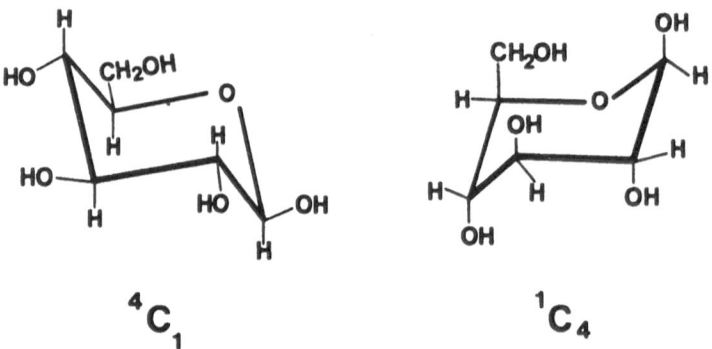

Fig. 3.1. Chair conformations of 6-membered sugar rings.

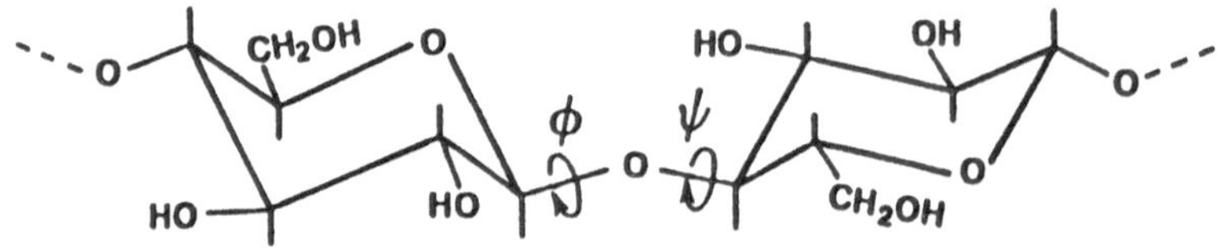

Fig. 3.2. Conformational variables in carbohydrate chains (illustrated for cellulose).

which all bonds are fully staggered. Substituents at each carbon atom may be present either in *equatorial* locations, widely spaced around the periphery of the ring, or in crowded *axial* positions above or below the ring. Interconversion between $^4C_1$ and $^1C_4$ chair forms has the effect of converting all equatorial substituents to axial, and vice versa. For all sugars encountered in food polysaccharides, the stable chair conformation is the one in which the bulky C-6 group is equatorial rather than in the sterically crowded axial location.

Linkage of sugars in carbohydrate chains occurs between the OH group at C-1 of one residue and any of the other OH groups of the next (O-2, O-3, O-4 or O-6), with formal elimination of water. Branching occurs by linkage at two (or more) of these positions on the same residue. In the stable chair form (C-6 equatorial) an axial linkage at O-1 is designated as a α and an equatorial linkage as β. O-2, O-3 and O-4 may be either axial or equatorial, depending on the specific sugar.

Since, as discussed above, the component monosaccharide units can be regarded as essentially locked in the chair conformation in which C-6 is equatorial, the overall shape of the polysaccharide chain (Rees et al., 1982) is determined by the dihedral angles between adjacent residues (Fig. 3.2). These may be either fixed, and have the same values at all positions along the polymer chain, to give ordered chain conformations, or constantly fluctuating, to give the overall "random coil" behaviour typical of polymer solutions.

Order and Disorder

Adoption of regular, ordered shapes that can pack together efficiently (Rees et al., 1982) is essential for assembly of polysaccharide chains into compact, unhydrated forms, such as cellulose fibrils or starch granules. Whether such ordered assemblies remain stable on exposure to excess water or dissociate into individual hydrated chains depends on the interplay of a number of different factors. The most obvious is charge. Many polysaccharides have charged groups (e.g. COO^- or SO_3^-) which repel one another, thus favouring expanded coil geometry in solution, rather than compact ordering. Less obviously, the presence of small co-solutes, such as sugars or salts, can alter the solvent quality of water and shift the balance between polymer–polymer interactions and polymer–solvent interactions, normally in the direction of decreased solubility.

Adoption of an ordered structure also entails considerable loss of mobility (i.e. entropy), which must be more than offset by favourable non-covalent interactions between the participating chains. Non-covalent bonds (such as hydrogen bonds, electrostatic attractions and van der Waals forces) are individually weak and are effective in stabilising polymer assemblies only when they act *co-operatively* in extended arrays, so that ordered structures have a minimum critical length, typically of about 10 residues in each chain. Thus changes in primary sequence (such as branching, irregularly spaced sidechains, or anomalous residues in the polymer backbone) can be an important drive to solubility if they occur at spacings less than the minimum sequence length for ordered association. The presence of sidechains can, in itself, promote solubility by providing an additional entropic contribution from freedom of rotation about the sidechain–mainchain linkage. Similarly, polysaccharides with flexible linkages in the polymer backbone are less likely to form stable, solvent-resistant assemblies than those that are inherently stiff.

Finally, temperature is an important determinant of solubility. The overall change in free energy (ΔG) on going from a compact, ordered structure to a disordered coil is related to the enthalpy change (ΔH) from loss of favourable non-covalent interactions and the entropy change (ΔS) from increased conformational mobility by:

$$\Delta G = \Delta H - T\Delta S \qquad\qquad (3.1)$$

Thus entopic effects, favouring solubility, become increasingly important with increasing temperature (T). Because of the simultaneous, co-operative involvement of large numbers of weak bonds, the formation and melting of polysaccharide ordered structures usually occur as sharp processes (in many ways analogous to phase transitions of small molecules), in response to comparatively small changes in temperature (or other external variables such as ionic strength or pH).

Inter-residue Linkage Patterns and Ordered Packing

A major difference between polysaccharides and most other types of polymer is that the same monomer unit can be linked together in different ways to give different macromolecular structures. Fig. 3.3 shows four polymers of glucose (cellulose, amylose, curdlan and dextran). Despite being built up from the same monomer, these materials all have very different physical properties.

Conversely, different sugars linked together in the same way often give polysaccharides with closely similar properties (Rees et al., 1982). For example,

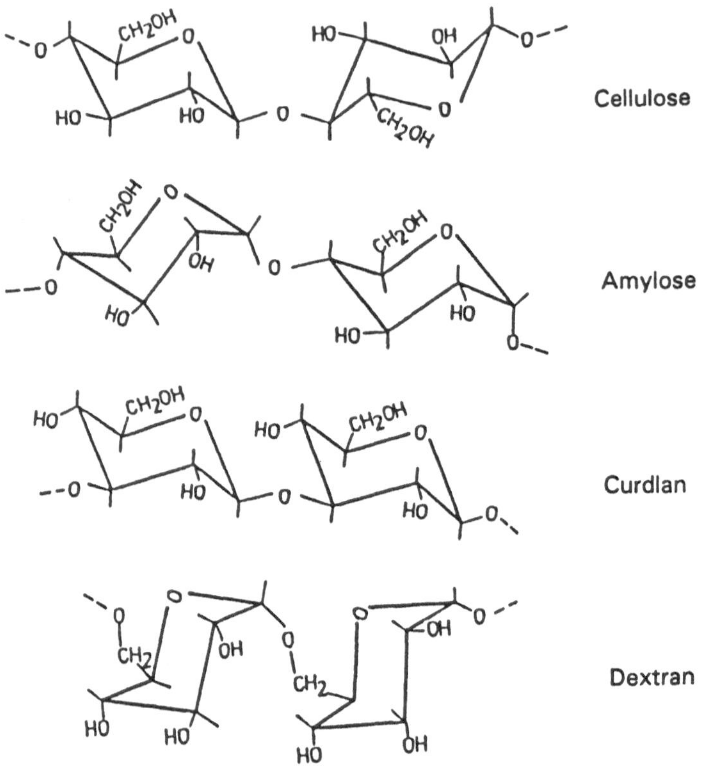

Fig. 3.3. Polymers of glucose, linked β-1,4 (cellulose), α-1,4 (amylose), β-1,3 (curdlan) and α-1,6 (dextran).

cellulose, chitin, mannan (the backbone of the galactomannan family of plant polysaccharides) and xylan (the backbone of arabinoxylans and related hemicelluloses) all form mechanically strong, solvent-resistant matrices, but are built up from different monomer units (glucose, N-acetylglucosamine, mannose and xylose respectively). In each case, however, the component residues are linked together through equatorial bonds diagonally opposite each other across the sugar ring (β-1,4 diequatorial), so that the bonds to and from each residue are parallel and almost co-linear. This linkage pattern (Fig. 3.4a) gives flat, ribbon-like structures that can pack into tough, fibrillar assemblies.

Other types of bonding pattern also give rise to characteristic ordered structures, with associated characteristic physical properties, largely indepen-dent of the nature of the component residues (unless gross changes, such as the presence or absence of charge, are also involved). For example, when the bonds to and from each residue are once more directly opposite one another but axial rather than equatorial, so that, although still parallel, they are now offset by the full width of the sugar ring, the resulting ordered structures are again ribbon-like, but highly buckled (Fig. 3.4b) and pack together with cavities which, when the chains are charged, can accommodate site-bound counterions. Dimeric "egg-box" structures of this type occur in the calcium-induced ordered

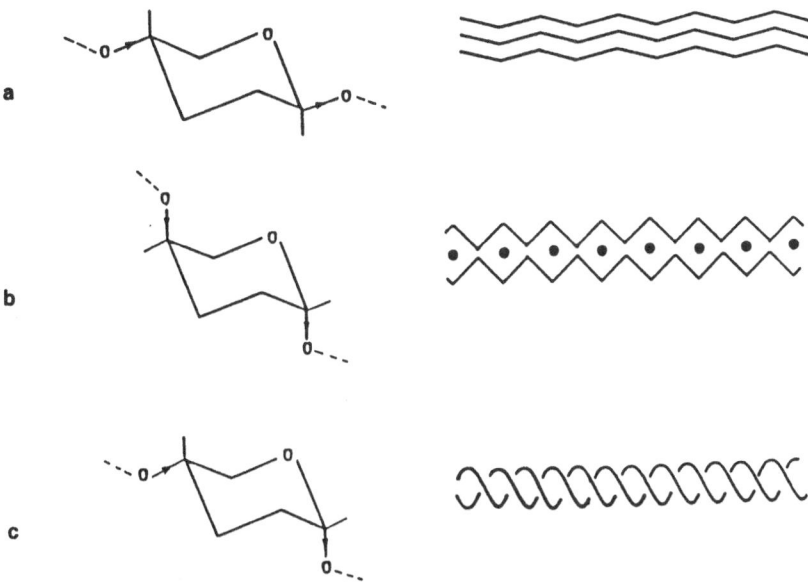

Fig. 3.4. Relationship between the ordered structures of polysaccharide chains and the relative orientation of bonds to and from component residues. **a** Extended ribbons; **b** buckled ribbons; **c** hollow helices.

assemblies of 1,4-diaxially linked polygalacturonate sequences (in pectin) and polyguluronate sequences (in alginate).

When the bonds to and from each residue are no longer parallel (Fig. 3.4c), a systematic "twist" in chain direction is introduced, giving helical ordered structures which are usually stabilised by packing together co-axially. This situation can arise from bonds which are no longer diagonally opposite each other (as in the curdlan structure shown in Fig. 3.3) or which are diagonally opposite, but with one axial and one equatorial (as in amylose). The ordered structures of amylose and curdlan (a gelling polysaccharide used widely in Japan, but not cleared for food use in the West) are double and triple stranded helices, respectively. Linkage outside the sugar ring (as in the dextran structure in Fig. 3.3) joins the component residues by three rather than two covalent bonds, giving additional entropic stability to the disordered form.

Hydrated Networks

One of the most characteristic features of many polysaccharides in vitro is their ability to form cohesive gels at low concentrations (typically around 1% w/v, although some polysaccharides gel at concentrations of 0.1% or less). The same behaviour often occurs in vivo in formation of hydrated tissue structure. Crosslinking of such networks (Fig. 3.5) involves extended "junction zones" in

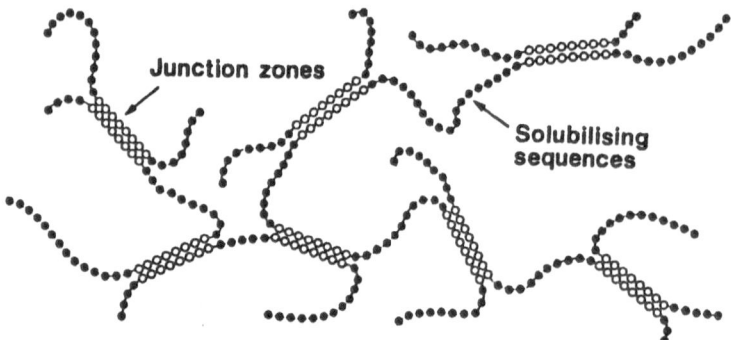

Fig. 3.5. Schematic representation of hydrated polysaccharide network.

which the participating chains pack together into ordered assemblies, which can be of any of the structural types shown in Fig. 3.4 (flat nested ribbons, buckled "egg-box" dimers or co-axial helices). Formation of a hydrated network rather than an insoluble precipitate, however, requires the junctions to be linked by interconnecting sequences that are conformationally disordered (as in solution), providing an entropic drive to solubilise the network.

Co-existence of ordered and disordered regions within the same polysaccharide system can occur in a number of ways (Rees et al., 1982). As a general mechanism, the presence of a small amount of residual disorder in an otherwise fully ordered polymer can lower the overall free energy by an entropic contribution that more than outweighs the enthalpic advantage of further ordering. In most polysaccharides, however, ordered association is limited by primary structure.

The simplest situation is where the polymer has a block structure, with regions that are soluble under the prevailing solvent conditions interspersed by regions capable of forming stable associations. A well-characterised example is the calcium alginate gelling system, where sequences of one type (1,4-diaxially linked polyguluronate) adopt a "buckled-ribbon" conformation and form junctions stabilised by site-bound calcium ions (Fig. 3.4b) and other sequences which cannot bind calcium in this way confer solubility (1,4-diequatorially linked polymannuronate, and heteropolymeric blocks incorporating both mannuronate and guluronate). In other systems, such as plant galactomannans (which include the food polysaccharides guar gum and locust bean gum), pendant sidechains limit association of the polymer backbone.

Inter-chain junctions can also be terminated by the occurrence in the primary sequence of anomalous residues that are geometrically incompatible with incorporation in the ordered structure. The structural properties of agar and carrageenan polysaccharides in algal tissue are regulated in this way. "Kinking" residues of 1,2-linked rhamnose have a similar role in pectin, and are spaced such that the 1,4-diaxially linked polygalacturonate sequences of the polymer chain have a regular length of approx. 25 residues. These sequences form calcium-mediated junctions in the same way as the polyguluronate regions of alginate, but the extent and stability of association may be modified by the occurrence of a proportion of the galacturonate residues as the methyl ester.

Polysaccharide "Weak Gels"

As discussed previously (see Equation (3.1)), conversion of a polysaccharide chain segment from a fluctuating, disordered state in solution to a rigid, ordered conformation in a gel junction zone involves substantial loss of entropy, and will therefore occur only if the compensating enthalpy advantage is sufficiently large. In other words, formation of a conventional hydrated network ("true" gel) requires comparatively strong non-covalent bonding between the participating chains. The force required to break the resulting network is therefore correspondingly large, giving structures that are cohesive and self-supporting under gravity.

Certain polysaccharides (notably the bacterial exopolysaccharide xanthan, which is now used extensively in food), however, exist in solution in a rigid, ordered chain conformation, rather than as disordered coils (Norton et al., 1984). Side-by-side association of such rigid structures involves little loss of entropy and can therefore occur even if the bonding is weak. The result is a three-dimensional network structure analogous to that indicated in Fig. 3.5 for "true gels", but with far less stable association between the chains (Ross-Murphy et al. 1983). Such "weak gel" networks are often sufficiently cohesive to hold particles in suspension or stabilise emulsions over long periods of time. They are not, however, strong enough to support their own weight under gravity, and therefore flow like normal polymer solutions, although, as discussed later, there are substantial quantitative differences in viscosity behaviour between "weak gels" and solutions of disordered polysaccharide chains.

Hydrodynamic Volume of Disordered Polysaccharide Chains

In contrast to the ordered structures of polysaccharides which, as outlined above, are critically sensitive to detailed primary structure, the properties of disordered chains in solution are dependent predominantly on molecular size (Morris et al., 1981), which in turn is therefore likely to be a crucial determinant of biological function.

The most direct index of the volume occupied by individual coils is the "limiting viscosity number" or "intrinsic viscosity", $[\eta]$. This is the fractional increase in viscosity per unit concentration of polymer, under conditions of extreme dilution (where there are no interactions between chains), and has units of reciprocal concentration (rather than units of viscosity). Intrinsic viscosity is related to molecular weight (M) by the Mark–Houwink relationship:

$$[\eta] = KM^a \tag{3.2}$$

Theoretically, a has a value of 2 for fully-extended rigid rods and 0.5 for freely-jointed coils. For most real disordered polysaccharides a is substantially higher (Morris and Ross-Murphy, 1981), often around one, so that intrinsic viscosity (coil volume) increases more or less linearly with increasing molecular weight.

The constant of proportionality (K) is largely dependent on the nature of the linkages between adjacent residues in the polysaccharide backbone (Rees et al., 1982). Linkage patterns (Fig. 3.4) giving extended, ribbon-like ordered structures (flat or buckled) also give rise to expanded coil dimensions in solution (i.e. high values of K), whereas the non-parallel linkages that promote helical ordered structures give small, compact coils (low values of K).

Short sidechains (such as the single-residue galactose substituents on plant galactomannans) have little, if any, effect on coil dimensions; the intrinsic viscosity of such materials is determined almost entirely by the length of the polymer backbone (McCleary et al., 1981). Extensive branching (as in amylopectin or gum arabic), however, gives rise to very compact coils (i.e. extremely low values of K) and to a decreased dependence of coil volume on molecular weight ($a < 0.5$).

In charged polysaccharides, coil dimensions can be altered substantially by changes in ionic strength (I). Electrostatic repulsions between chain segments increase coil volume, but can be screened out by addition of salt, allowing the coil to contract towards the dimensions it would have adopted if uncharged. Quantitatively, intrinsic viscosity decreases linearly with $1/\sqrt{I}$ (Smidsrød and Haug, 1971), extrapolating at infinite ionic strength ($1/\sqrt{I} = 0$) to the intrinsic viscosity of a neutral polysaccharide of the same primary structure and chainlength.

Coil Overlap and Entanglement

As the concentration (c) of a solution of disordered polysaccharide chains is increased, a stage is reached at which the individual coils are forced to interpenetrate one another to form an entangled network (Graessley, 1974). The concentration at which this occurs is known as c^*. Below c^*, where individual coils are free to move through the solvent with little mutual interference, viscosity is virtually independent of shear rate (this is known as "Newtonian" behaviour). Above c^*, where chains can move only by the much more difficult process of "wriggling" (reptating) through the entangled network of neighbouring chains, viscosity (η) becomes highly dependent on shear rate ($\dot{\gamma}$). At low shear rates, where there is sufficient time for entanglements pulled apart by the flow of the solution to be replaced by new entanglements between different chains, with no net change in "crosslink density", η remains constant at the maximum "zero shear" value, η_0. With increasing shear rate, however, the rate of re-entanglement falls behind the rate of forced disentanglement, and viscosity falls (Fig. 3.6).

The transition from a dilute solution of independently moving coils to an entangled network is also accompanied by a very marked change in the concentration-dependence of viscosity. At concentrations below c^*, the main effect of the polysaccharide coils is to perturb the flow of the solvent by tumbling around and setting up "countercurrents" which increase the overall viscosity.

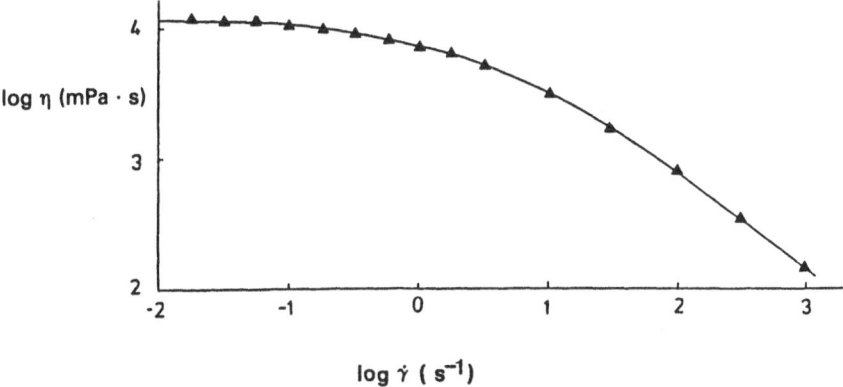

Fig. 3.6. Decrease in viscosity (η) with increasing shear rate ($\dot{\gamma}$) for a typical solution of entangled polysaccharide coils ($c > c^*$).

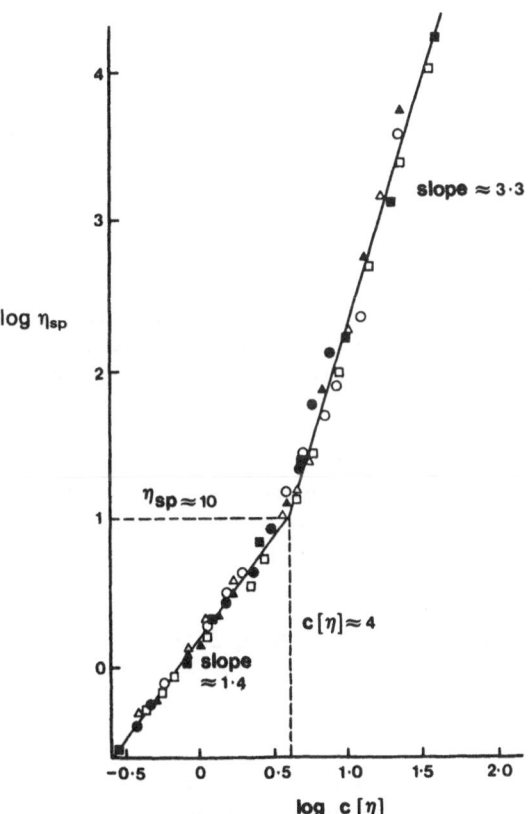

Fig. 3.7. Variation of maximum "zero shear" viscosity with degree of space-occupancy for various disordered polysaccharides (shown by different symbols). From Morris et al. (1981), with permission.

The fractional increase in viscosity due to the presence of the polymer (the "specific viscosity", $\eta_{sp} = (\eta - \eta_s)/\eta_s$, where η_s is the viscosity of the solvent) is roughly proportional to the number of chains present, but second-order effects due to mutual interference of countercurrents from neighbouring molecules increase the concentration-dependence to approx. $c^{1.3}$, so that doubling concentration increases η_{sp} by a factor of approx. 2.5. At higher concentrations, where the chains are entangled, "zero shear" viscosity increases much more steeply with increasing concentration, varying as approx. $c^{3.3}$ (so that doubling concentration gives about a ten-fold increase in viscosity). At the onset of entanglement, polysaccharide solution viscosity (Morris et al., 1981) is usually about 10 mPa·s (i.e. about ten times the viscosity of water), so that almost all practical food applications involve entangled networks at higher concentrations.

For any specific polysaccharide sample the onset of coil overlap is determined by two things: the number of chains present (proportional to concentration) and the volume that each occupies (proportional to intrinsic viscosity $[\eta]$). Coil volume can vary widely from sample to sample, with corresponding variation in the critical concentration (c^*) at which entanglement begins. However, when viscosity is plotted as a function of the extent of space-occupancy by the polymer, characterised by the "coil overlap parameter' $c[\eta]$, rather than against concentration alone, then results for most "random coil" polysaccharides superimpose closely (Fig. 3.7), irrespective of primary structure and molecular weight (Morris et al., 1981), with the onset of entanglement (c^* transition) occurring when $c[\eta] \approx 4$.

Shear-Rate Dependence of Viscosity

In dilute solutions of disordered coils ($c < c^*$), viscosity (η) shows only a slight dependence on shear rate ($\dot{\gamma}$), typically less than 30% over several decades of $\dot{\gamma}$, due to individual coils being stretched out by the flow and offering less resistance to movement. In entangled networks ($c > c^*$), however, the reduction in η with increasing $\dot{\gamma}$ ("shear-thinning") can be very large, with viscosities often dropping by several orders of magnitude. For samples with a high polydispersity of chain length (which is invariably the case for food polysaccharides) the form of shear-thinning at concentrations above c^* is entirely general and can be fitted (Morris, 1990) with good precision by:

$$\eta = \eta_0/[1 + (\dot{\gamma}/\dot{\gamma}_{1/2})^p] \tag{3.3}$$

where $\dot{\gamma}_{1/2}$ is the shear rate required to reduce viscosity to $\eta_0/2$, and $p = 0.76$ (the absolute value of the slope of log η vs. log $\dot{\gamma}$ at high shear rate). Rearrangement of Equation (3.3) gives:

$$\eta = \eta_0 - (1/\dot{\gamma}_{1/2})^p \eta \dot{\gamma}^p \tag{3.4}$$

Thus plotting η against $\eta\dot{\gamma}^{0.76}$ gives a straight line of intercept η_0 and gradient $-(1/\dot{\gamma}_{1/2})^{0.76}$. For any given solution, viscosity (η) at any shear rate ($\dot{\gamma}$) can therefore be defined completely (Equation (3.3)) by two parameters, η_0 and $\dot{\gamma}_{1/2}$, both of which can be derived from a simple linear plot.

It should be noted that the common practice of fitting shear-thinning data to a "power-law" of the form:

$$\eta = k\dot{\gamma}^{(n-1)} \tag{3.5}$$

where n is the so-called "pseudoplasticity index", is equivalent to treating double-logarithmic plots of η vs. $\dot{\gamma}$ (such as that shown in Fig. 3.6) as straight lines, and is therefore totally invalid for entangled coils.

The shear-thinning behaviour of "weak gels" is quite different from that of entangled coils (Morris, 1984). In particular, since a finite stress is required to rupture the network, the viscosity (defined as the ratio of stress applied to shear rate generated) increases progressively with decreasing shear rate, rather than reaching a maximum equilibrium value (as in Fig. 3.6 for entangled coils). Indeed, for most "weak gel" systems, double-logarithmic plots of η vs. $\dot{\gamma}$ are linear (so that in this case the power law analysis of Equation (3.5) is valid), and have a slope greater than the maximum value of -0.76 for disordered polysaccharides.

Implications for Digesta Viscosity

To a first approximation, chyme may be considered as a biphasic system consisting of solid particles dispersed in a solution of soluble polymeric material. The viscosity generated by solid particles (see, for example, Everett, 1988) is largely independent of their size, but is directly related to the fraction of the total volume that they occupy (phase volume, ϕ). At low phase volumes:

$$\eta_{sp} \approx k\phi \tag{3.6}$$

The constant of proportionality, k, has a value of 2.5 for spherical particles, increasing to around 4 for elongated "rods". Since the density of food materials is usually close to that of water, ϕ is approximately equal to $c/100$, where c is the concentration of the particulate phase in per cent w/v. Thus:

$$[\eta] = \eta_{sp}/c \approx k/100 \tag{3.7}$$

In other words, dispersed solids have intrinsic viscosities in the range 0.025–0.04 dl/g. By comparison, the intrinsic viscosities of soluble polysaccharides (Morris and Ross-Murphy, 1981) range typically from about 1 dl/g for compact coils to around 20 dl/g for commercial thickeners (such as guar gum) and can reach values of at least 70–80 dl/g for rigid, rod-like molecules such as xanthan.

It is clear, therefore, that in fluid digesta with any significant content of dissolved polysaccharides, these will dominate the overall viscosity. The same is not, however, true at higher solids content (as in faeces). With decreasing water content, and thus increasing phase volume of particulate material, the viscosity generated by the particles increases very steeply as they approach close packing

(Everett, 1988). This is analogous to the sharp increase in concentration-dependence of viscosity for disordered coils when they reach full space-occupancy at c^*, but is an even more dramatic effect since, unlike polymer coils, solid particles cannot interpenetrate one another. The precise volume fraction at which close packing is reached depends on the shape of the particles and their size distribution, but in general, development of significant viscosity by undissolved food particles is unlikely to occur until they occupy about half the total volume ($\phi \approx 0.5$).

The viscosities generated by soluble dietary fibre constituents in more dilute digesta (in the stomach and small intestine) will follow the generalities of concentration dependence and shear rate dependence detailed in previous sections for isolated polysaccharides in vitro, with some obvious caveats for designing and reporting animal trials and clinical studies of the physiological action of soluble fibres in vivo.

In particular, the crucial importance of molecular size is often ignored (Ellis et al., 1986). As illustrated in Fig. 3.7, the viscosity generated by disordered coils has little to do with their chemical composition, but is directly dependent on the degree of space-occupancy by the polymer, characterised by the (dimensionless) product of concentration (proportional to the number of chains present) and intrinsic viscosity (proportional to the volume which each occupies). It is therefore just as essential when documenting studies of physiological activity to give an indication of molecular size as it is to report concentration and structure. A particular danger is that apparent differences in the effectiveness of different soluble fibres may be due simply to differences in the molecular weights of the particular samples used, rather than reflecting a genuine dependence of physiological activity on chemical composition.

The most direct index of molecular size is intrinsic viscosity, whose determination is described in detail elsewhere (Morris, 1984). An acceptable alternative would be to measure viscosities at a few concentrations in the range of practical usage. In view of the extreme shear-thinning of polysaccharide solutions, it is virtually useless to report viscosity to a single shear rate (particulary if the rate is not specified). Measurements at a few different shear rates, however, can be used to construct a linear plot of η vs. $\eta\dot{\gamma}_{0.76}$ and hence derive the values of η_0 and $\dot{\gamma}_{1/2}$ which define completely the viscosity at all shear rates (Morris, 1990). For "weak gel" systems the equivalent parameters are k and n (Equation 3.5) from a linear plot of $\log \eta$ vs. $\log \dot{\gamma}$.

A complication in interpreting results from clinical studies of soluble fibre is that concentrations in the lumen may be quite different from those ingested. In particular, recent studies using a pig model (Roberts et al., 1990) have shown a substantial increase in the total volume of digesta passing through the small intestine with increasing concentration and molecular weight of soluble polysaccharide in the feed (thus partially offsetting the initial differences in viscosity). The mechanism of this feedback process is not yet fully understood, but it is clearly of importance in defining optimum levels and types of soluble fibre for clinical use.

A further obvious consideration is that soluble polysaccharides can confer viscosity only once they have dissolved. This may explain conflicting reports on the effectiveness of guar gum in reducing postprandial hyperglycaemia, since different commercial guar granulates dissolve at quite different rates (Peterson and Ellis, 1988).

Transport and Release of Nutrients

The ability of guar gum and other viscous polysaccharides to reduce postprandial concentrations of blood glucose, with associated reduction in insulin levels, is one of the most extensively documented aspects of the physiological action of dietary fibre. Two mechanisms bring nutrients into contact with the mucosal surface of the gut. Intestinal contractions create turbulence, allowing digesta from the centre of the lumen to be transported close to the epithelium. Nutrients then have to diffuse across the thin, relatively unstirred layer of fluid immediately adjacent to the intestinal mucosa.

An increase in the viscosity of the luminal contents will obviously impair the peristaltic mixing process, and this is likely to be the dominant mechanism by which soluble fibres retard the release of small molecules into the bloodstream. Hindered mixing of luminal contents may also slow the overall digestive process by decreasing the rate of transport of enzymes to their substrates and bile acids to unmicellised fat. A further effect of dissolved polysaccharides may be to inhibit diffusion of nutrients across the unstirred layer, by presenting a physical obstacle to movement of small species (Häglund et al., 1988), but this is likely to be significant only at very high polymer concentrations.

As discussed in the previous section, insoluble fibres may also contribute to digesta viscosity and hence to the restriction of peristaltic mixing. More directly, however, nutrients trapped within the particles must first be released into the surrounding intestinal fluid before they can be absorbed through the gut wall. The rate of release will obviously be directly proportional to the total surface area of the solid particles, and hence increase with decreasing particle size. It will also be affected by, for example, the physical state of the solute (e.g. whether it is present in solid form or is already dissolved in water trapped within the particle), the physical structure of the particle (e.g. whether it is readily deformable, like a sponge, so that dissolved solids can be squeezed out by peristaltic contractions, or rigid, so that solutes must diffuse out), and by the surface properties of the particle (e.g. surface tension effects).

The concentration of nutrients within the continuous aqueous phase will be constantly depleted by enteric absorption, and replenished, as outlined above, by release of material from food particles. The progress of these sequential release processes will, of course, also be influenced by transit times (i.e. the duration of exposure to a particular absorptive surface or digestive environment).

Finally, increased dietary intake of charged polysaccharides may have implications for the availability of essential mineral nutrients. Tight site-binding of counterions within the ordered structure of charged polysaccharides such as pectin has been detailed above. Weaker "atmospheric" binding can occur around disordered polyelectrolyte chains in solution or at the surface of insoluble fibres.

In all cases, electrostatic binding will, of course, occur only when the ionic substituents of the polysaccharide retain their charge. Sulphate groups (as in carrageenan) remain charged to very low pH, but the pKa of carboxyl groups in, for example, pectin and alginate is around 3.4. Thus at gastric pH these materials may become partially un-ionised and shed their bound counterions, while at higher pH in the small intestine they will regain their charge and once more participate fully in electrostatic binding, perhaps with ions different from those with which they were initially associated.

Susceptibility to Digestive Enzymes and Colonic Fermentation

Although the potential susceptibility of polysaccharides to cleavage by specific enzymes is, of course, dependent on their primary sequence, the extent of hydrolysis which occurs in practice can be drastically reduced by conformational ordering and packing.

For example, xanthan, which has a cellulosic backbone, can be degraded by cellulase enzymes when it is in a disordered coil form, but on conversion to the rigid, ordered structure (which gives rise to its characteristic "weak gel" properties) it is almost entirely resistant (Rinaudo and Milas, 1980). Similarly, the ordered (double helical) structures of amylopectin in ungelatinised (native) starch granules, and of amylose after retrogradation, constitute the "resistant" starch which survives digestion by human enzymes in the foregut.

The same considerations will obviously apply to degradation of dietary fibre constituents by bacterial enzymes in the colon, with soluble, disordered chains being much more susceptible to cleavage than packed, ordered assemblies, provided that the appropriate enzymes are generated by the bacterial flora.

Conclusions

Since the physical properties of polysaccharides are determined more by the way in which the component residues are linked together than by the nature of the residues, analysis of dietary fibre for the types and proportions of sugars present is unlikely, in itself, to give much indication of function. Perhaps the only useful generality is that charged polysaccharides are usually more readily soluble than neutral chains, although even here the presence of a sufficient concentration of appropriate counterions can promote stable association of polyelectrolytes into solvent-resistant assemblies.

Determination of the linkages between adjacent residues in the polysaccharide repeating sequence is, of course, a substantial improvement, but is still an incomplete description since, as detailed earlier, minor departures from structure regularity (e.g. branching; anomalous residues; sidechains) can have a major influence on physical properties. When the spacing of these interruptions is larger than the critical sequence length for ordered association, their effect is to promote formation of hydrated networks rather than insoluble aggregates. At shorter spacings they may completely abolish interchain association and solubilise an otherwise insoluble primary sequence.

Characterisation of the distribution of structural irregularities along the polymer chain (i.e. determination of "fine structure") has been achieved for some polysaccharide systems, by selective chemical or enzymatic degradation, but this is a highly skilled, lengthy undertaking that could certainly not be adopted for routine analysis of dietary fibre. Progress in understanding the mechanism of action of insoluble fibre or swollen, hydrated networks is therefore more likely to come from relating physiological effects to the macroscopic properties of these materials rather than to their chemical composition.

References

Ellis PR, Morris ER, Low AG (1986) Guar gum: the importance of reporting data on its physico-chemical properties. Diabetic Med 3:490–491

Everett DH (1988) Basic principles of colloid science. Royal Society of Chemistry, London

Graessley WW (1974) The entanglement concept in polymer rheology. Springer, Berlin, Heidelberg, New York (Advances in polymer science, vol 16)

Häglund B-O, Ellison M, Sundelöf L-O (1988) Diffusion permeability in concentrated polymer solutions. Chem Scripta 28:129–131

McCleary BV, Amado R, Waibel R, Neukom H (1981) Effect of galactose content on the solution and interaction properties of guar and carob galactomannans. Carbohydr Res 92:269–285

Morris ER (1984) Rheology of hydrocolloids. In: Phillips GO, Wedlock DJ, Williams PA (eds) Gums and stabilisers for the food industry 2: Pergamon Press, Oxford, pp 57–78

Morris ER (1990) Shear-thinning of "random coil" polysaccharides: characterisation by two parameters from a simple linear plot. Carbohydr Polym 13:85–96

Morris ER, Ross-Murphy SB (1981) Chain flexibility of polysaccharides and glycoproteins from viscosity measurements. In: Techniques in carbohydrate metabolism. Elsevier, London (chapter B310)

Morris ER, Cutler AN, Ross-Murphy SB, Rees DA, Price J (1981) Concentration and shear rate dependence of viscosity in random coil polysaccharide solutions. Carbohydr Polym 1:5–21

Norton IT, Goodall DM, Frangou SA, Morris ER, Rees DA (1984) Mechanism and dynamics of conformational ordering in xanthan polysaccharide. J Mol Biol 175:371–394

Peterson DB, Ellis PR (1988) Misconceptions about the clinical use of guar. Pract Diabetes 5:133

Rees DA, Morris ER, Thom D, Madden JK (1982) Shapes and interactions of carbohydrate chains. In: Aspinall GO (ed) The polysaccharides, vol 1. Academic Press, New York, pp 195–290

Rinaudo M, Milas M (1980) Enzymic hydrolysis of the bacterial polysaccharide xanthan by cellulase. Int J Biol Macromol 2:45–48

Roberts FG, Smith HA, Low AG, Ellis PR (1990) Influence of wheat breads containing guar flour supplements of high and low molecular weights on viscosity of jejunal digesta in the pig. In: Southgate DAT et al. (eds) Dietary fibre: chemical and biological aspects. Royal Society of Chemistry, London, pp 164–168 (Special publication no. 83)

Ross-Murphy SB, Morris VJ, Morris ER (1983) Molecular viscoelasticity of xanthan polysaccharide. Faraday Symp Chem Soc 18:115–129

Smidsrød O, Haug A (1971) Estimation of the relative stiffness of the molecular chain in polyelectrolytes from measurements of viscosity at different ionic strengths. Biopolymers 10:1213–1227

Stoddart JF (1971) Stereochemistry of carbohydrates. Wiley, New York

Commentary

Southgate: This paper provides a useful account of the physico-chemical properties of food polysaccharides focusing especially on the properties of isolated soluble polysaccharides, principally those used as polysaccharide additives. As such it provides a background to understanding the way in which these polysaccharides behave in solution and in colloidal systems. The information is very relevant to the role of isolated polysaccharides in food systems especially food functionality and texture. It may well be that more careful consideration of these properties in the design of physiological studies may advance understanding of structure/physiological effects. It may also advance the pharmacological use of polysaccharides as cholesterol-lowering agents or agents for improving dietetic control of diabetes mellitus. I strongly support the concept that measurement of physical properties is essential for understanding the physiological effects, which cannot come from chemical analysis of the polysaccharides alone.

I think that the term "dietary fibre" is inappropriate for describing an isolated polysaccharide when its structure is known, and "non-starch polysaccharides" should be the preferred terminology for the group and the trivial names for an individual polysaccharide, e.g. guar gum or pectin.

It is not made clear in the introduction that the pectin added to foods is substantially depolymerised when compared with pectic substances in foods and has lost many sidechains. Also, the etherification of the hydroxyl groups of cellulose with methyl or carboxymethyl groups makes radical changes to physical properties, and comparison with native cellulose is possibly slightly misleading.

Author's reply: I am pleased that Professor Southgate shares my view of the importance of relating physiological action to physical properties. My personal opinion is that the term "dietary fibre" is so diffuse that it hinders rational discussion (the same might be said of the equally unhelpful term "food additive"!). "Non-starch polysaccharide" is not much better because of (a) the issue of resistant starch, and (b) the huge range of physical properties spanned by different polysaccharides. The main thrust of my chapter (as indicated in the opening paragraph) is to suggest that we should really focus on different states of molecular organisation and packing, rather than on the source and chemical composition of the materials.

The intention of the third paragraph of the Introduction was to make the point that "industrial" polysaccharides and "natural" polysaccharides form part of the same spectrum of chemical structures and physical properties, so that general principles established for one can be applied to the other. I certainly did not intend to imply that extraction and, particularly, chemical derivatisation have no effect on physical properties; indeed much of the later discussion is devoted to describing and explaining the type of changes that can occur.

Chapter 4

Dietary Fibre Analysis

N.-G. Asp, T.F. Schweizer, D.A.T. Southgate and O. Theander

Classification of Carbohydrates in Foods as Related to Dietary Fibre Analysis

Whichever definition is used for dietary fibre the major components are polysaccharides and the classification of these carbohydrates in foods provides the background for the analytical strategies.

It is possible to classify the carbohydrates in the diet in several different ways depending, for example, on their sources, their role in the foods themselves, their chemical structures and reactivity, their physical properties or according to their nutritional and physiological effects (British Nutrition Foundation, 1990). In the nutritional context one is seeking to distinguish substances or groups of substances that have specific nutritional or physiological effects when consumed. This is especially true in the case of dietary fibre where we are concerned with the postulated effects that relate to protection from chronic disease (Southgate, 1988; Southgate and Englyst, 1985). The quantification of these effects depends on measurement of the specific groups of substances. Since this measurement will depend primarily on chemical properties it is appropriate to make the basis of the classification a chemical one (Southgate, 1976a), although even on this basis there are a number of different schemes that can be used.

Classification and terminology are so closely related that they cannot be separated. The different classes or sets of carbohydrates must be named in some way so that they can be distinguished. The choice of analytical strategy then depends on which classification is relevant for the purposes for which the analyses are required (Southgate, 1976b; Southgate et al., 1978; Asp and Johansson, 1984; Schweizer, 1989, 1990), although it is important to note at this stage that practical considerations will often determine which analytical strategy is acceptable (Southgate, 1969a, b). Thus, classification of all the types of non-cellulosic polysaccharides present in foods is entirely feasible at several different levels of complexity (Selvendran, 1984); analytical separation and analysis is likewise feasible but impractical when one of the constraints on analysis is time.

Principal Criteria for Classification

Most of the chemical reactions of the carbohydrates are general rather than specific and do not lend themselves to form the basis for classification, with the possible exception of reducing and non-reducing sugars, and structural features provide the most acceptable characteristics to use.

Degree of Polymerisation

The precise boundary between the oligosaccharides and the polysaccharides is difficult to define with rigour and the limit of 10 residues as used by IUPAC for inclusion as polysaccharides is arbitrary. A higher number of residues may be required for the development of tertiary configuration (British Nutrition Foundation, 1990). Insolubility in 80% v/v ethanol, retention by dialysis tubing or an ultrafiltration membrane, however, forms the practical basis for the boundary. A range of factors other than degree of polymerisation including the type of linkages, extent of branching and bonding with non-carbohydrate components also act as determinants.

Oligosaccharides with more than five monosaccharide residues are uncommon naturally. Higher oligosaccharides are formed during the preparation of starch or gum hydrolysates and may occur in foods where these materials are used as ingredients, or may be formed as a result of the processing of starchy foods. Higher oligosaccharides of fructose are also present in foods where fructans are the principal storage polysaccharide.

This primary classification divides the food carbohydrates into three major categories. "Sugars" (mono- and disaccharides), oligosaccharides and polysaccharides (Table 4.1). The latter corresponds to the "Complex Carbohydrates" used in the McGovern Report (US Senate Select Committee on Nutrition and Human Needs, 1977). Thus, it includes both starch and dietary fibre, although the term has also been used to differentiate "available" polysaccharides as opposed to simple sugars.

Classification of the Polysaccharides

In classifying the polysaccharides further, the degree of polymerisation is of less value because most food polysaccharides appear to be polydisperse, which may be exaggerated by the methods of extraction. Classification systems that rely on one set of criteria invariably produce a series of overlapping sets and a number of different criteria are required. This is illustrated in Table 4.1 (British Nutrition Foundation, 1990) which lists the major classes of polysaccharides in foods. The first column considers the groups of polysaccharides according to their role in the plant food.

There are three major categories of intrinsic (occurring naturally in foods) polysaccharides; the storage polysaccharides of which the starches are

Table 4.1. Classification of polysaccharides

Source in diet	Major types	Polysaccharide species	Monosaccharide backbone	Bonds in backbone
Intrinsic				
Storage	Starch	Amylose	Glucose	Linear 1-4α
		Amylopectin	Glucose	Branched 1-4α
	Fructans	E.g. inulin	Fructose	
	Galactomannans	E.g. guar, locust-bean gum	Mannan	Linear 1-4β
Plant cell wall	Non-cellulosic	Pectin components	Galacturonic acid	Linear 1-4α
		Arabino-galactans	Galactose	Linear 1-4α
		Arabino-xylans	Xylans	Linear 1-4β
		Gluco-xylans	Xylans	Linear 1-4β
		β-glucans	Glucose	Mixed 1-3, 1-4β
	Cellulosic	Cellulose	Glucose	Linear 1-4β
Non-structural soluble components	Gums Mucilages	Many heteropolysaccharides	Very diverse	Non-α-glucosidic bonds
Extrinsic				
Ingredients and food additives	Starch	Esters, ethers,	Glucose	1-4/1-6α
	Modified Cellulose	Ethers	Glucose	1-4β
	Pectins	Amidated	Galacturonic acid	1-4α
	Alginates		Guluronic/mannuronic	
	Gums storage		Mannan	
	Gums exudate		Wide range	

quantitatively the more important; the structural materials of the plant cell walls and those polysaccharides that serve to protect the plant from desiccation, i.e. gums and mucilages. The extrinsic polysaccharides (added to foods during preparation or formulation) are a diverse group of polysaccharide ingredients and food additives used primarily to modify or control the physical characteristics of foods. These extrinsic components are almost invariably derived from plant tissues and therefore share many features of chemical structure with the intrinsic components (Southgate, 1976a). The boundaries between these categories are not absolute. Each of the primary categories can be subdivided into subgroups on the basis of type of molecular structures: the component monosaccharides forming the backbone of the polymer and the types of branching present. The configuration of the glycosidic linkages in the backbone of the polymer is extremely important because it determines the tertiary structure of the molecule, which in turn determines the physical properties of the polysaccharides and their capacity to associate with other polysaccharide chains and with proteins. Thus linear molecules with a 1-4 beta configuration and equatorial O(4) as in glucose and mannose are capable of associating and hydrogen-bonding to form fibrillar insoluble crystalline structures such as cellulose fibrils.

The capacity to bind to proteins is especially important physiologically, since it determines susceptibility to enzymatic hydrolysis. Polysaccharides with 1-4 and 1-6 alpha glucosidic bonding can be hydrolysed by the amylase in the mammalian salivary and pancreatic secretions to give glucose, maltose, isomaltose and malto-oligosaccharides and thus can be hydrolysed and absorbed within the small intestine. Together with mono- and disaccharides, they formed the "available" carbohydrates of McCance and Lawrence (1929). This criterion divides the polysaccharides into two distinct groups, the alpha glucans (the starches and glycogen) and other polysaccharides (the non-starch polysaccharides). Physical and chemical modifications of the alpha-linked glucans also determine the extent of enzymatic hydrolysis with amylases.

No enzymes capable of hydrolysing the non-alpha glucans have been demonstrated in mammalian small intestinal secretions and this group of polysaccharides is therefore non-digestible (in this context it is proposed that the term "small intestinal digestible" be used to describe components that are hydrolysed and absorbed in the small intestine and "digestion" the process of hydrolysis and absorption in the small intestine. The term "apparent digestibility" is widely used in animal nutrition to describe the overall disappearance of nutrients during gastro-intestinal transit as judged by measurement of faecal excretion: this is the combined effect of small intestinal digestion and bacterial degradation in the large intestine).

Table 4.2. Alternative classifications of food polysaccharides

Role in the plant or food	Types of polysaccharides	Analytical classification	Sites of digestion	Products of digestion	Physiological classification
Storage polysaccharides	Starch amylose amylopectin	α-glucans _____	Small intestine (enzymatic)	Mono and disaccharides	Available carbohydrates
	Fructans			— — — — — — — — —	
— — — — —	Galactomannans				
Structural components of the plant cell walls	Non-cellulosic pectins hemicullose Cellulose		Large intestine (Microbial)	Short chain fatty acids acetate propionate butyrate	Unavailable carbohydrates
— — — — —		Non-α-glucans			
Isolated polysaccharides					
Natural occurring	Gums Mucilages Pectin	Non-starch polysaccharides		Carbon dioxide Hydrogen Methane	
— — — — —					
Polysaccharide food additives	Gums Algal polysaccharides Modified celluloses Modified starches				
	Bacterial polysaccharides (xanthan gum)				

Dashed line denotes boundaries not absolute.

Further classification in terms of physical characteristics is of limited value for several reasons. Many physical properties are shared within the various groupings so far proposed, particularly in the case of solubility.

Many polysaccharides do not produce true aqueous solutions but sols and this property is shared by both linear and branched molecules and both alpha- and beta-linked polymers. Solubility is often pH and ionic strength dependent and, furthermore, can be dependent on the specific cations present in the solution; solubility is therefore useful and valid as a criterion for classification only when the conditions under which it was measured are closely defined. The classification proposed can be related to physiological properties as is shown in the Table 4.2. In almost every case it is evident that the boundaries between observed effects are not absolute and do not correspond precisely.

The fact that the physiological boundaries do not correspond precisely with classification based on chemical structural grounds has important implications for the choice of analytical procedures. In addition, the physiological boundaries are subject to biological variation which imposes additional limitations on the capacity of an analytical procedure to be consistent with physiological and nutritional effects. The factors involved in the delineation of these boundaries are intrinsic, relating to the location and physical state of the polysaccharides in the food (and therefore may be dependent on the type of processing the food has received), or extrinsic, depending on the variables associated with the person or group of people eating the food. Thus the delineation of the physiological boundary depends on the integration of all these factors. Chemical analysis of foods can only address some of these factors but for nutritional purposes, the analytical objective is to produce a value or values that match the physiological boundary with a high degree of confidence.

Recommendations for Nomenclature for use in the Classification of Carbohydrates in Nutritional Studies

Polysaccharides. Polymers with 11 or more monosaccharides (including uronic acid residues, IUPAC).

Starches. Homopolysaccharides from plants made up of α-(1,4):α-(1,6)-linked glucosyl units.

Non-starch Polysaccharides. Plant polysaccharides that are not α-glucans.*

Plant Cell Walls. The sum of all the structural components present in the plant cell wall including non-carbohydrate materials, protein, lignin and inorganic constituents.

---

* In practice, the delimitation between starch and non-starch polysaccharides is defined by the conditions of solubilisation and the enzymic hydrolysis. Enzyme resistant starch may therefore remain in the non-starch polysaccharide fraction, unless special measures are taken to solubilise such starch before the amylase treatment.

Plant Cell Wall Polysaccharides. Polysaccharides that are present in foods in the form of intact cell walls or cell wall fragments.

Associated Substances. Non-carbohydrate components of plant cell walls.

Lignin.[†] Polymers of phenylpropan laid down in the plant cell wall matrix.

Available Carbohydrates.[‡] Those carbohydrates that can be digested and absorbed as carbohydrate from the small intestine. The sum of glucose, fructose, sucrose, lactose, maltose, the malto-oligosaccharides and starches.

Apparently Digestible Carbohydrates. The sum of sugars and polysaccharides that disappear during transit through the gastro-intestinal tract.

The Definition of Dietary Fibre: A Determinant of Analytical Strategy

The definition of dietary fibre has been a matter of some confusion because the original derivation of the term was imprecise and difficult to formalise in a precise legalistic sense. A precise definition is only necessary for those who need a rigid framework for action; this includes those who have to enforce regulation or comply with it. For legislative purposes, therefore, there must be a definition which in effect will be related to the methods used. Fig. 4.1 summarises the analytical terminologies that have been used in relation to dietary fibre analysis.

Dietary fibre was used by Hipsley (1953) as a "shorthand" term for the constituents of the plant cell wall. It was used again by Trowell (1972) to describe the components of diets that were rich in plant foods where the cell wall material was present intrinsically in the foods which were therefore relatively unrefined (Burkitt and Trowell, 1975; Trowell et al., 1985). Therefore the measurement of dietary fibre, as originally defined, requires the measurement of the plant cell walls in foods and the diet. The composition of the plant cell wall is such (Siegel, 1968; Southgate, 1975, 1976a, b, c; Selvendran, 1984) that measurement of the plant cell wall polysaccharides and lignin provides a good index. The definition proposed by Trowell et al. (1976) was specifically chosen so that polysaccharides that were structurally related to the plant cell wall polysaccharides would be included in the definition because these isolated polysaccharides were being used experimentally as models for components of the plant cell wall. More pragmatically the isolated polysaccharides were also analytically indistinguishable from the corresponding plant cell wall components.

[†] Materials with some physical characteristics of lignin, i.e. insolubility in 72% sulphuric acid, may be formed in foods by processing and contribute to "Klason lignin".

[‡] When available carbohydrate values are estimated "by difference" i.e. by deducting "dietary fibre" values from total carbohydrate "by difference", other substances such as sugar alcohols and undigestible oligosaccharides are included in addition to errors arising from the measurement of water, protein, fat, dietary fibre and ash.

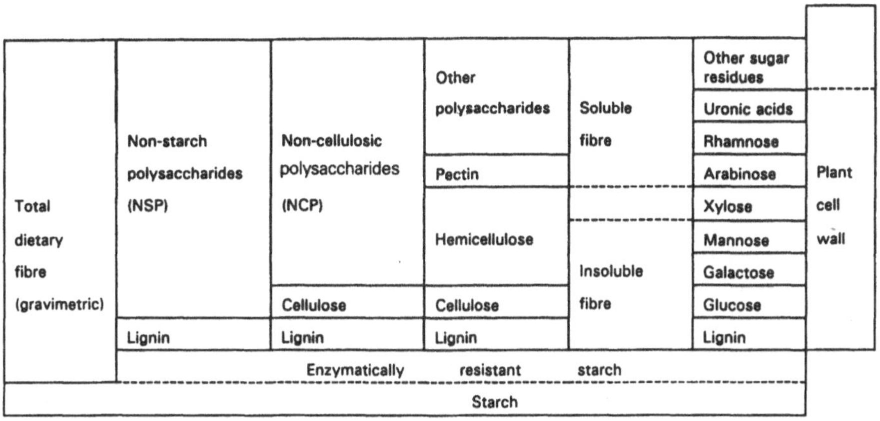

Total dietary fibre (gravimetric)	Non-starch polysaccharides (NSP)	Non-cellulosic polysaccharides (NCP)		Soluble fibre	Other sugar residues	Plant cell wall
			Other polysaccharides	Soluble fibre	Uronic acids	
					Rhamnose	
			Pectin		Arabinose	Plant
					Xylose	cell
			Hemicellulose		Mannose	wall
				Insoluble fibre	Galactose	
	Cellulose	Cellulose		Glucose	
Lignin	Lignin	Lignin		Lignin	
	Enzymatically resistant starch					
	Starch					

Fig. 4.1. The relationship between the different ways of measuring "dietary fibre". Broken lines indicate boundaries that are not absolute. (Modified from Asp and Johansson (1984) and British Nutrition Foundation (1990)).

Main Features of Analytical Strategies

The Trowell et al. (1976) definition formed the basis for the development of analytical strategies based on the measurement of dietary fibre as plant cell wall polysaccharides (and related polysaccharides) plus lignin (Southgate, 1976b, c). Some principles of dietary fibre analysis are common to most methods now in use.

The first stage is the removal of sugars and oligosaccharides. This may be carried out as a separate stage or combined with the removal of starch. Starch is present in many foods in much higher concentrations than cell wall polysaccharides and if it is not removed effectively the value for the other polysaccharides will be inflated. Enzymatic hydrolysis is the approach adopted in all methods. Different enzyme preparations are used and these determine the pre-treatment of the samples and hydrolysis conditions.

All amylolytic enzymes require the starch to be partially gelatinised so a gelatinisation stage is included in the pre-treatment. In some foods, especially those that have been thermally processed, some parts of the starches become resistant to enzyme hydrolysis; precise measurement of the plant cell wall material and non-starch polysaccharides requires that these fractions are treated to make them hydrolysable. The polysaccharides not hydrolysed by the selected amylolytic enzymes are usually recovered by precipitation with ethanol by bringing the concentration to 80% v/v and recovering the polysaccharides either by filtration or centrifugation. Some polymers are soluble in this strength of aqueous ethanol and recovery of these requires other techniques (Selvendran and Du Pont, 1984).

The residual polysaccharides can be measured gravimetrically, although when this is done separate values for lignin are not obtained without further analysis.

The residual polysaccharides can be measured gravimetrically, although when this is done separate values for lignin are not obtained without further analysis. The residues always contain protein and mineral matter and separate analyses of these are required; small amounts of other materials such as cutin, suberin and polyphenolic substances may also be included in the residue.

Other procedures hydrolyse the residue and measure the monosaccharides and uronic acids present, thus obtaining the total polysaccharide values by summation. Klason lignin and permanganate lignin values can be obtained by gravimetric methods on the residue. Hydrolysis may be sequential, i.e., dilute acid hydrolysis of the more labile non-cellulosic components followed by 12 mol/l hydrolysis, or use the Seaman method, i.e. dispersion in 12 mol/l sulphuric acid followed by dilution to 0.4–2 mol/l and heating. The individual monosaccharides can be measured after separation by gas-liquid chromatography (GLC) after derivatisation, or directly by high-performance liquid chromatography (HPLC). Values for major classes of monosaccharides or total monosaccharides can also be obtained colorimetrically.

The various methods differ in their technical details but the principles have a great deal in common. In view of the emphasis on the plant cell wall in dietary fibre definitions, an important feature of analytical methods is their ability to provide an index of the plant cell wall. The direct measurement of plant cell walls in foods is, however, very time-consuming and two principal analytical strategies have developed: one is based on the measurement of non-starch polysaccharides, which are the major components of the plant cell wall; the second strategy measures the undigestible polysaccharides (non-starch polysaccharides plus resistant starch) plus lignin which stems from the physiological properties of plant cell wall material. The evolution of these two strategies is discussed in following sections of this chapter.

Implications for the Choice of Analytical Methods for the Carbohydrates in Foods

This introductory discussion concerns principles because the individual methods are described below. It is also important to focus on analysis for nutritional purposes. This can be defined as analysis designed to measure the nutritional attributes of a foodstuff, or more usually a diet, so that the analytical values relate to the nutritional effects or consequences when the food, or diet, is eaten. Analyses undertaken for regulatory purposes have traditionally been concerned with protecting the consumer with regard to the identity and purity of a foodstuff. They have only recently become concerned with informing the consumer about both what a food contains in the way of ingredients and also its nutritional composition, the primary objective being to enable the consumer to make an informed choice about his or her diet. Thus nutritional labelling should give the consumer some information about the nutritional effects that the food will have when consumed. For example, it will provide so much metabolisable energy, so much of the different vitamins and minerals, etc. Analyses for nutritional labelling should therefore be based on the objectives given above.

Criteria for the Choice of Method: The Conflict Between the Requirements of Research and Regulation

Although, as argued above, regulatory analyses should be nutritionally relevant, nevertheless there are areas where the needs of nutritional research on dietary fibre and regulatory analyses for nutritional labelling diverge and these must be recognised.

Firstly, for research purposes the method must provide sufficiently detailed information and should be amenable to extension and modification by the individual researcher as determined by the needs of the research. This may demand, for example, complete separation of the non-cellulosic polysaccharides to understand specific effects in the small intestine. Other characteristics may seem to be more important, i. e. more predictive than chemical analysis, for example, viscosity in the study of effects on nutrient absorption, or particle size for determining extent of fermentation. Thus research demands an open-ended choice of methods, the time spent on measurement is judged on the capacity of the results to predict nutritional effects. In some cases a simpler method may suffice but this is again judged on the predictive value of the results.

A regulatory method, on the other hand, must usually be closely defined so that any competent worker can perform the method in the same way and obtain the results that are comparable within the accepted limits of the performance of the method. The analyst may have to defend the values obtained in a legal context. In addition the regulatory analysis must be carried out routinely in the laboratories of food producers who wish, or are required by law, to label their products. These requirements impose severe constraints on the choice of method. A time-consuming method will add to the cost of a product and may not be able to keep pace with production and create delays that further increase costs. The need for a closely defined protocol for a method has the effect of favouring a simple, robust method because this is more likely to be performed in a reproducible fashion.

In any debate about the most appropriate method it is important to recognise those constraints which do not impinge on the scientific issues of what is the most conceptually correct technique. Finally, it must be recognised that reliance on a single analytical technique will not detect systematic analytical bias unless there exists an absolute standard. This condition is not the case for dietary fibre, nor indeed for many nutrients, and the ideal is to have two and preferably more methods using different basic principles that give comparable analytical results.

Development of Crude Fibre, Detergent Fibre and Enzymatic Methods

The development of gravimetric methods for the measurement of "undigestible" fractions of forages, feed and food has taken place over a long period of time. Very early in the last century attempts were made to measure fibre in feeds after maceration and extraction with various agents. The analysis of crude fibre by

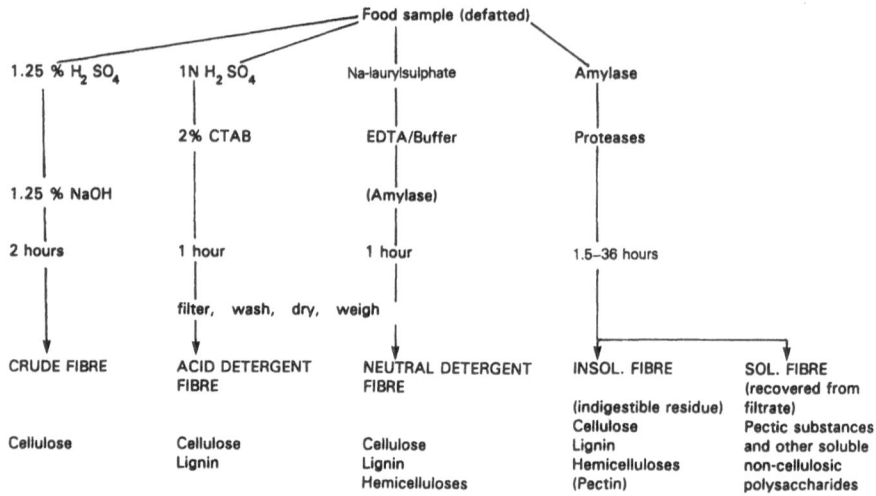

Fig. 4.2. Principles of gravimetric methods and main components measured (CTAB = cetyltrimethylammonium bromide).

sequential extraction of plant materials with diethyl ether, dilute acid and alkali goes back to the procedure developed in Weende by Henneberg and Stohmann (1859).

Nearly 30 years later Stutzer and Isbert (1888) published a study on digestion of carbohydrates in feed and food by intestinal juices which together with the studies of Remy (1931) and Williams and Olmstedt (1935) may be considered as the earliest enzymatic method for the measurement of fibre. All gravimetric methods described since then, schematically outlined in Fig. 4.2, have evolved from either of these basic approaches.

Crude Fibre

The Weende crude fibre procedure has found widespread application in the evaluation of animal feed as an index of the least digestible matter. Its main advantage is the use of only three cheap and generally available reagents. However, the simplicity of the method is superficial and reproducibility is only possible with rigid attention to the protocol. Even so, variable proportions of lignin and hemicelluloses are solubilised, and the residues contain variable amounts of nitrogen including Maillard-type artefacts in heated materials.

The severe limitations of the crude fibre procedure were recognised early on, and they led to the development of many modifications which have been thoroughly reviewed (Thomas, 1972; Thomas and Elchazly, 1976; Southgate, 1976b, c). Probably the most serious drawback of the crude fibre procedure was the loss of the majority of the cell wall fractions hemicellulose and lignin due to solubility in alkali (Thomas, 1972). However, crude fibre methods without an alkali step (Kühl, 1936; Walker and Hepburn, 1955) or using oxidative conditions (Scharrer and Kürschner, 1931) did not gain wide acceptance, mainly because the residues contained too much nitrogen. Thus, the Weende procedure which appeared as an official AOAC method already in 1916 remained unchanged in its principles until now (Anonymous, 1990).

Detergent Fibre Methods

With the introduction of detergents, Van Soest (1963a) achieved major progress in the analysis of feeds, and two standard procedures rapidly gained wide acceptance, namely an acid detergent fibre (ADF) method (Van Soest, 1963b) and a neutral detergent fibre (NDF) method (Van Soest and Wine, 1967), as outlined in Fig. 4.2. Both ADF and NDF residues can be further fractionated so that separate values for cellulose, insoluble hemicelluloses, lignin, cutin and silica can be determined (Robertson and Van Soest, 1981).

The detergent in the ADF method reduced the problem of residual nitrogen in acid fibre residues without compromising the recovery of lignin, and was therefore advocated for the evaluation of ruminant feed. The milder NDF method was recommended (Van Soest and Wine, 1967) to measure "the insoluble organic matter indigestible by animal enzymes" in feed for non-ruminants. This made the NDF method attractive as a rapid measure of dietary fibre in food, at a time when the measurement of "indigestible residues" by enzymic gravimetric methods was not very practicable. However, adequate starch removal by the NDF procedure could only be achieved when incorporating an enzymatic step for amylolysis (Schaller 1976). A number of variants including pre-incubation, post-incubation and inclusion of heat-stable amylases in the NDF reagent have been described for this modification (Robertson and Van Soest, 1981; Horvath and Robertson, 1986) and are still being developed (Jeraci and Van Soest, 1990). Amylase-modified NDF procedures were adopted as official methods for foods by the AACC (AACC method 32-20) and a few national food authorities (Anonymous, 1982, 1983).

In comparison with the recent enzymatic methods the NDF methods can be criticised for not measuring soluble polysaccharides, especially the pectic substances, escaping digestion in the human small intestine. Indeed, soluble components cannot be at present recovered satisfactorily from the detergent solution and have to be measured in a separate assay, as discussed below. In the future this could limit the further use for food analysis of this method which had been developed originally for feed analysis.

Enzymatic Methods

Until about 10 years ago the enzymatic methods could not successfully compete with the crude fibre and detergent fibre procedures, although it was well known that these latter methods measured only parts of the indigestible polysaccharides. The missing parts were erroneously counted as digestible carbohydrates, either in the so-called nitrogen-free extract of animal feed or as carbohydrate-by-difference in human food. However, the older enzymatic methods, which have been comprehensively reviewed (Asp and Johansson, 1984; Thomas and Elchazly, 1976), determined only insoluble fibre as indigestible residues and were more laborious and time-consuming than the simple empirical methods (Fig. 4.2).

Williams and Olmsted (1935) developed a procedure using enzymes to remove protein and starch and more recently Hellendoorn et al. (1975) used mammalian enzymes, pepsin and pancreatin; Hellendoorn (1983) regarded it an advantage to include also undigestible protein and starch fractions in the dietary fibre, and preferred the term "indigestible residue" because it was more explicit. As one of the first to recognise the importance of fermentation for the physiological activity of the undigestible residue of food, he expressed the definition of dietary fibre analytically as "the part of the food which is not solubilised after the most energetic enzymatic treatment".

The first gravimetric procedures accounting for both insoluble and soluble parts of dietary fibre (Fig. 4.3) were developed at about the same time but independently by Furda (1977, 1981), Schweizer and Würsch (1979, 1981), and Asp and Johansson (1981). These authors isolated soluble fibres from the enzymic digests by precipitation with four volumes of ethanol. It could also be shown that the insoluble and soluble residues were amenable to detailed characterisation by acid hydrolysis and analysis of the carbohydrate monomers (Schweizer and Würsch, 1979, 1981; Asp and Johansson, 1981). In principle this made these procedures the most complete of gravimetric methods allowing the determination of a global total fibre value and of separate values for insoluble

	Asp et al. 1983	AOAC Prosky et al. 1988 Schweizer et al. 1988	AOAC modified Lee et al. 1992
Sample	1 g*	1 g*	1 g*
Buffer Enzyme step 1	Na-phosphate pH 6 Termamyl 100°C, 15′	Na-phosphate pH 6 Termamyl 100°C, 15 (~30)′	MES/TRIS pH 8.2 Termamyl 95-100°C, 35′
pH adjustment Enzyme step 2	to pH 1.5 Pepsin 40°C, 60′	to pH 7.5 Protease 60°C, 30′	Protease 60°C, 30′
pH adjustment Enzyme step 3	to pH 6.8 Pancreatin 40°C, 60′	to pH 4.0-4.6 Amyloglucosidase 60°C, 30′	to pH 4.1-4.7 Amyloglucosidase 60°C, 30′
pH adjustment	to pH 4.5		
Alcohol precipitation with 4 vol 95% ethanol** Volume required	400 ml	280 ml	225ml
Filtering aid	Celite 545	Celite 545	Celite
Protein correction Ash correction	N x 6.25 (optional) Incineration 525°C	N x 6.25 Incineration 525°C	N x 6.25 Incineration 525°C

*   Smaller samples can be analysed if samples are difficult to filter
**   The enzyme digest can be filtered before the alcohol precipitation to recover insoluble fibre separately.

The soluble fibre is then precipitated from the filtrate and recovered in a separate filtration. Alternatively, soluble fibre can be obtained as the difference between total and insoluble fibre as approved by the AOAC.

Fig. 4.3. Main steps and comparison of enzymatic–gravimetric methods.

and soluble parts, with the options of getting their detailed chemical composition and of measuring physiologically relevant physical properties (Schweizer et al., 1983).

Subsequent efforts of Asp, Furda and Schweizer were mainly directed towards making these methods more precise, robust, fast and reproducible, and hence suitable for routine analysis.

The Method of Asp et al.

The development of the Hellendoorn method by Asp et al. (1983) led to the shortening of incubation times and a practicable way of separating the dietary fibre, i.e. filtration through glass crucibles with Celite as a filtering aid (Fig. 4.3). Ultrafiltration and dialysis for recovery of the soluble components were considered too slow, although these techniques have been successfully applied by Meuser et al. (1983) and Arrigoni et al. (1984), respectively. In order to make the starch removal more rapid and complete, the heat stable amylase Termamyl® was used in the gelatinisation step, as introduced earlier by Theander and Åman (1979). The sequential treatment with amylase–protease–amylase would also be expected to facilitate the hydrolysis of starch that might initially be encapsulated in, for example, cell structures.

The appearance of inorganic material especially due to co-precipitation in the alcohol precipitation step was recognised early and subject to thorough studies by Schweizer et al. (1984) and Frölich et al. (1984). Incineration of the residue is a pragmatic way to correct for this ash. Correction for protein (Kjeldahl nitrogen × 6.25) associated with the residue was left optional by Asp et al. (1983), but is generally applied to obtain dietary fibre estimates compatible with the requirements of component analysis.

The AOAC Method

The AOAC method for total dietary fibre (TDF; Prosky et al., 1984, 1985) was developed from the joint experience of Asp, Furda and Schweizer. The method was finally approved by the AOAC in November 1985 after two collaborative studies (see below). The initial gelatinisation/Termamyl step and the filtration with Celite were adopted from the method of Asp et al. (1983), whereas the enzymes of Furda (1977, 1981) were used. Slight modifications regarding buffer strength and pH adjustment were introduced in a later version tested in the Swiss collaborative study (Schweizer et al., 1988) and also adopted by the AOAC (Prosky et al., 1988). The main steps of the AOAC method and the method of Asp et al. are shown in Fig. 4.3.

In addition to the AOAC approval, the method obtained official status in Switzerland, Germany and in the Nordic countries. In the Netherlands a method similar to that of Asp et al. (1983) with mammalian enzymes is approved.

Lee and Hicks (1990) developed a further simplified version of the AOAC method, involving replacement of the initial phosphate buffer with a MES/TRIS

(2(N-morpholino)ethanesulphonic acid/tris hydroxymethyl aminomethane) buffer to diminish co-precipitation, elimination of one pH adjustment and some further reduction in volumes.

The Various Steps in Enzymatic Gravimetric Methods

Sample Preparation

A simple extraction of the bulk of the fat with petroleum spirit is recommended in the AOAC method when the fat content is more than 5% (first version) or 10% (second version) on a dry matter basis. Asp et al. (1983) showed that mixed diets with up to 20% fat could be analysed without fat extraction. The exact limit above which fat extraction is necessary cannot be given since it depends on the nature of the samples. Residues of fat are removed by the alcohol and acetone washings of the fibre residues after filtration. In the Swiss version of the AOAC method an additional washing with petroleum ether is prescribed because the initial fat removal is not considered necessary for samples which can be milled without it. This eliminates a possible source of error.

Milling to particle size <0.5 mm is recommended after fat extraction if necessary. In samples which are difficult to mill particle size <1 mm may be acceptable.

Starch gelatinisation close to 100 °C in the presence of Termamyl is preferable to autoclaving for two reasons: it diminishes the risk of (1) retrogradation of starch at cooling, and (2) degradation of heat-labile dietary fibre polysaccharides. Using this procedure, Asp et al. (1983) found only traces of starch in the fibre residues of starch-rich materials such as uncooked wheat flour.

Resistant Starch

When analysing bread, Johansson et al. (1984) found higher dietary fibre values both in the crust and crumb than expected from the raw materials. This was due to the formation of resistant starch as originally defined by Englyst et al. (1982), i.e. a starch fraction available to amylase degradation only after solubilisation in 2 mol/l potassium hydroxide (KOH) or dimethylsulphoxide (DMSO). Some of the starch in the fibre residues was available to glucoamylase without solubilisation and referred to as residual starch. Prolonged baking, storage at room temperature or freezing did not influence the level of resistant starch (Siljeström and Asp, 1985), and there is no published evidence from studies using the AOAC method that the sample preparation would generate resistant starch. The contribution of resistant starch can be determined by starch analysis of the gravimetric fibre residue.

The resistant starch in the gravimetric residue is mainly retrograded amylose (Berry et al., 1988; Siljeström et al., 1989; Sievert and Pomeranz, 1989; Sievert et al., 1991). It is resistant to degradation in the small intestine of rats (Björck et al., 1986) and man (Englyst and Cummings, 1985, 1987, 1988; Schweizer et al.,

1990), and constitutes a major fraction of the total malabsorbed starch in foods, such as bread, cornflakes and beans, but not in cooked potatoes and green unripe bananas.

Protein Degradation

The originally very acid pH of around 1 suggested by Hellendoorn et al. (1975) was changed to 1.5 in the methods using mammalian enzymes. With the short incubation time used at this pH, there was no evidence of losses of acid-labile dietary fibre components (Asp et al., 1983). Nevertheless, the AOAC method employed a neutral protease mainly to avoid the risk of such losses.

Complete removal of protein is not achieved, but part of the residual protein is cell wall material which some have considered as a component of the dietary fibre complex (Saunders and Betschart, 1980; Trowell, 1988).

The protein correction with Kjeldahl nitrogen $\times$ 6.25 is arbitrary, since the exact conversion factor is not known. In samples such as protein concentrates or isolates, in which most of the residue is protein, or samples containing aminopolysaccharides the use of a standard factor may introduce an error. On the other hand, routine GLC methods for dietary fibre analysis do not account for aminosugars. In analysis of most foods and diets, the error introduced by the protein correction is insignificant. Maillard reaction products, that retain most of their nitrogen content even in advanced stages (Theander, 1987) generally do not contribute to gravimetric dietary fibre estimates corrected for protein (Siljeström et al., 1986) although they may contribute to Klason lignin (Theander, 1987).

Recently Nishimune et al. (1991) published TDF values for 231 Japanese foods and 21 groups of mixed foods. A few minor modifications of the AOAC method were introduced for some foods. Thus analysis of undigestible protein in animal foods was performed with the Biuret colorimetric method to avoid deducting the values for aminopolysaccharides. Shrimps (without shell) were reported to have 5.5% TDF (wet weight basis) with this method. An extra pepsin step was introduced to diminish the protein correction when analysing animal foods.

Alcohol Precipitation

Addition of four volumes of 95% ethanol yields a final ethanol concentration of 78%. Increase of the ethanol concentration to 85% did not increase the yield of soluble fibre. Ethanol concentrations around 80% are used in all dietary fibre methods for recovery of soluble fibre and are generally regarded to precipitate saccharides with a degree of polymerisation (DP) of 10 or more. As mentioned above, highly branched polysaccharides may be soluble at considerably higher DP, as is the case with, for example, arabinans in sugar beet fibre (Asp, 1990). It has also been shown for maltodextrins that about 40% of DP 10 and still 20% of DP 11 were not precipitated from an aqueous solution by four volumes of pure ethanol. Conversely, lower DPs were not totally soluble (Schweizer and Reimann, 1982).

Polydextrose is not measured as dietary fibre, because most of it is soluble in 80% ethanol. However, it can be measured by HPLC after starch degradation with Termamyl and amyloglucosidase according to the AOAC method (Kobayashi et al., 1989).

Correction for Minerals

Correction for minerals associated with the dietary fibre or co-precipitated is carried out by incineration. The organic part of phytic acid, that is recovered mainly in the soluble fraction, will give a small but usually insignificant contribution. Some caution is needed when analysing materials high in organic acids (such as oxalic acid) that may co-precipitate. Whenever such co-precipitation is suspected, the assay should be repeated after extraction of such compounds.

Comparison of Methods

The method of Asp et al. (1983) and the AOAC method have been repeatedly shown to give similar values for total dietary fibre (Asp, 1986, 1990). Advantages with the AOAC method are smaller volumes and shorter incubation times. The modifications of Lee and Hicks (1990) and Lee et al. (1992) imply further simplifications. The less expensive and more generally available physiological enzymes are an advantage of the method of Asp et al.

In both raw and variously processed wheat samples the total fibre assayed according to Asp et al. agreed very well with values according to the Uppsala Method C (Siljeström et al. 1986). Theander et al. (1990), however, reported lower values with the Uppsala method in some samples. When gravimetric residues from cereals (Nyman et al., 1984), and vegetables (Nyman et al., 1987) have been analysed with GLC according to the Uppsala methodology, recovery figures are generally close to 100%. Lower recoveries are obtained for some materials and can be due to incomplete hydrolysis as for Sterculia gum (Nyman and Asp, 1985) or residues of tannins (Saura-Calixto, 1988).

Other Current Gravimetric Methods

This section on gravimetric methods would be incomplete without an assessment of the so-called plant cell wall methods. Most of these methods were not designed for food analysis in a nutritional context, but rather aimed at obtaining highly purified cell wall preparations for biochemical studies (Selvendran et al., 1987). The analytical schemes are usually time-consuming and delicate, not adapted to mixed and processed foods, and may not include soluble fibre components. Recently, a new method for measuring cell walls in foods has been proposed which addresses the above difficulties (Brillouet et al., 1988). The scheme provides cell wall residues after removal of protein with protease and detergent, and of starch with dimethylsulphoxide and amylases. Soluble fibres are recovered from the combined proteolysis and amylolysis liquors after dialysis and analysed by GLC and colorimetry. Unfortunately, the authors had to conclude that this part of the procedure was not satisfactory.

Recently, two other gravimetric methods have been proposed claiming conceptual and practical advantages, especially for the purpose of routine analysis and labelling (Mongeau and Brassard, 1986; Jeraci et al., 1989). Mongeau and Brassard (1986) revived the NDF procedure and combined it with a separate determination of hot water-soluble (SOL) fibre. The values for NDF + SOL are claimed to be in agreement with the TDF measured by the AOAC method. However, performing the analysis of insoluble and soluble fibre on two different samples and under different solubilisation conditions is conceptually unsatisfactory because of the inherent risk of analysing some components twice or not at all. A further disadvantage is that separate analysis of insoluble and soluble fibres is obligatory, without being necessarily meaningful. The urea enzymatic dialysis method of Jeraci et al. (1989) is based on starch and protein solubilisation with 8 mol/l urea in a dialysis tube, addition of bacterial amylase and protease, followed by in situ dialysis and recovery of dietary fibre residue precipitated with ethanol. The main advantages over the AOAC method described by thee authors of this new approach were improved starch removal, smaller ash and protein corrections, no heat exposure of the samples and less reagents needed. The method has also been proposed for separate determination of insoluble and soluble fibre (Jeraci et al. 1990). It remains to be seen whether the handling of dialysis tubings will not be an obstacle in collaborative studies.

The Southgate Method for Unavailable Carbohydrates

During the analytical work for the preparation of the third edition of *The Composition of Foods* (McCance and Widdowson, 1960) W.I.M. Holman and D.A.T. Southgate made some methodological studies on the measurement of the sugars and starches in foods in an effort to apply some newer techniques to the measurement of available carbohydrate values for inclusion in the new edition. Alongside this work Southgate also began to review the developing analytical literature on the polysaccharide components of the plant cell wall and in the summer of 1959 began experimental work in connection with the experimental re-evaluation of the calorie conversion factors for mixed diets (Durnin, 1961; Southgate, 1961; Southgate and Durnin, 1970). In these studies it was desirable to be able to measure all the energy yielding components in the diet and especially important to have sound estimates of both available and unavailable carbohydrates because of the controversy relating to the use of the Atwater factors (Maynard, 1944; Widdowson, 1955).

On the basis of studies of the techniques in use at that time (Southgate, 1981) it was decided to follow McCance and Widdowson's principles and seek to measure the available and unavailable carbohydrates directly as carbohydrate. It was also desirable to analyse the components sequentially on the same analytical sample to avoid both double-counting and missing fractions. In the present context only the methods for unavailable carbohydrates are directly relevant but the extraction of sugars and hydrolysis of starch need to be considered. A detailed account and critique of the method was published in James and Theander (1981) and these details need not be repeated here.

Principles

The free sugars and oligosaccharides were extracted from the sample of mixed diet, food or faeces with hot aqueous methanol (85% v/v) and the alcohol-insoluble residue further extracted with diethyl ether and allowed to dry in air. The air-dried residue was used for the measurement of starch and the unavailable carbohydrates. The boundary between the polysaccharides hydrolysed in the small and the large intestine was taken as hydrolysis with a Takadiastase preparation (Parke Davis; Takadiastase for analysis on talc) in acetate buffer. The unhydrolysed polysaccharides were recovered by precipitation with ethanol (4 vols) and dried with acetone. The residue was then heated with 1 mol/l sulphuric acid at 100 °C for 2.5 hours. The hydrolysate was filtered or centrifuged and the filtrate used for the analysis of the components of the non-cellulosic polysaccharides; the residue was dispersed in 12 mol/l sulphuric acid and left overnight at 0–4 °C, rapidly diluted and filtered. The filtrate was analysed for sugars and the residue filtered off, washed, dried and weighed as a measure of lignin. Hexoses were measured by the anthrone method (Roe, 1955), pentoses by the method of Albaum and Umbreit (1947) and uronic acids by the carbazole reaction (initially Dische, 1955; later Bitter and Muir, 1962).

Performance

The procedure was time-consuming and the manipulations required skill and practice, especially the colorimetric methods using strong acid which are difficult to automate and prone to interference from organic dust material. However, with training several laboratories achieved satisfactory within-laboratory results especially if they adopted regular use of in-house reference materials and suitable quality assurance procedures (Southgate, 1987). In collaborative studies performance was not satisfactory primarily because a new protocol was introduced without proper testing and because the conditions of the study did not permit a pre-trial test sample. In addition several modifications that had not been evaluated were introduced.

Comparisons with the detergent fibre procedures showed that these underestimated unavailable carbohydrates and that some gravimetric procedures for indigestible material gave higher values (Greenberg, 1976). Comparisons with the non-starch polysaccharide procedures of Englyst (Englyst et al., 1982) showed that in processed cereal foods the Southgate method gave higher values because of the inclusion of undigested starch and lignin. In foods where these two components are not present agreement was usually good (Southgate and Englyst, 1985). It should be remembered that the original Southgate method (1969b) was designed to measure unavailable carbohydrates, as defined by McCance and Lawrence (1929), not NSP, so this difference should be expected in the light of current knowledge about the extent of starch digestion in the small intestine.

Limitations

The major limitation of the procedure as originally described was the reliance on colorimetric procedures that were only semi-specific and in addition were technically exacting and relatively non-robust. The delineation of the boundary between starch and the unavailable "small intestinal indigestible" polysaccharides using Takadiastase is subject to the same criticism as the choice of any in vitro system using any combination of enzymes.

The Southgate method was concerned with the measurement of "unavailable carbohydrates", i.e. those polysaccharides that are not hydrolysed and absorbed in the small intestine, and therefore to exclude starch which was considered an available carbohydrate. The non-carbohydrate lignin was included in this grouping as originally defined.

Analysis of Individual Components of Dietary Fibre

A meeting in 1977 organised by the EEC and the International Agency for Research on Cancer (WHO) in Lyon marked the starting point for efforts to introduce more modern and informative analytical methods in the field of dietary fibre (Theander and James, 1979). In 1979 a GLC method for the characterisation of gravimetrically determined insoluble and soluble dietary fibre residues was published (Schweizer and Würsch, 1979) which combined advantages of the procedures of Hellendoorn et al. (1975) and Southgate (1969b). In the same year the carbohydrate group in Uppsala published a gas chromatographic method (GLC) for the analysis and characterisation of dietary fibre (DF) as the sum of polysaccharides and Klason lignin after starch removal (Theander and Åman, 1979). The latest modification of this GLC method was recently presented at a meeting in Dallas as the Uppsala method for rapid analysis and characterisation of individual constituents of DF (Theander et al. 1990).

The method of Englyst (Southgate et al., 1978; Englyst, 1981) was originally based upon that of Southgate (1969b), GLC replacing the colorimetric methods for determination of neutral sugar constituents. This method has also undergone a number of developments described below, and a colorimetric variant was published (Englyst and Hudson, 1987) for routine analysis. Both the original Uppsala method and the first Englyst method were used to determine the DF content in different types of food samples in a collaborative study presented in Cambridge in 1978 (James and Theander, 1981).

Table 4.3. Comparison of main steps in total dietary fibre determination by GLC with the latest modifications of the Uppsala method (Theander et al., 1990) and the Englyst method (Englyst and Cummings, 1990)

Procedure	Uppsala method	Englyst method
Sample size (dry matter)	250–500 mg	50–300 mg
Fat removal	Extraction with petroleum ether when content exceeds 6%	Extraction with acetone when content exceeds 5%
Starch removal	(1) Termamyl (0.5 hours; 96 °C) in acetate buffer (0.1 mol/l, pH 5) (2) Amyloglucosidase (16 hours, 60 °C)	(1) Dimethylsulphoxide (DMSO) (0.5 hours, boiling water bath) (2) Termamyl (10 min, boiling water bath) in acetate buffer (0.08 mol/l, pH 5.2) (3) Pancreatin and pullulanase (0.5 hours, 50 °C + 10 min, boiling water bath)
Precipitation of soluble fibre	80% (v/v) ethanol (1 hour, 4 °C)	80% (v/v) ethanol (0.5 hours, ice water)
Drying of the fibre residues	45 °C overnight	Acetone washing, 80 °C until dry
Analysis of neutral sugars	(1) 12 mol/l H_2SO_4 (1 hour, 30 °C) (2) Addition of internal standard *myo*-inositol (3) 0.4 mol/l H_2SO_4 (1 hour, 125 °C) (4) Alditol acetate preparation by sodium borhydride reduction and 1-methylimidazole/acetic anhydride (5) Individual correction factors regularly determined for each sugar	(1) 12 mol/l H_2SO_4 (1 hour, 35 °C) (2) 2 mol/l H_2SO_4 (1 hour, 100 °C) (3) Addition of internal standard (allose) (4) Alditol acetate preparation by sodium borohydride reduction and 1-methylimidazole/acetic anhydride (5) Individual standard correction factors for acid hydrolysis losses (introduced in the instructions for the MAFF IV study 1989)
Analysis of uronic acids	Stoichometric decarboxylation or colorimetry with 3,5-dimethylphenol (Scott, 1979). Calibration based on galacturonic acid	Scott procedure with 3,5-dimethylphenol Calibration based on galacturonic acid
Lignin	Gravimetrically as Klason (sulphuric acid) lignin	Not determined

The effective heat-stable amylase (Termamyl) step developed in Uppsala for enzymatic removal of starch without degrading the fibre polysaccharides has been incorporated into gravimetric methods for determination of DF (Asp et al., 1983; Prosky et al., 1984) and also in the latest version of the Englyst method (Englyst and Cummings, 1990).

To determine pectic substances, a stoichiometric decarboxylation for the determination of uronic acid residues was introduced in the Uppsala method, whereas Englyst used a colorimetric assay with a 3,5-dimethylphenol reagent (Scott, 1979).

A brief summary on problems related to specific analysis of dietary fibre components is given below. For more details, the reader is referred to James and Theander (1981), Englyst and Cummings (1984, 1988, 1990), Theander and Westerlund (1986a, b) and Theander et al. (1990). An extensive publication by Selvendran et al. (1989) dealing with methods for analysis of DF is also recommended. The main steps of the most recent versions of the Uppsala method and the Englyst method are summarised and compared in Table 4.3.

Determination and Chemical Characterisation of Total Dietary Fibre by the Uppsala Methodology

The principles for the analysis of total DF and individual DF components by the Uppsala method (Theander et al., 1990) are presented in Fig. 4.4. Representative samples of dry materials are ground to pass a 0.5 mm screen, whereas samples with higher water contents are freeze-dried and then ground, or homogenised directly. If samples contain more than 6% fat pre-extraction with petroleum ether is recommended.

Starch is removed by incubations with a thermostable α-amylase (Termamyl) and amyloglucosidase. This enzyme system has proved to be very effective for various types of starch containing fibre sources and products. The Termamyl-enzyme incubation in a boiling water bath causes simultaneous gelatinisation and hydrolysis of the starch. However, retrograded amylose ("resistant starch") is not removed unless it is first solubilised with alkali or DMSO.

It is imperative that the enzymes used for starch degradation are free from fibre-degrading activity. Unfortunately it would appear that many commercial amyloglucosidase preparations at present have, for example, β-glucanase activity and will thus give low values for the fibre contents in, for example, cereal samples. All enzyme batches should therefore be checked for such activities prior to use for fibre analysis.

After the completion of enzymic removal of starch, soluble fibres are precipitated with 80% ethanol and the DF residue containing soluble as well as insoluble fibres is obtained by centrifugation (Fig. 4.4). The content of neutral DF polysaccharides is then determined by GLC, after acid hydrolysis and preparation of alditol acetates. So far, uronic acids are determined on a separate sample of the original material using the decarboxylation procedure (Theander and Åman, 1979). As an alternative a simpler method (Scott, 1979) for

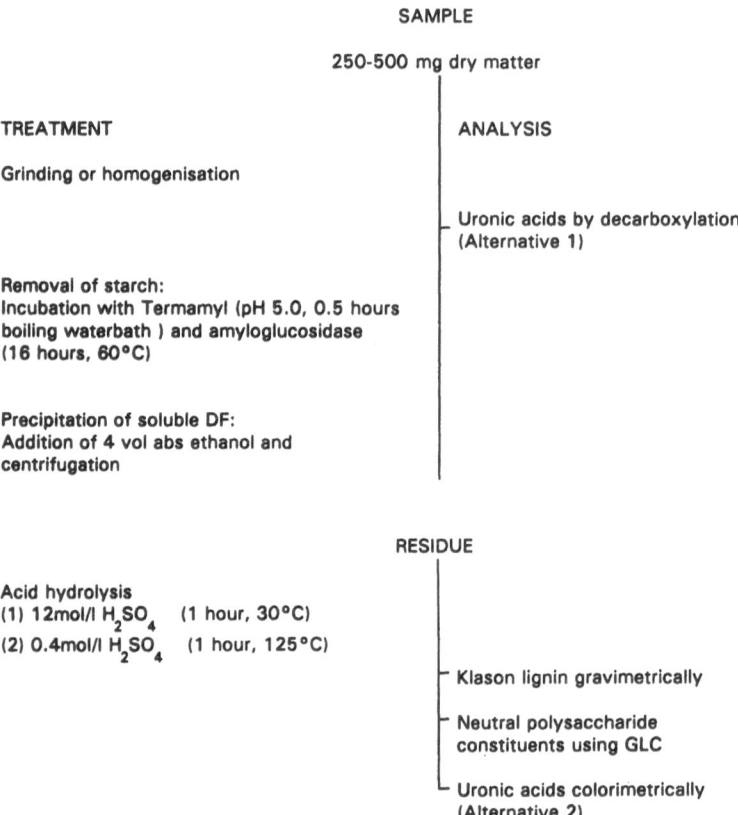

Fig. 4.4. Rapid analysis of dietary fibre by the Uppsala method.

colorimetric determination of uronic acids (in the hydrolysate) will probably be used in future studies (Table 4.3).

The lignin content is measured gravimetrically as Klason (sulphuric acid) lignin, obtained after acid treatment and ashing of the insoluble residue. The Uppsala method has been applied to a number of divergent samples, including foods, feeds, digesta and faeces, and a skilled analyst can run over 40 samples per week by this improved procedure. During 1991 the method will be evaluated for various types of fibre sources (cereals, vegetables and fruits) in a collaborative AOAC study, in which O. Theander is an associated referee. In connection with this a detailed manual of the method will be published.

Another more rapid modification has also been published (Method B, Theander and Åman 1982) which is suitable when dealing with samples with low contents of starch. It is based on removal of 80% ethanol extractives followed by direct analysis of the DF constituents in the manner described above. The DF glucan content is obtained as the difference between the total glucan content (determined by GLC) and the starch content which is analysed enzymically.

Analysis and Characterisation of Soluble and Insoluble Dietary Fibre

DF includes a mixture of water-soluble and insoluble components mainly from cell wall materials, but there is no sharp borderline between the two categories. The yield of the respective fraction can vary considerably with the fractionation conditions used (physical pre-treatment, enzymatic treatment, temperature, time and pH). Thus recent studies (Schweizer and Würsch, 1979; Englyst et al., 1982, Englyst, 1985; Graham et al., 1988; Marlett et al., 1989; Englyst and Cummings, 1990) have shown that the yield and composition of soluble fibres were very dependent on the extraction conditions used.

The first GLC method for analysis of DF by the Uppsala group (Method A) was based on separate analysis of soluble and insoluble DF constituents (Theander and Åman, 1979). After removal of 80% ethanolic extractives and of starch enzymatically, the soluble fibre fraction was isolated by dialysis and the insoluble one by centrifugation. The fractions were then analysed for the content of DF essentially as described above for the Uppsala method. This method has been used in two collaborative studies (Theander and Åman, 1981; Varo et al., 1983). At present a more rapid method for routine analysis of soluble fibre is under development. In this method it is a keypoint to reach as complete a recovery as possible of soluble fibre components when these are precipitated by 80% (v/v) ethanol. It has been previously shown (Theander and Westerlund, 1986a) that such losses did not exceed 3% of the total DF polysaccharides for samples of wheat flour, raw potato, carrot and wheat bran. Recently in a detailed study using gel filtration (Theander et al., 1990) of the ethanolic supernatant, the polysaccharide fraction (DP > 10) escaping precipitation was analysed in various foods. The amounts of soluble fibre polysaccharides not recovered were low, corresponding to 1%–6% of the total fibre content of the original sample. The highest values were found for the most severely heat-treated sample (bread crust). This indicates that the solubility of DF polysaccharides may be changed by thermal treatment, for instance by depolymerisation as shown previously for cereals (Siljeström et al., 1989; Westerlund et al., 1989).

Main Features of the Method of Englyst et al.

The method of Englyst et al. (Southgate et al., 1978; Englyst, 1981; Englyst et al., 1982; Englyst and Cummings, 1984, 1988, 1990) for determination of non-starch polysaccharides (NSP) emerged from the Southgate method (Southgate, 1969b), using GLC for specific determination of neutral sugar constituents. Colorimetric methods are used for uronic acids, originally carbazol (Englyst, 1981) and in later versions a Scott type procedure (3,5-dimethylphenol). Lignin is not determined (Fig. 4.5).

In the version of Englyst et al. (1982), three parallel samples were analysed for determination of total NSP, insoluble NSP and cellulose, respectively. Soluble NSP is calculated as the difference between total and insoluble NSP. The

Table 4.4. Modifications of steps in the GLC method of Englyst et al. used in various collaborative studies by the Ministry of Agriculture, Fisheries and Food (MAFF)

	MAFF II (Englyst et al., 1987a)	MAFF III (Englyst et al., 1987b)	MAFF IV (methods as described by Englyst and Cummings, 1990)
Starch removal	(1) Dimethylsulphoxide (DMSO) 1 hour, boiling water bath (2) Pancreatic α-amylase + pullulanase 16–18 hours, 42 °C	(1) DMSO 1 hour, boiling water bath (2) Pancreatin + pullulanase 16–18 hours, 42 °C	(1) DMSO 0.5 hour, boiling water bath (2) Termamyl, 10 min, boiling water bath (3) Pancreatin + pullulanase 0.5 hour, 50 °C + 10 min boiling water bath
Analysis of neutral sugars	(1) 12 mol/l H_2SO_4, 35 °C, 1–1.25 hours (2) Dilution to 1.4 mol/l. Internal standard added (erythritol and myoinositol), 2 hours, boiling water bath (3) Drying before acetylation (4) Average correction for hydrolysis losses by 0.9, 2 × correction for rhamnose	(1) 12 mol/l H_2SO_4, 35 °C, 1–1.25 hours (2) Dilution to 0.8 mol/l, 2–2.5 hours' boiling water bath. Addition of internal standard (allose) after cooling (3) 1-Methylimidazole catalysed derivatisation (4) Average correction for hydrolysis losses by 0.9, 2 × correction for rhamnose	(1) 12 mol/l H_2SO_4, 35 °C, 1 hour (2) Dilution to 2 mol/l, 1 hour boiling water bath (3) 1-Methylimidazole catalysed derivatisation (4) Individual standard correction factors for each sugar
Uronic acid determination	3,5-dimethylphenol Glucuronic acid standard	3,5-dimethylphenol Glucuronic acid standard	3,5-dimethylphenol Galacturonic acid standard

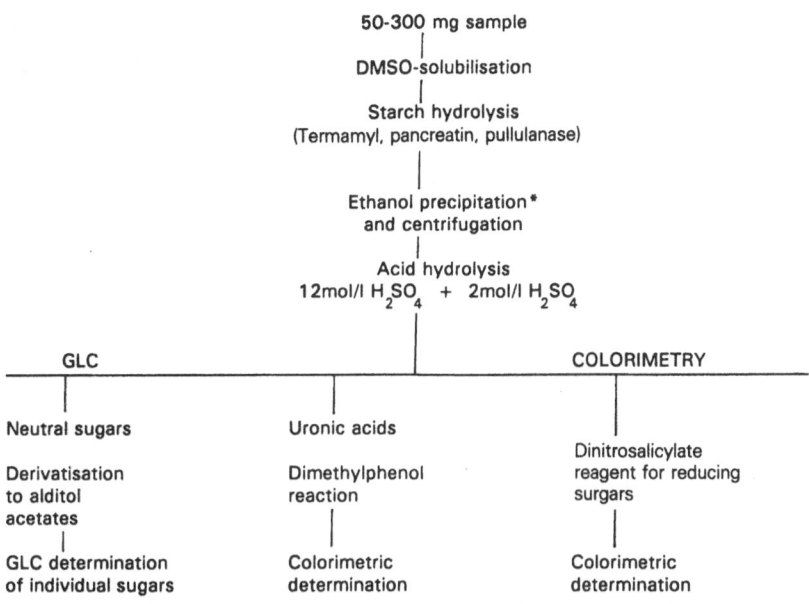

Fig. 4.5. Main steps of the Englyst method for dietary fibre determination (Englyst and Cummings, 1990)

insoluble NSP is prepared by extraction with a phosphate buffer pH 7 at 100 °C. Direct determination of soluble fibre has not been reported.

The method uses a relatively small sample (50–300 mg) with the advantage that it is essentially a one tube procedure. On the other hand, this requires a very homogeneous sample milled to small particles.

As shown in Table 4.3, there are many similarities between the most recent modifications of the Uppsala method and the Englyst method for total dietary fibre determination, but also significant differences. The different modifications of the Englyst method regarding starch removal and hydrolysis/derivatisation are shown in Table 4.4.

A most important difference is the solubilisation of "resistant starch" (Englyst et al. 1982) with DMSO. The use of DMSO can be expected to increase the solubility of DF, since this reagent is a solvent for hemicellulose polysaccharides (Hägglund et al., 1956; Gruppen et al., 1991). The possibility that DMSO influences the recovery of dissolved polysaccharides by the ethanol precipitation must also be considered. However, Englyst and Cummings (1984) found that DMSO did not significantly reduce the values for NSP as used in their method.

The hydrolysis of starch was originally carried out with overnight incubations with a mixture of pancreatic amylase and pullulanase. In the latest version (Englyst and Cummings, 1990) a Termamyl step at 100 °C was adopted, allowing shortening of the amylase treatment to less than 1 hour. The Englyst method uses Seaman hydrolysis with 12 mol/l sulphuric acid to disperse the cellulose, with conditions similar to those of the Uppsala method. The final hydrolysis is carried out in 2 mol/l sulphuric acid in a boiling waterbath for 1 hour, whereas the Uppsala method uses 0.4 mol/l acid for 1 hour at 125 °C.

In the analysis of the neutral sugar composition with GLC it is important to use correction factors for each neutral sugar constituent in order to correct for hydrolytic losses, derivatisation yields and GLC-response (Theander and Westerlund, 1986a; Theander et al., 1990). An internal standard that is resistant to acidic treatment, such as *myo*-inositol used in the Uppsala method and in the earlier versions of the Englyst method (Englyst, 1981, Englyst et al., 1987a), can be added before the hydrolysis step, which is advantageous. The most recent modifications of the Englyst method (Englyst et al., 1987b; Englyst and Cummings, 1990) employ D-allose added after hydrolysis as standard. Phytic acid which is present in significant amounts in various foods has been shown to give no traces of free *myo*-inositol during the hydrolysis conditions used in the Uppsala method. Originally hydrolysis losses were supposed to correspond to about 10% (Englyst et al., 1982) but in the latest version of the method individual correction factors have finally been introduced for the various neutral sugar monomers (instructions for the MAFF IV study, 1989).

A simplified version of the Englyst method using colorimetric determination of reducing sugars with dinitrosalicylate (Englyst and Hudson, 1987) was introduced as an alternative for NSP determination when information on the monomeric composition is not required. The method has been tested collaboratively and compared with the original GLC approach (Englyst et al., 1987b) as reported below.

Alternatives for the Determination of Dietary Fibre Constituents

Analysis of Neutral DF Constituents

As discussed above, determination of neutral DF polysaccharides is generally based on acid hydrolysis of polysaccharides and subsequent GLC analysis of monosaccharides released.

Acid hydrolysis of insoluble fibre polysaccharides requires a two-step procedure involving treatment with 12 mol/l sulphuric acid and post-hydrolysis with dilute acid, particularly because of crystalline cellulose. It is important that the conditions used are sufficiently rigorous to effect complete hydrolysis of the polysaccharides, and sulphate ester groups formed during treatment with 12 mol/l sulphuric acid must be hydrolysed by the post-hydrolysis step (Theander and Westerlund, 1986a). The effect of particle size and pre-hydrolysis time to achieve optimum hydrolysis yield has recently been investigated (Hoebler et al., 1989). On the other hand, soluble fibre polysaccharides can be hydrolysed directly by dilute sulphuric acid or trifluoroacetic acid.

The monosaccharides in the acid hydrolysates may be quantified by GLC or HPLC. So far GLC, particularly on capillary columns, is recommended for efficient separation and accurate determination of the monosaccharides. The monosaccharides are usually converted to volatile alditol acetate derivatives before quantification by GLC but other derivatives have also been used with success (Schweizer and Würsch, 1979, 1981; Neeser and Schweizer, 1984). The use of 1-methylimidazole as a powerful catalyst of acetylation was introduced by Connors and Pandit (1978). This technique, modified by Englyst and Cummings in 1984, has proved to be very valuable and is in use in several procedures, including analysis of DF with the Uppsala method and the Englyst method. As a result derivatisation becomes much faster and easier and can be performed in the presence of borate without interference. Correction factors covering hydrolysis losses, derivatisation yields, and GLC responses for the individual sugars are necessary for accurate quantification and these are determined by subjecting reference sugar mixtures to similar treatment as the DF samples (Theander and Westerlund, 1986a). Due to differences in columns as well as aging of columns, the correction factors may change and should therefore be re-checked regularly. It is also recommended to analyse a standard fibre sample regularly to check the reproducibility of the method. For instance, eight totally independent analyses of purified cotton linter were found to give an average cellulose content of 99.0% (SD 1.3) and a xylan content of 0.25% (Theander et al., 1990).

Recently a procedure for direct acetylation of aldoses in the acidic hydrolysate (without previous reduction) has been developed (Hämäläinen et al., 1990). So far this procedure has only been tested on a limited number of samples but the agreement is good compared with the Uppsala method.

HPLC offers an alternative procedure for analysis of aldoses in polysaccharide hydrolysates, but has not so far proved to be as powerful a technique as GLC. Comprehensive reviews on HPLC with various applications in the carbohydrate field have been published (Honda, 1984; Hicks, 1988; Lee, 1990) and the use of amperometric determination of monosaccharides seems promising (Lee, 1990). An advantage with using HPLC for analysis of monosaccharides compared with GLC is that preparation of derivatives is not required.

Determination of Uronic Acid Constituents

Analysis of uronic acids by GLC is more difficult than of neutral sugar constituents. The release of these acids in acceptable yields from the polymers is complicated by the high stability of glycosyl uronic acid linkages towards acid hydrolysis, resulting in formation of aldobiuronic acids. Further, the monomeric uronic acids are more rapidly degraded to non-carbohydrate products than the neutral sugars under the acidic conditions prevailing. Several workers in the DF field have, therefore, used colorimetric assays (Bitter and Muir, 1962; Blumenkrantz and Asboe-Hansen, 1973; Scott, 1979). A common disadvantage with colorimetric methods is the sensitivity to the reaction conditions, and the interference from other compounds such as, for example, neutral sugars, proteins, and phenols. The introduction of 3,5-dimethylphenol by Scott (1979) who also compared the use of different phenol derivatives for colorimetric determination of uronic acids in plant materials, offers certain advantages. One of the modifications of the Scott procedure is used for the measurement of uronic acids in the Englyst method (Englyst et al., 1982). This reagent seems to be less affected by hexoses present and have a greater sensitivity than the carbazole reaction (Bitter and Muir, 1962).

Theander and Åman (1979) have shown that the decarboxylation method, developed by Bylund and Donetzhuber (1968) for analysis of uronic acid contents in woods and pulps, is also a rapid, accurate and reproducible method for analysis of DF samples. The decarboxylation in hydroiodic acid is stoichiometric and different types of uronic acids have the same response. This method, like the colorimetric methods, does not estimate the amount of individual constituents but only the sum of uronic acids. At present the procedure of Scott (1979) is investigated as an alternative to the decarboxylation procedure with respect to the Uppsala method. The rate of formation of 5-folmyl-2-furancarboxylic acid, on which the colorimetric determination is based, was shown by Scott to be faster for galacturonic than for glucuronic acid.

The uronic acids partly occur esterified with methanol or acetic acid, which has to be taken into account when measuring them quantitatively. However, these substituents do not interfere with the determination of the total uronic acid content, neither with the decarboxylation method, nor with colorimetric methods. Acetyl substituents can be quantified as 1-acetylpyrrolidine by HPLC (Månsson and Samuelsson, 1981).

Determination of Lignin

There is no specific method for the determination of lignin (the complex polymer of phenylpropane units) which is not time-consuming. A colorimetric acetylbromide method developed by Johnson et al. (1961) and later modified by Morrison (1972) can be useful when comparing lignin contents in similar plant species (Selvendran et al., 1989). Lignin can also be estimated by a procedure involving oxidation with potassium permanganate (Robertson and Van Soest, 1981; Theander et al., 1977). The Uppsala group, like many others working with lignified plant materials, prefers a sulphuric acid method (Theander and Westerlund, 1986a) for gravimetric estimation of lignin as so-called Klason lignin. This lignin method is conveniently combined with the determination of the neutral DF polysaccharides. When human foods are analysed the lignin values obtained by this method partly represent not only native lignin but also tannins, cutins and some proteinaceous products. Some ash is always present in the residue but in the Uppsala method this is corrected for. From heat-treated foods the residue may also contain undigestible Maillard reaction products and it has been proposed (Theander and Westerlund, 1986a) that the Klason lignin value should be designated the "non-carbohydrate" part of the DF. The increase of nitrogen content in the Klason lignin residue during thermal food processing is a suitable marker for the extent of Maillard reactions.

Other Constituents of Dietary Fibre

Phenolic acids which are present as ester-linked substituents to DF poly-saccharides and/or lignin may be included in this group. In some cases these components may contribute significantly to the dietary fibre content (Theander et al., 1990) as found for samples of maize bran and sugar beet fibre. Phenolic acids can be measured after release by alkaline treatment, by HPLC (Ternrud et al., 1987).

Collaborative Studies

Attempts to identify through collaborative studies the most appropriate approaches to the comprehensive analysis of dietary fibre go back to 1977. At the meeting in Lyon, France, held to explore the relationship between diet and cancer incidence, it was decided to test fibre measurement methodologies by inter-laboratory study of reference materials. One year later, the results of this exercise were assessed at a meeting held in Cambridge, UK and later published in book form (James and Theander, 1981).

Nineteen laboratories participated in this inter-laboratory study, and four different approaches were used, namely the colorimetric Southgate method, GLC methods, detergent methods and enzymatic–gravimetric methods. Although great variations – both within and between methods – were noticed, this collaboration resulted in the identification of most major difficulties in dietary fibre analysis, including such central issues as resistant starch or the method dependence of the separation of dietary fibre into insoluble and soluble fractions. These same two points also became evident in a follow-up study on processing effects on dietary fibre and starch values analysed with different methods (Varo et al., 1983).

The Cambridge meeting was an important step for future method developments. Unfortunately, it also initiated unnecessary polarisation between the methods aiming at the measurement of dietary fibre as the undigestible polysaccharides and lignin and those attempting to measure non-starch polysaccharides (NSP) as an index of plant cell wall. Some preferred to measure carbohydrates directly, whereas others could see that under certain circumstances simpler gravimetric approaches would be adequate.

Studies under Review and Performance Criteria

Until now, most collaborative studies have dealt with the Englyst procedure for NSP (Englyst et al., 1982) or the enzymatic–gravimetric AOAC method (Prosky et al., 1984) and subsequent modifications of these (Englyst and Cummings, 1984; 1988; Englyst and Hudson, 1987; Prosky et al., 1985, 1988). The NDF method combined with a measurement of SDF was also tested (Mongeau and Brassard, 1986, 1990) but other promising methods (Asp et al., 1983; Theander and Westerlund, 1986b) have not yet been studied collaboratively.

Table 4.5 gives an overview of the various studies for TDF of which the results are presently available. Table 4.6 summarises the studies with separate determinations of IDF and SDF. These tables have been arranged to make the main studies comparable and to give objective criteria for method performance evaluation. In particular, all repeatability and reproducibility data have been converted to r_{95} and R_{95}, respectively. An R_{95} value of 2.0 at a TDF content of 10 g per 100 g means that 19 out of 20 single determinations coming from various laboratories would fall in the range 9–11 g per 100 g.

Table 4.5. Summary table of main collaborative studies of methods for total dietary fibre (TDF) or non-starch polysaccharides (NSP)[a]

Trial name	Number of samples[b]	Number of results (Labs)	Outliers %[c]	Range of total dietary fibre contents (% d.b.)	Repeatability r_{95} Mean	(Range)	Reproducibility R_{95} Mean	(Range)	Main foods studied
AOAC method									
AOAC 84	13	750 (32)	2	3–89	2.39	(1.3–3.8)	5.43	(1.7–8.8)[d]	As for 85 and 88 plus lettuce, raisins, diets
AOAC 85	9	160 (9)	9	1–87	1.26	(0.4–2.8)	2.00	(0.8–3.8)[e]	Flours, breads, brans, potatoes, rice, oats, soy isolate
AOAC 88	10	172 (9)	5	1–87	1.78	(1.0–2.7)	2.68	(1.3–4.0)[f]	
Swiss 87	3 (P)	90 (15)	4	2–20	0.73	(0.3–1.1)	1.07	(1.0–1.1)	Milk cereal with fruits, cereal mix, vegetable mix
AOAC/ AACC 90	8 (P)	160 (10)	3[g]	13–72	2.49	(1.1–4.0)	3.33	(2.2–6.7)	Cereals, brans, dry fruits, dry vegetables
Neutral detergent fibre plus soluble fibre estimate									
Canada 90	5 (P)	98 (10)	8[g]	1–46	1.99	(0.5–2.9)	3.60	(0.6–5.8)	Rice, bread, beans, turnip, wheat bran
Englyst method[h]									
MAFF II	7	238 (17)	13	3–10	1.48	(0.6–2.3)	6.04	(3.7–8.7)	Breads
MAFF III									
GLC	7 (P)	266 (19)	10	1–10	1.67	(0.7–3.1)	2.62	(1.2–3.8)	Breads, cornflakes, oats
Colorim	7 (P)	266 (19)	11	1–12	1.77	(0.9–2.7)	3.20	(1.1–5.2)	

a Precision data calculated according to ISO-DIN-5725.
b (P) denotes trials in which pre-trial samples were given.
c Dixon and Cochran outliers (p < 0.05) unless otherwise noted. Precision data were calculated without these outliers.
d Without soy isolate (R = 21.2).
e Without soy isolate (R = 2.67).
f Without Fabulous Fiber (R = 5.33) and soy isolate (R = 3.89).
g Grubb's and Cochran's test used.
h Only NSP data shown, precision measures for the sum of NSP and resistant starch were less good.

Table 4.6. Collaborative studies with separate IDF/SDF[a]

Trial name		Number of samples	Number of results (Labs)	Outliers[a] %	Fibre range (% d.b.)	I95 Mean	(Range)	R95 Mean	(Range)
AOAC 88	IDF	10	208 (11)	4	1–87	1.30	(0.1–3.6)	2.20	(0.9–4.0)[b]
	SDF	10	208 (11)	2	0–9	1.05	(0.5–2.0)	1.47	(0.7–3.2)[c]
AOAC/ AACC 90	IDF	8	172 (11)	5	8–65	2.16	(1.3–2.9)	3.16	(1.8–5.8)
	SDF	8	174 (11)	2	3–31	1.68	(0.9–2.6)	3.33	(1.6–6.7)
Canada 90	NDF	5	98 (10)	10	1–40	1.44	(0.3–2.3)	2.34	(0.8–4.4)
	SOL	5	100 (10)	6	0–10	1.19	(0.3–2.2)	2.34	(0.7–4.5)

[a] Statistical calculations from original reports (Cochran's and Grubb's outliers).
[b] Without soy isolate (R95 = 5.10) and Fabulous Fiber (R95 = 12.60).
[c] Without Fabulous Fiber (R95 = 11.32).

Note to Tables 4.5 and 4.6

The different studies conducted for the Association of Official Analytical Chemists were published in the following references: AOAC 84, Prosky et al., 1984; AOAC 85, Prosky et al., 1985; AOAC 88, Prosky et al., 1988) AOAC/AACC 90 denotes the study of Lee et al. (1992) with a modified AOAC method for soluble, insoluble and total dietary fibre. This modification obtained official first action status as an alternative AOAC method in August 1991. Swiss 87 denotes the Swiss study with the AOAC method, published by Schweizer et al. (1988). Canada 90 is a collaborative study with a method based on a neutral detergent fibre analysis and separate measurement of soluble fibre (Mongeau and Brassard, 1990). The collaborative studies of the Ministry of Agriculture, Fisheries and Food, UK, using the Englyst method, were published as follows: MAFF II, Englyst et al., 1978a; MAFF III, Englyst et al., 1987b.

Relative standard deviations RSD(r) and RSD(R), i.e. coefficients of variation, are related with r and R through the standard deviations s(r) and s(R) and the average fibre content X, e.g. for reproducibility:

$$\% \; RSD(R) \; = \; (s(R)/X) \times 100$$

$$R_{95} \; = \; s(R) \times 2.8$$

It is important to recognise that both types of measures of precision can be misleading when considered in isolation. Thus, at 25% RSD(R) can correspond to a good R_{95} of 2.1 (at 3 g TDF per 100 g) but also to a very poor R_{95} of 21 (at 30 g TDF per 100 g). Conversely, an excellent R_{95} of 1.0 may stand for a 36% RSD(R) at 1 g per 100 g TDF as well as for a 0.7% RSD(R) at 50 g TDF per 100 g. Therefore, Figs. 4.6 and 4.7 represent the R values of Tables 4.5 and 4.6, respectively, as a function of the actual fibre contents.

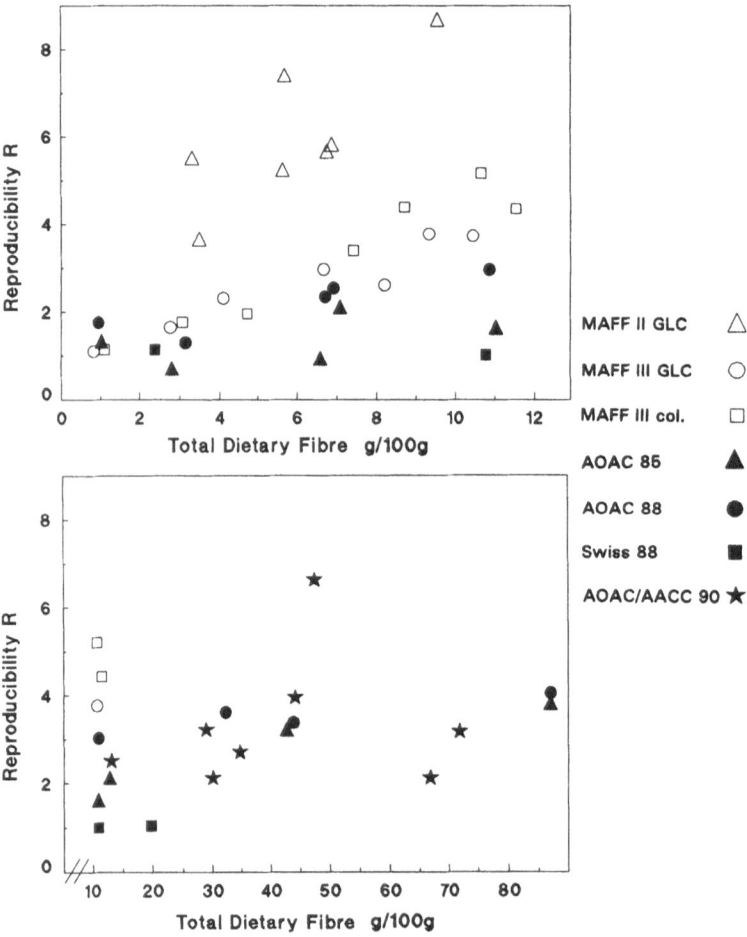

Fig. 4.6. Relation between total dietary fibre and reproducibility R from seven collaborative studies. The upper panel gives fibre contents between 0 and 12 g/100 g, the lower panel between 10 and 90 g/100 g. Study names are as in Table 4.5. Open symbols used for Englyst procedures, closed symbols for gravimetric methods.

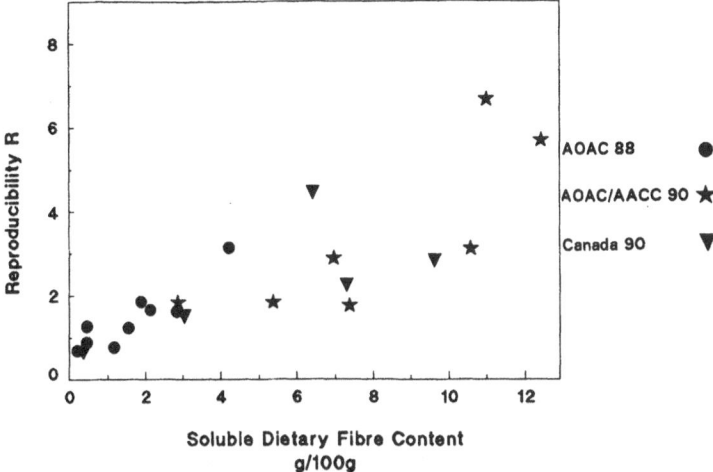

Fig. 4.7. Relation between soluble dietary fibre and reproducibility R from three collaborative studies with gravimetric methods. Study names are as in Table 4.5.

Total Dietary Fibre with Gravimetric Methods

The first inter-laboratory study with the AOAC method, AOAC 84 in Table 4.5 (Prosky et al., 1984), was the biggest collaborative effort reported up to now, but the results varied within wide limits, as revealed by both r_{95} and R_{95}. However, this initial trial allowed identification of the main problems of the procedure:

Too high a final phosphate concentration and hence variable ash contents of the gravimetric residues
Bad control of residual protein determination, as revealed by the soy isolate sample
Variable starch removal because of insufficient milling and too short an incubation time, as revealed by the rice sample.

After correction of these shortcomings, the second study (Prosky et al., 1985) resulted in much improved precision data and in more accurate values for the rice and soy isolate sample. The procedure has been accepted as official by the AOAC and several national bodies. Meanwhile, there was an increasing desire, especially in the USA, to measure IDF and SDF separately, even in routine and for food labelling. Therefore, a third trial was organised in which TDF was also measured and compared with the sum of IDF and SDF (Prosky et al., 1988). For this trial the initial phosphate buffer concentration was again increased to improve buffer capacity without, however, raising the final phosphate concentration. This AOAC 1988 trial gave slightly higher average r and R for TDF than AOAC 1985 (Table 4.5), probably due to the heavier workload involved, three times as many crucibles being handled in that study.

Using the same method as in the AOAC 1988 trial, a Swiss study (Schweizer et al., 1988) gave the best precision measures reached so far (Table 4.5). Three main factors may have contributed to this, namely the pre-trial sample with a target value for training, a more detailed description of the procedure and, third, the participating laboratories which were mostly government laboratories without experience in fibre analysis. Especially the two latter factors can be assumed to minimise the danger of free interpretations of a method description which of course would result in mediocre reproducibilities.

More recently two other studies with gravimetric procedures have become available. The trial called Canada 90 in Table 4.5 (Mongeau and Brassard, 1990) involving five samples and ten collaborators reached as good reproducibilities for rice (R = 0.62) and bread (R = 2.24) as the AOAC method, but somewhat poorer data for the other three samples. In any case it does not seem attractive to determine TDF as sum of NDF and SOL, i.e. two different procedures, when only TDF is needed.

The AOAC/AACC 90 trial used a modification of the official AOAC method (Lee et al., 1992). A Tris/Mes buffer is used instead of phosphate with the advantage of one pH adjustment less and of a slightly reduced alcohol consumption for precipitation of SDF. The precision measures reached with this method are similar as with the unmodified method (Fig. 4.6). However, only fibre contents above 10 g per 100 g have been included, so that the performance in the lower range of fibre contents remains to be seen.

Non-starch Polysaccharides (NSP) with the Englyst Procedures

The Englyst procedures have been collaboratively studied in four trials coordinated by the UK Ministry of Agriculture, Fisheries and Food (MAFF) of which three have now been published. The first study, MAFF I, compared five different methods and found considerable inter-laboratory variation with all methods, but only the Englyst procedure was selected for further study (Cummings et al., 1985). This study is not included in Table 4.5 because no common statistical treatment was made for the various methods under investigation.

In the MAFF II study (Englyst et al., 1987a) seven breads were analysed by the GLC procedure. The trial resulted in acceptable repeatabilities but unsatisfactory reproducibilities. The need for special expertise and equipment and the lack of experience were identified as underlying causes for this. One reason for the problems was later identified as the distribution of an incorrect column packing material for GLC (Englyst et al., 1987a).

In the MAFF III study (Englyst et al., 1987b) similar samples were analysed by a modified GLC procedure and two colorimetric procedures. However, only one of the colorimetric methods (Englyst and Hudson, 1987) would be applicable to all food types and is therefore included here. This study produced considerably improved R values, with only minor differences between GLC and colorimetry (Table 4.5). The trial was specifically concerned with the measurement of NSP in cereals with fibre contents below 12%. There was a considerable number of outliers and the need for further study was apparent, especially if these methods were to be advocated for routine use.

In the MAFF III study there was an average 15% difference between the average GLC and colorimetric results of a same sample with the colorimetric methods giving the higher results. It has been speculated (Schweizer, 1989, 1990) that this could be due to incomplete acid hydrolysis which would affect dietary fibre values from GLC methods more than from colorimetric methods. Interestingly, in the MAFF II study the mean results obtained by the GLC procedure for the sum of NSP and resistant starch were about 20% lower than TDF analysed by one laboratory with enzymatic–gravimetric methods (Englyst et al., 1987a). This could well mean that the two approaches agree better than thought by Englyst et al. (1987a), as also supported by inter-method comparisons. It would, however, also mean that the GLC method could not serve without modification as the reference method for the colorimetric procedure intended for quality control.

Separate Measurement of Insoluble and Soluble Dietary Fibre

Considerable interest in the distinct physiological effects of certain sources of soluble fibres have resulted, especially in North America, in a desire to validate collaboratively separate determinations of IDF and SDF. This has led to three collaborative studies which are summarised in Table 4.6. From the 10 samples in the AOAC 88 study (Prosky et al., 1988) four only had more than 10% of TDF as SDF and simultaneously more than 1.5% total dietary fibre. For three of these samples (oats, potatoes and rye bread) satisfactory results were obtained for both IDF and SDF. The fourth sample, a psyllium preparation, posed problems. All other samples had only insignificant amounts of SDF. However, because there was a good agreement in this study between the sum of IDF and SDF and of separately determined TDF, it was concluded that SDF could be measured by the difference (TDF−IDF) until further improvement in direct SDF measurement would be achieved.

In the meantime two other studies covering a broader range of SDF contents with normal foods were accomplished (Mongeau and Brassard, 1990; Lee et al., 1992). When comparing Figs. 4.5, 4.6 and 4.7 it seems that the precision of SDF measurement could almost reach the one of TDF. Fig. 4.7 also shows that the apparently disappointing RSD(R) precision data for SDF in the AOAC 88 trial may well have been due to sample choice only.

Before undertaking new collaborative studies on SDF it seems advisable to await further investigations focusing on improved and physiologically more sound separations between IDF and SDF (Schweizer, 1989, 1990). On the other hand, however, the pressure from consumers and legislators for having SDF values labelled cannot be ignored.

Inter-method Comparisons

Formal collaborative studies covering more than one method have been rare (Englyst et al., 1987b), but several studies have included analyses by at least one laboratory of the same samples with a different method (James and Theander,

1981; Prosky et al., 1984; Englyst et al., 1987a). Although such complementary data can give much valuable information concerning method accuracy, they do not contribute to objective judgement of precision data.

A recent preliminary study which was co-ordinated by the EC Bureau of Reference (P. Wagstaffe, personal communication) is therefore very timely, because it compared for the first time the method performance of the Englyst GLC and the AOAC method. Three reference materials (wheat flour, rye flour and haricot beans) were analysed in 10 laboratories by the AOAC method and in 5 laboratories by the GLC method. As Fig. 4.8 shows, the AOAC method gave clearly smaller intra- and inter-laboratory variability. Consequently, the TDF content in these samples will be certified according to results obtained with

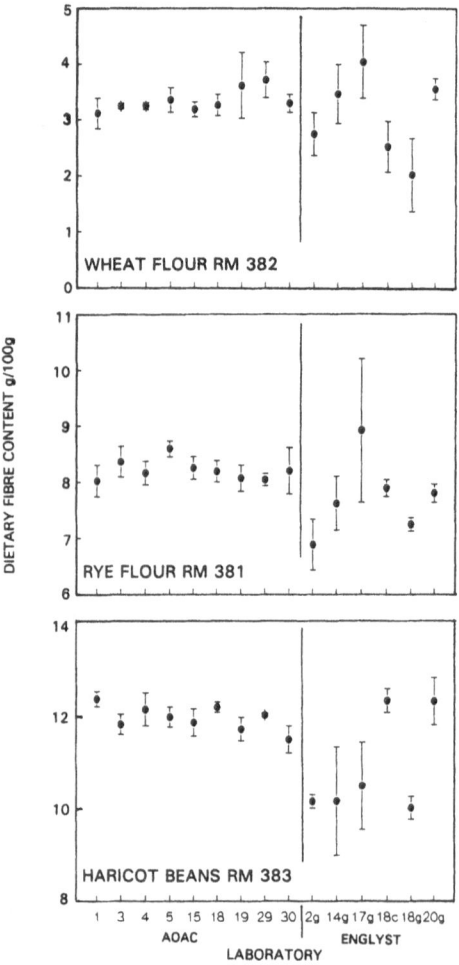

Fig. 4.8. Results of a European collaborative study of reference materials (Community Bureau of Reference, BCR). Laboratories 1–30 (left side) used the AOAC methods, 2–20 (right side) the Englyst methods (g = GLC; c = colorimetric). Bars denote 1 S.D.

the AOAC method. Indicative values will be given for the Englyst-type methods. Furthermore, Fig. 4.8 seems to reveal that the mean values for TDF and NSP are quite similar. This could indicate that for many foods the two parameters may not be as different as previously thought. In any case, the ranges of TDF and NSP values reported are clearly overlapping each other.

Summary and Conclusions

Methods for dietary fibre analysis have developed along two principally different lines:

1. Gravimetric methods in which the fibre is isolated and weighed
2. Component analysis methods in which dietary fibre constituents are determined more or less specifically

Both types of methods are needed for various purposes. Regarding wealth of details and need for laboratory equipment and skill, the gravimetric methods are comparable with Kjeldahl nitrogen for protein estimation or total fat determination, whereas the component analysis methods are comparable with amino acid or fatty acid determinations.

Gravimetric methods involve the risk of determining non-fibre constituents contaminating the fibre residue whereas component analysis methods based on specific determination of monomers require complete hydrolysis and predictable hydrolysis losses.

Most current methods use 78%–80% (v/v) ethanol for precipitation of water-soluble dietary fibre components and thus for delimitation of fibre polysaccharides from oligosaccharides and starch hydrolysis products. Usually this limit corresponds to about 10 monomeric units, but occasionally considerably larger polysaccharides may be soluble in 80% (v/v) ethanol. The delimitation between water-"soluble" and water-"insoluble" fibre is method-dependent and the physiologically most relevant delineation is not yet established.

With enzymatic–gravimetric methods, such as the method of Asp et al. and the AOAC method, both soluble and insoluble dietary fibre components can be recovered. Corrections for protein and ash associated with the fibre residue are applied. The AOAC method has been subject to a number of collaborative studies with results satisfactory enough for approval for total dietary fibre determination by the AOAC and several national bodies. More recently it was approved for insoluble fibre determination, which means that soluble fibre can be obtained as the difference between total and insoluble fibre. A modification has been approved also for direct soluble fibre determination.

Two main component analysis methods have been developed using GLC for neutral sugar determination: the Uppsala method by Theander et al. and the Englyst method by Englyst et al. In many respects recent developments have caused these methods to converge. The most important remaining differences regard:

1. Solubilisation of starch with DMSO in the Englyst method implying that a resistant starch fraction mainly consisting of retrograded amylose is included in

dietary fibre assayed with the Uppsala method – as in gravimetric methods – but not in the NSP assay with the Englyst method. Amyloglucosidase 16 hours (Uppsala) vs. pancreatin plus pullulanase 0.5 hours (Englyst) for starch hydrolysis after the initial Termamyl treatment.

2. Acid hydrolysis conditions (post-hydrolysis with 0.4 mol/l sulphuric acid 1 hour at 125 °C in the Uppsala method vs. 2 mol/l 1 hour at 100 °C in the Englyst method).

3. Inclusion of Klason lignin in the Uppsala method but not in the Englyst method.

4. Soluble fibre determination directly in the Uppsala method, but as the difference between total and insoluble fibre in the Englyst method.

The Englyst method has been tested in collaborative studies with gradually improved performance. A simplified version using a colorimetric determination of sugars in the acid hydrolysates has been developed and also tested collaboratively. An AOAC collaborative study with the Uppsala method is under way.

The limited data available for inter-method comparisons generally indicate a good agreement between total dietary fibre estimates of foods with gravimetric methods and with the Uppsala method. Lower values are obtained with the Englyst method in foods containing resistant starch and/or lignin. The range of estimates in different laboratories using the same method, however, is generally wider than differences of means obtained with different methods.

References

Albaum HG, Umbreit WW (1947) Differentiation between ribose-3-phosphate and ribose-5-phosphate by means of the orcinol-pentose reaction. J Food Sci 45:336–340

Anonymous (1982) Schweiz. Lebensmittelbuch, 2. Band, Kapitel 22, Methode 8.1. Eidg. Drucksachen und Materialzentrale, Bern

Anonymous (1983) Amtliche Sammlung 35 LMBG, Methode 00.00-7

Anonymous (1990) Official methods of analysis. AOAC, Arlington, VA, sec.973.18

Arrigoni E, Caprez A, Amadò R, Neukom H (1984) Gravimetric method for the determination of insoluble and soluble dietary fibres. Z Lebensm Unters Forsch 178:195–198

Asp N-G (1986) Enzymatic gravimetric methods: The suggested AOAC method and related techniques. In: Spiller G (ed) CRC handbook on dietary fiber in human nutrition. CRC Press, Boca Raton, pp 45–55

Asp N-G (1990) Delimitation problems in definition and analysis of dietary fiber. In: Furda I, Brine CJ (eds) New developments in dietary fiber. Plenum Press, New York, pp 227–236

Asp N-G, Johansson C-G (1981) Techniques for measuring dietary fiber. In: James WPT, Theander O (eds) The analysis of dietary fiber in food. Marcel Dekker, New York, pp 173–189

Asp N-G, Johansson C-G (1984) Dietary fibre analysis. Nutr Abstr Rev 54:735–752

Asp N-G, Johansson C-G, Hallmer H, Siljeström M (1983) Rapid enzymatic assay of insoluble and soluble dietary fiber. J Agric Food Chem 31:476–482

Berry CS, I'Anson K, Miles MJ, Morris VJ, Russel PL (1988) Physical-chemical characterization of resistant starch from wheat. J Cereal Sci 8:203–206

Bitter T, Muir HM (1962) A modified uronic acid carbazole reaction. Anal Biochem 4:330–334

Björck I, Nyman M, Pedersen B, Siljeström M, Asp N-G, Eggum B (1986) On the digestibility of starch in wheat bread. J Cereal Sci 4:1–11

Blumenkrantz N, Asboe-Hansen G (1973) New method for quantitative determination of uronic acids. Anal Biochem 54:484–489

Brillouet JM, Rouau X, Hoebler C, Barry JL, Carré B, Lorta EA (1988) A new method for determination of insoluble cell walls and soluble non-starchy polysaccharides from plant materials. J Agric Food Chem 36:969–979

British Nutrition Foundation (1990) Complex carbohydrates in foods. Chapman and Hall, London

Burkitt DP, Trowell HC (eds) (1975) Refined carbohydrate foods and disease. Some implications of dietary fibre. Academic Press, New York

Bylund M, Donetzhuber A (1968) Semimicro determination of uronic acids. Svensk Papperstidn 15:505–508

Connors KA, Pandit NK (1978) N-methyl-imidazole as a catalyst for analytical acetylations of hydroxy compounds. Anal Chem 50:1542–1545

Cummings JH, Englyst HN, Wood R (1985) Determination of dietary fibre in cereals and cereal products – collaborative trials. Part I: Initial trial. J Assoc Off Anal Chem 23:1–35

Dische Z (1955) New color reactions for determination of sugars in polysaccharides. In: Glick D (ed) Methods of biochemical analysis, vol II. Interscience, New York, pp 313–358

Durnin JVGA (1961) The availability of nutrients in diets containing differing quantities of unavailable carbohydrate: a study on young and elderly men and women. I. General description and proportionate losses of calories. Proc Nutr Soc 20:ii

Englyst HN (1981) Determination of carbohydrate and its composition in plant materials. In: James WPT, Theander O (eds) The analysis of dietary fiber. Marcel Dekker, New York, pp 71–93

Englyst HN (1985) Dietary polysaccharide breakdown in the gut of man. PhD thesis, University of Cambridge, UK

Englyst HN, Cummings JH (1984) Simplified method for the measurement of total non-starch polysaccharides by gas-liquid chromatography of constituent sugars as alditol acetates. Analyst 109:937–942

Englyst HN, Cummings JH (1985) Digestion of the polysaccharides of some cereal foods in the human small intestine. Am J Clin Nutr 42:778–787

Englyst HN, Cummings JH (1987) Digestion of polysaccharides of potato in small intestine of man. Am J Clin Nutr 45:423–431

Englyst HN, Cummings JH (1988) Improved method for measurement of dietary fiber as non-starch polysaccharides in plant foods. J Assoc Off Anal Chem 71:808–814

Englyst HN, Cummings JH (1990) Non-starch polysaccharides (dietary fiber) and resistant starch. In: Furda I, Brine CJ (eds) New developments of dietary fiber. Plenum Press, New York, pp 205–225

Englyst HN, Hudson G (1987) Colorimetric method for routine measurement of dietary fibre as non-starch polysaccharides. A comparison with gas-liquid chromatography. Food Chem 24:63–76

Englyst HN, Wiggins HS, Cummings JH (1982) Determination of the non-starch polysaccharides in plant foods by gas-liquid chromatography of constituent sugars as the alditol acetates. Analyst 107:307–318

Englyst HN, Cummings J, Wood R (1987a) Determination of dietary fibre in cereals and cereal products – Collaborative trials. II. Study of a modified Englyst procedure. J Assoc Publ Analysts 25:59–71

Englyst HN, Cummings JH, Wood R (1987b) Determination of dietary fibre in cereals and cereal products – collaborative trials. III. Study of further simplified procedures. J Assoc Publ Analysts 25:73–110

Frölich W, Schweizer TF, Asp N-G (1984) Minerals and phytate in the analysis of dietary fibre from cereals. II. Cereal Chem 61:357–359

Furda I (1977) Fractionation and examination of biopolymers from dietary fiber. Cereal Foods World 22:252–254

Furda I (1981) Simultaneous analysis of soluble and insoluble dietary fiber. In: James WPT, Theander O (eds) The analysis of dietary fiber in food. Marcel Dekker, New York, pp 163–172

Graham H, Grön Rydberg M-B, Åman P (1988) Extraction of soluble fiber. J Agric Food Chem 36:494–497

Greenberg CJ (1976) Studies on the fibre in human diets. PhD thesis. University of Cambridge, UK

Gruppen H, Hamer RJ, Voragen AGJ (1991) Barium hydroxide as a tool to extract pure arabinoxylans from water-insoluble cell wall material of wheat flour. J Cereal Sci 13:275–290

Hägglund E, Lindberg B, McPherson J (1956) Dimethylsulphoxide, a solvent for hemicellulose. Acta Chem Scand 10:1160–1164

Hämäläinen M, Theander O, Nordkvist E, Ternrud IE (1990) Multivariate calibration in the determination of acetylated aldoses by g.l.c. Carbohydr Res 207:167–175

Hellendoorn EW (1983) Fermentation as the principal cause of the physiological activity of indigestible food residue. In: Spiller GA (ed) Topics in dietary fiber research. Plenum Press, New York, pp 127–168

Hellendoorn EW, Noordhoff MG, Slagman J (1975) Enzymatic determination of the indigestible residue (dietary fibre) content of human food. J Sci Food Agric 26:1461–1468

Henneberg W, Stohmann F (1859) Ueber das Erhaltungsfutter volljährigen Rindviehs. J Landw 3:485–551

Hicks KB (1988) High-performance liquid chromatography of carbohydrates. Adv Carbohydr Chem Biochem 46:17–72

Hipsley EH (1953) "Dietary fibre" and pregnancy toxaemia. Br Med J ii:420–422

Hoebler C, Barry JL, David A, Delort-Laval J (1989) Rapid acid hydrolysis of plant cell wall polysaccharides and simplified quantitative determination of their neutral monosaccharides by gas-liquid chromatography. J Agric Food Chem 37:360–367

Honda S (1984) High-performance liquid chromatography of mono- and oligosaccharides. Anal Biochem 140:1–47

Horvath PJ, Robertson JB (1986) Detergent analysis of food. In: Spiller GA (ed) Handbook of dietary fiber in human nutrition. CRC Press, Boca Raton, pp 37–40

James WPT, Theander O (eds) (1981) The analysis of dietary fibre in food. Marcel Dekker, New York

Jeraci JL, Van Soest PJ (1990) Improved methods for analysis and biological characterization of fiber. In: Furda I, Brine CJ (eds) New developments in dietary fiber. Plenum Press, New York, pp 245–263

Jeraci JL, Lewis BA, Van Soest PJ, Robertson JB (1989) Urea enzymatic dialysis procedure for determination of total dietary fiber. J Assoc Off Anal Chem 72:677–681

Jeraci JL, Lewis BA, Robertson JB, Van Soest PJ (1990) Analysis of foodstuffs for dietary fiber by the urea enzymatic dialysis method. In: Furda I, Brine CJ (eds) New developments in dietary fiber. Plenum Press, New York, pp 311–320

Johansson C-G, Siljeström M, Asp N-G (1984) Dietary fibre in bread and corresponding flours – formation of resistant starch during baking. Z Lebensm Unters Forsch 179:24–28

Johnson DB, Moore WE, Zank LC (1961) The spectrophotometric determination of lignin in small wood samples. Tappi 44:793–796

Kobayashi T, Yoshino H, Mori B (1989) Determination of polydextrose. Nippon Nögeikagaku Kaishi 63:1611–1613

Kühl H (1936) Die Rohfaser und ihre Bestimmung Pharm. Zentralhalle 77:249–253

Lee SC, Hicks VA (1990) Modifications of the AOAC total dietary fiber method. In: Furda I, Brine CJ (eds) New developments in dietary fiber. Plenum Press, New York, pp 237–244

Lee S, Prosky L, DeVries J (1992) Determination of total, soluble and insoluble dietary fiber in foods: Collaborative study. J Assoc Off Anal Chem (in press)

Lee YC (1990) High-performance anion-exchange chromatography for carbohydrates analysis. Anal Biochem 189:151–162

Månsson P, Samuelsson B (1981) Quantitative determination of O-acetyl and other O-acryl groups in cellulosic material. Svensk Papperstidning 84:R15–R16, R24

Marlett JA, Chesters JG, Longaere MJ, Bodganske JJ (1989) Recovery of soluble dietary fiber is dependent on the method of analysis. Am J Clin Nutr 50:479–485

Maynard LA (1944) The Atwater system of calculating the caloric value of diets. J Nutr 28:443–452

McCance RA, Lawrence RD (1929) The carbohydrate content of foods. HMSO, London (Medical Research Council special report series no. 135)

McCance RA, Widdowson EM (1960) The composition of foods. HMSO, London (Medical Research Council special report series no. 297)

Meuser F, Suckow P, Kulikowski W (1983) Analytische Bestimmung von Ballaststoffen in Brot, Obst und Gemüse. Getreide, Mehl und Brot 37:380–383

Mongeau R, Brassard R (1986) A rapid method for the determination of soluble and insoluble dietary fiber: Comparison with AOAC total dietary fiber procedure and Englyst's method. J Food Sci 51: 1333–1336

Mongeau R, Brassard R (1990) Determination of insoluble, soluble, and total dietary fiber: Collaborative study of a rapid gravimetric method. Cereal Foods World 35:319–324

Morrison IM (1972) Improvements in the acetyl bromide technique to determine lignin and digestibility and its application to legumes. J Sci Food Agric 23:1463–1469

Neeser JR, Schweizer TF (1984) A quantitative determination by capillary gas-liquid chromatography of neutral and amino sugars (as O-methyloxime acetates) and a study on the hydrolytic conditions for glycoproteins and polysaccharides in order to increase sugar recoveries. Anal Biochem 142:58–67

Nishimune T, Sumimoto T, Yakusiji T et al. (1991) Determination of total dietary fiber in Japanese foods. J Assoc Off Anal Chem 74:350–359

Nyman M, Asp N-G (1985) Bulk laxatives. Their dietary fibre composition, degradation and faecal bulking capacity in the rat. Scand J Gastroenterol 20:887–895

Nyman M, Siljeström M, Pedersen B et al. (1984) Dietary fiber content and composition in six cereals at different extraction rates. Cereal Chem 61:14–19

Nyman M, Pålsson KE, Asp N-G (1987) Effects of processing on dietary fibre in vegetables. Lebensm Wiss Technol 20:29–36

Prosky L, Asp N-G, Furda I, DeVries JW, Schweizer T, Harland B (1984) Determination of total dietary fiber in foods, food products, and total diets: Inter-laboratory study. J Assoc Off Anal Chemists 67:1044–1052

Prosky L, Asp N-G, Furda I, DeVries JW, Schweizer TF, Harland B (1985) Determination of total dietary fiber in foods and food products: Collaborative study. J Assoc Off Anal Chem 68:677–679

Prosky L, Asp N-G, Schweizer TF, DeVries JW, Furda I (1988) Determination of insoluble, soluble and total dietary fiber in foods and food products: Inter-laboratory study. J Assoc Off Anal Chem 71:1017–1023

Remy E (1931) Experimentelle Studien zur Biochemie und Biologie der Rohfaser. Biochem Z 236: 1–18

Roe JH (1955) The determination of sugar in blood and spinal fluid with anthrone reagent. J Biol Chem 212:335–343

Robertson JB, Van Soest PJ (1981) The detergent system of analysis and its application to human foods. In: James WPT, Theander O (eds) The analysis of dietary fiber in food. Marcel Dekker, New York, pp 123–158

Saunders RM, Betschart AA (1980) The significance of protein as a component of dietary fiber. Am J Clin Nutr 33:960–961

Saura-Calixto F (1988) Effects of condensed tannins in the analysis of dietary fiber in carob pods. J Food Sci 53:1769–1771

Schaller DR (1976) Analysis of dietary fiber. Food Prod Dev 11(9): 70

Scharrer K, Kürschner K (1931) Ein neues, rasch durchführbares Verfahren zur Bestimmung der Rohfaser in Futtermitteln, Biedermanns Zentralblatt, B. Tierernährung 3:302–310

Schweizer TF (1989) Dietary fibre analysis. Lebensm Wiss Technol 22:54–59

Schweizer TF (1990) Dietary fiber analysis and nutrition labelling. In: Furda I, Brine CJ (eds) New developments in dietary fiber. Plenum Press, New York, pp 265–272

Schweizer T, Reimann S (1982) Beitrag zur Analytik von Stärkehydrolysaten. Z Lebensm Unters Forsch 174:23–28

Schweizer TF, Würsch P (1979) Analysis of dietary fibre. J Sci Food Agric 30:613–619

Schweizer TF, Würsch P (1981) Analysis of dietary fibre. In: James WPT, Theander O (eds) The analysis of dietary fiber in food. Marcel Dekker, New York, pp 203–216

Schweizer TF, Bekhechi AR, Koellreutter B, Reimann S, Pometta D, Bron BA (1983) Metabolic effects of dietary fiber from dehulled soybeans in humans. Am J Clin Nutr 38:1–11

Schweizer TF, Frölich W, Del Vedovo S, Besson R (1984) Minerals and phytate in the analysis of dietary fiber from cereals I. Cereal Chem 61:116–119

Schweizer TF, Walter E, Venetz P (1988) Collaborative study for the enzymatic, gravimetric determination of total dietary fibre in foods. Mitteilungen aus dem Gebiete der Lebensmitteluntersuchung und Hygiene 79:57–68

Schweizer TF, Andersson H, Langkilde AM, Reimann S, Torsdottir I (1990) Nutrients excreted in ileostomy effluents after consumption of mixed diets with beans or potatoes. II. Starch, dietary fibre and sugars. Eur J Clin Nutr 44:567–576

Scott RW (1979) Colorimetric determination of hexuronic acids in plant materials. Anal Chem 51:936–941

Selvendran RR (1984) The plant cell wall as a source of dietary fiber: chemistry and structure. Am J Clin Nutr 39:320–327

Selvendran RR, Du Pont MS (1984) Analysis of dietary fibre. In: King RD (ed) Developments in food analysis techniques. Applied Science, London, pp 1–68

Selvendran RR, Stevens BJH, Dupont MS (1987) Dietary fiber: chemistry, analysis and properties. Adv Food Res 31:117–209

Selvendran RR, Verne AVFV, Faulks RM (1989) Methods for analysis of dietary fibre. In: Lindskens HF, Jackson JF (eds) Plant fibers. Springer, Berlin, Heidelberg, New York, pp 234–259 (Modern methods of plant analysis. New series, vol 10)

Siegel SM (1968) The biochemistry of the plant cell wall. In: Florkin M, Stoz EH (eds) Comprehensive biochemistry, vol 26A, Elsevier, Amsterdam, pp 1–51

Sievert D, Pomeranz Y (1989) Enzyme resistant starch. I. Characterization and evaluation by enzymatic, thermoanalytical, and microscopic methods. Cereal Chem 66: 342–347

Sievert D, Czuchajowska Z, Pomeranz Y (1991) Enzyme resistant starch. III. X-Ray diffraction of autoclaved amylomaize VII starch and enzyme resistant starch residues. Cereal Chem 68:86–91

Siljeström M, Asp N-G (1985) Resistant starch formation during baking – effect of baking time and temperature and variations in the recipe. Z Lebensm Unters Forsch 181:4–8

Siljeström M, Westerlund E, Björck I, Holm J, Asp N-G, Theander O (1986) The effects of various thermal processes on dietary fibre and starch content of whole grain wheat and white flour. J Cereal Sci 4:315–323

Siljeström M, Eliasson AC, Björck I (1989) Characterization of resistant starch from autoclaved wheat starch. Starch/Staerke 41:147–151

Southgate DAT (1961) The availability of nutrients in diets containing differing quantities of unavailable carbohydrates: a study of young and elderly men and women. 2. Nitrogen, fat, carbohydrates and some inorganic constituents. Proc Nutr Soc 20:iii

Southgate DAT (1969a) Determination of carbohydrates in food. I. Available carbohydrates. J Sci Food Agric 20:326–330

Southgate DAT (1969b) Determination of carbohydrates in foods. II. Unavailable carbohydrates. J Sci Food Agric 20:331–335

Southgate DAT (1975) Fibre in human nutrition. Bibltheca Nutr Dieta 22:109–124

Southgate DAT (1976a) The chemistry of dietary fibre. In: Spiller GA, Amen RJ (eds) Fiber in human nutrition. Plenum Press, New York, pp 31–72

Southgate DAT (1976b) The analysis of dietary fibre. In: Spiller GA, Amen RJ (eds) Fiber in human nutrition. Plenum Press, New York, pp 73–107

Southgate DAT (1976c) Determination of food carbohydrates. Applied Science, London

Southgate DAT (1981) Use of the Southgate method for unavailable carbohydrates in the measurement of dietary fiber. In: James WPT, Theander O (eds) The analysis of dietary fiber in foods. Marcel Dekker, New York, pp 1–19

Southgate DAT (1987) Reference materials for improving the quality of nutritional data for foods. Fresenius Zeitschrift Analytische Chemie 26:660–664

Southgate DAT (1988) Dietary fibre and the diseases of affluence. In: Dobbing J (ed) A balanced diet? Springer, Berlin Heidelberg London, pp 117–139

Southgate DAT, Durnin JVGA (1970) Calorie conversion factors: and experimental reassessment of the factors used in calculation of the energy value of human diets. Br J Nutr 24:517–535

Southgate DAT, Englyst HN (1985) Dietary fibre: chemistry, physical properties and analysis. In: Trowell H, Burkitt D, Heaton K (eds) Dietary fibre, fibre-depleted foods and disease. Academic Press, London, pp 31–55

Southgate DAT, Hudson GJ, Englyst H (1978) The analysis of dietary fibre: the choices for the analyst. J Sci Food Agric 29:979–988

Stutzer A, Isbert A (1888) Untersuchungen über das Verhalten der in Nahrungs- und Futtermitteln enthaltenen Kohlenhydrate zu den Verdauungsfermenten. Z Physiol Chem 12:72–130

Ternrud IE, Lindberg JE, Theander O (1987) Continuous changes in straw carbohydrate digestion and composition along the gastrointestinal tract of ruminants. J Sci Food Agric 41:315–324

Theander O (1987) Chemistry of dietary fibre components. Scand J Gastroenterol 22(Suppl. 129):21–28

Theander O, Åman P (1979) Studies on dietary fibres. I. Analysis and chemical characterization of water-soluble and water-insoluble dietary fibres. Swed J Agric Res 9:97–106

Theander O, Åman P (1981) Analysis of dietary fibers and their main constituents. In: James WPT, Theander O (eds) The analysis of dietary fiber. Marcel Dekker, New York, pp 51–70

Theander O, Åman P (1982) Studies on dietary fibre. A method for the analysis and chemical characterisation of total dietary fibre. J Sci Food Agric 33:340–344

Theander O, James P (1979) European efforts in dietary fiber characterization. In: Inglett GE, Falkehag I (eds) Dietary fibers, chemistry and nutrition. Academic Press, New York, pp 245–249

Theander O, Westerlund E (1986a) Determination of individual components of dietary fiber. In: Spiller G (ed) CRC handbook of dietary fiber in human nutrition. CRC Press, Boca Raton, pp 57–75

Theander O, Westerlund E (1986b) Studies on dietary fiber 3. Improved procedures for analysis of dietary fiber. J Agric Food Chem 34:330–336

Theander O, Åman P, Miksche G-E, Yasuda S (1977) Carbohydrates, polyphenols and lignin in seed hulls of different colors from turnip rapeseed. J Agric Food Chem 25:270–273

Theander O, Åman P, Westerlund E, Graham H (1990) The Uppsala method for rapid analysis of total dietary fiber. In: Furda I, Brine CJ (eds) New developments in dietary fiber. Plenum Press, New York, pp 273–281

Thomas B (1972) Beiträge zur Nomenklatur und Analytik pflanzlicher Zellwandsubstanzen. Gertreide, Mehl und Brot 26:158–165, 168–169

Thomas B, Elchazly M (1976) Zur Problematik der Rohfaserbestimmung. Getreide, Mehl und Brot 30:252–255

Trowell H (1972) Ischemic heart disease and dietary fiber. Am J Clin Nutr 25:926–932

Trowell H (1988) Dietary fiber definitions. Am J Clin Nutr 48:1079–1080

Trowell HC, Southgate DAT, Wolever TMS, Leeds AR, Gassull MA, Jenkins DJA (1976) Dietary fibre redefined. Lancet i:967

Trowell H, Burkitt D, Heaton K (eds) (1985) Dietary fibre, fibre-depleted foods and disease. Academic Press, London

US Senate Select Committee on Nutrition and Human Needs (1977) Dietary goals for the United States. US Government Printing Office, Washington

Van Soest PJ (1963a) Use of detergents in the analysis of fibrous feeds. I. Preparation of fiber residues of low nitrogen content. J Assoc Offic Agric Chemists 46:825–829

Van Soest PJ (1963b) Use of detergents in the analysis of fibrous feeds. II. A rapid method for the determination of fiber and lignin. J Assoc Offic Agric Chemists 46:829–835

Van Soest PJ, Wine RH (1967) Use of detergents in the analysis of fibrous feeds. IV. Determination of plant cell wall constituents. J Assoc Off Anal Chem 50:50–55

Varo P, Laine R, Koivistoinen P (1983) Effect of heat treatment on dietary fiber: inter-laboratory study. J Assoc Off Anal Chem 66:933–938

Walker DM, Hepburn WR (1955) Normal-acid fibre: A proposed analysis for the evaluation of roughages. I. The analysis of roughages by the normal-acid fibre method and its use for predicting the digestibility of roughages by sheep. Agric Prog 30:118

Westerlund E, Theander O, Andersson R, Åman P (1989) Effects of baking on polysaccharides in white bread fractions. J Cereal Sci 10:149–156

Widdowson EM (1955) Assessment of the energy value of human foods. Proc Nutr Soc 14:142–145

Williams RD, Olmstedt W (1935) A biochemical method for determining indigestible residue (crude fibre) in faeces: lignin, cellulose, and non-water soluble hemicelluloses. J Biol Chem 108:653–666

Note Added in Proof

The MAFF IV Study

Results from the fourth collaborative study of the Ministry of Agriculture, Fisheries and Food, UK, the MAFF IV study, were released in preliminary form recently (MAFF Information Bulletin for Public Analysts on EC methods of analysis and sampling for foodstuffs, No. 117, Ministry of Agriculture, Fisheries and Food, Norwich, UK). This trial investigated soluble, insoluble and total non-starch polysaccharide determination (S-NSP, I-NSP and T-NSP, respectively) with the GLC and colorimetric varieties of the Englyst method and soluble, insoluble and total dietary fibre (SDF, IDF and TDF, respectively) with the AOAC method.

Comparison of mean and ranges of the NSP and fibre estimates shows that soluble components constitute a larger proportion of the total with both Englyst methods than with the AOAC method. As in the MAFF III study, the colorimetric Englyst method gave consistently higher NSP estimates than the GLC variety. TDF values with the AOAC method were generally higher than T-NSP estimates, that constituted on an average 88% and 83% of the TDF values for the colorimetric and GLC Englyst methods, respectively.

The preliminary statistical analysis of the MAFF IV study indicates similar between-laboratory reproducibility for soluble and insoluble components determined with the Englyst colorimetric method and the AOAC method, and somewhat better reproducibility for the Englyst GLC estimates. Reproducibility figures for T-NSP were similar to those reported in earlier studies with the Englyst method (Table 4.5). For TDF with the AOAC method, however, the reproducibility seemed less good than in earlier studies (Table 4.5). There are at least two probable explanations for this: (1) no kits or enzymes were distributed for the AOAC method, which was the case for the Englyst methods; and (2) TDF was obtained as the sum of SDF and IDF, which is not the approved procedure.

From the practical point of view, the MAFF IV study supports that for most food samples, the between-laboratory variation in TDF or NSP determinations is still larger than differences of means obtained with the AOAC or Englyst methods. This means that single estimates with the two methods are generally not significantly different.

The AOAC Method

The modified AOAC method of Lee et al. (1992) for soluble, insoluble and total dietary fibre obtained official first action status by the AOAC on 10 August 1991. Preliminary results from the latest collaborative study with the original AOAC method for insoluble, soluble and total dietary fibre (Prosky et al., 1988) indicate similar reproducibility figures to those obtained for the modified method of Lee et al. (AOAC/AACC 90; Tables 4.5 and 4.6; L. Prosky, personal communication).

Commentary

Morris: This is a very useful and balanced account of the progress that has been made in fibre analysis and the problems that remain. It is, of course, unfortunate that the original intention of including Dr. Englyst in the author list was not realised.

The reasoning behind the assertion that "classification in terms of physical characteristics is of limited value" is not convincing. I fully agree that the distinction between soluble and insoluble materials is not an absolute one, but depends on the nature of the solvent, which must therefore be clearly defined (and, of course, physiologically relevant). That, however, is a practical issue tractable to experimental investigation, not an insurmountable problem.

I also fully agree that polysaccharides with very different chemical structures can have similar physical properties (and, indeed, that polysaccharides of similar chemical composition can have very different physical properties). All that says, however, is that there is no simple relationship between composition and physical properties; it does not say that the former is more important than the latter. Some aspects of physiological response are clearly dependent on chemical structure: the obvious example is potential susceptibility to specific enzymes (although, even here, physical form may have a significant effect, as in resistant starch). Conversely, however, it may be argued that the physiological effects of dietary fibre as "roughage" and in retarding absorption are determined mainly by physical properties and that it is then the chemical characterisation that is of limited value.

The distinctions in Table 4.2 between "isolated polysaccharides", "natural occurring" and "food additives" seem strange. They are all "natural" (apart from chemically modified materials), and whether or not they are consumed in situ or extracted and added back depends on local technology and tradition. For example, the Japanese eat seaweed, whereas in the West algal polysaccharides are predominantly consumed as purified extracts.

Authors' reply: We agree that physical properties are at least as important as the chemical ones. Our remark on "limited value" only related to the extension of classifications of such properties at the present time.

Chapter 5

Gastro-intestinal Physiology and Function

N.W. Read and M.A. Eastwood

Introduction

The presence of non-starch polysaccharides in a meal may reduce postprandial sugar and lipid levels, reduce the bio-availability of micronutrients, assist weight reduction and increase stool output and the expulsion of gas from the colon. These effects can be explained by the physiological actions of non-starch polysaccharides, in particular their ability to displace nutrients from the diet, the dilution and sequestration of nutrients within the polysaccharide matrix, the imparting of viscous properties to gastro-intestinal contents and the provision of substrate for colonic fermentation.

Not all non-starch polysaccharides have the same effects or physiological actions. Guar gum, for example, reduces postprandial glycaemia, but has little effect on stool bulking. Other substances, such as wheat bran and cellulose may be better as laxative agents. The physiological action depends to a large extent on the physical and chemical properties of the individual non-starch polysaccharides, and these can vary quite considerably between different polymers or different molecular weights of the same polymer.

This chapter attempts to rationalise the effects of non-starch polysaccharides in health and disease by relating their physiological effects to their physical properties.

How Do Non-starch Polysaccharides Reduce Absorption of Nutrients in the Small Intestine?

How Does Increasing the Viscosity of Gastro-intestinal Contents Delay Absorption?

Most studies have concentrated on the relationship between viscous properties and absorption. Viscosity equals resistance to flow. In the gastro-intestinal tract, viscous solutions are anti-motility; they impair the propulsive and mixing effects of gastro-intestinal contractions (Blackburn et al., 1984a). When gastro-intestinal contents are rendered viscous by the incorporation of soluble non-starch polysaccharides, they trap complex food molecules within the matrix hindering their access to digestive enzymes and to the intestinal epithelium. Some polysaccharides can form gels rather than viscous solutions, especially when the concentration is increased. Gels are solid-like, but unlike viscous solutions, they can be irreversibly disrupted by the large shear forces that may occur in the mouth and in the stomach.

The anti-motility actions of viscous solutions can influence absorption by delaying gastric emptying, impairing convection or mixing in the upper small intestine, altering the absorptive site and delaying small bowel transit time.

Gastric Emptying

The addition of viscous polysaccharides to solutions of glucose delays gastric emptying, and may limit the absorption of glucose by slowing its delivery to the absorptive site in the small intestine. Several studies have shown an association between gastric emptying and postprandial blood levels of glucose or other rapidly absorbed materials (Holt et al., 1979; Schwartz and Levine, 1980), but is gastric emptying the major influence on absorption? In a study to elucidate the action of guar gum, we could find no correlation between the half-time for the emptying of glucose from the stomach and the degree of postprandial glycaemia (Blackburn et al., 1984a; Rainbird and Low, 1986). This suggested to us that the effects of viscosity in the small intestine may play a more dominant role.

Studies of the dynamics of gastric emptying have shown that the emptying of viscous solutions are associated with much higher antral pressures than the emptying of watery solutions (Bueno et al., 1981), but antral contractions indent the gastric lumen to a lesser extent during the emptying of viscous solutions (Prove and Ehrlein, 1982). These two sets of observations can be reconciled by proposing that viscous solutions resist the effect of antral contractions. The pressure recorded in the gastric lumen is a function of the power of the contraction and the resistance of the gastric contents to flow. Thus higher pressures are recorded in the presence of viscous solutions because they resist propulsion through the pylorus, and the same resistance would logically result in a reduction in antral indentation.

Viscous polysaccharides can have a different action on the gastric emptying of solids and liquids. The addition of guar gum to meals that consist of discrete solid and liquid components delays the emptying of liquids, but can accelerate the emptying of solid particles (Meyer et al., 1986). How can this come about?

Under normal circumstances, solids are retained in the fundus of the stomach until the majority of liquid has emptied. They then enter the antrum where they are disrupted by abrupt acceleration and deceleration forces produced by antral propulsion and pyloric closure until they are light enough to enter the axial stream and be propelled through the pylorus ahead of the advancing antral contraction (Meyer et al., 1986). Increasing the viscosity of gastric contents prevents the separation into discrete solid and liquid components. Solids are no longer retained in the fundus, and gravity does not cause them to settle out. Thus solids and liquids leave the stomach together in the viscous matrix. To put it another way, viscous polysaccharides "stabilise" the gastric contents, in an analogous manner to their action in stabilising emulsions in the preparation of ice creams.

The accelerated emptying of solids does not increase the absorption of the nutrients in the solids, if anything, it would inhibit it. This is because when gastric contents are viscous, solids are no longer disrupted by antropyloric contractions; they enter the duodenum in larger lumps (Meyer et al., 1986) and digestion is impaired by the reduction in surface area.

Reduction of Intestinal Mixing

Mixing of intestinal contents releases material trapped in the polysaccharide matrix, increases the interaction between digestive enzymes and the complex macromolecules in food and facilitates the access of the digestive products to the intestinal epithelium. Mixing is brought about by intestinal contractions. After a meal, the motor activity of the small intestine is changed to a pattern that consists of frequent brief contractions that are propagated for very short distances downstream. Radiological examination of intestinal contents gives the impression of chyme being milked for a few centimetres downstream and then flowing back to be milked by the next contraction. This type of activity would optimise mixing and reduce propulsion.

Viscous polysaccharides impair the digestion of starch in vitro, presumably by impairing the interaction with amylase (Isaksson et al., 1982; Dunaiff and Schneeman, 1981). Studies carried out in vivo have not necessarily demonstrated any impairment of digestion, perhaps because the reduced access of the products of digestion to the epithelium reduces the release of hormones that suppress pancreatic secretion (Scarpello et al., 1982; Isaksson et al., 1983b).

Perfusion of loops of small intestine of the rat or human in vivo with glucose solutions have shown that viscous polysaccharides reduce glucose absorption and the reduction in absorption is directly related to the viscosity of the solutions (Johnson and Gee, 1981; Elsenhans et al., 1981; Blackburn et al., 1984a). These experiments have been explained on the basis of an increase in the thickness of the unstirred water layer that lies immediately adjacent to the intestinal epithelium (Johnson and Gee, 1981). The concept of the unstirred water layer proposes that water becomes more structured and less mobile very close to solid–liquid interfaces as if the molecules line up in conformation to the solid surface. Thus in the small intestine, the unstirred layer is envisaged as a kind of water membrane across which substances have to diffuse before reaching the cell membrane. This unstirred layer is often measured by recording the time it takes the potential difference to change when the sodium in the lumen is rapidly changed to one of a different osmolality or sodium concentration (Read et al., 1977). The measurement relies on rapid changes of solution and clearly there are practical difficulties in achieving this in vivo when the solutions are viscous.

We believe that the unstirred water layer should be viewed more as a functional concept related to intestinal mixing than an anatomical entity with fixed dimensions. Vigorous stirring immediately adjacent to the epithelium, such as could be produced by contractions of the villi and microvilli, would minimise the influence of the unstirred layer on absorption. In contrast, if there were no forces causing mixing, then the unstirred layer would assume the dimensions of the intestinal lumen. Thus, by reducing mixing in the intestinal lumen, viscous polysaccharides would increase the dimensions of a less stirred layer. Our point is that reduction of mixing and increase of unstirred layer are two ways of describing the same thing. The only way in which the concepts might differ is if adherence of viscous polysaccharides to the epithelial surface caused persistence of an epithelial coating, which impaired the absorption of a subsequent meal which did not contain viscous polysaccharides. Histological evidence in the rat offers some support for this notion (Johnson and Gee, 1981).

Even if effects of viscous polysaccharides on the unstirred layer could be distinguished from effects on luminal mixing, they may not indicate a different mechanism. By measuring conductance of ionic solutions in the presence of viscous polysaccharides, Edwards and colleagues (1988) could find no evidence for any hindrance of ionic diffusion, whereas the mixing of two different solutions was markedly impaired if both were made viscous by the addition of guar gum. In a further experiment, they showed that viscosity inhibited the movement of glucose out of a tube of dialysis membrane that was sealed at either end only if the luminal contents were subjected to mixing by means of mechanical paddles. Phillips (1986), however, has suggested that viscous polysaccharides could delay the diffusion of larger molecular complexes of micelles to the absorptive surface.

Effects on Intestinal Transit and Absorptive Site

In general, the addition of viscous polysaccharides to liquid meals delays mouth to caecum transit time of the head of a meal. This effect is only partly explained by the delay in gastric emptying; there is evidence for an additional delay in small bowel transit (Bueno et al., 1981; Blackburn et al., 1984a; Brown et al., 1988). The delay in small bowel propulsion made us consider the possibility that viscous polysaccharides could reduce glucose absorption by confining the glucose solution to a smaller area of small intestine instead of allowing it to spread down the small intestine and be exposed to larger absorptive surface. Scintigraphic imaging of the small intestinal contents did not support this possibility (Blackburn et al., 1984b). Moreover, studies in rats gavaged with baked beans and different concentrations of guar gum (Brown et al., 1988) showed that the delay in small bowel transit was associated with hold up of the meal at two sites, the stomach and the terminal ileum. Transit through the proximal small intestine was very rapid probably because the viscosity was reduced at that site by dilution with digestive juices, and delayed in the ileum after much of the fluid had been reabsorbed.

Does this mean that the site of absorption is shifted downstream in the presence of viscous polysaccharides? One study has addressed this question and showed that after administration of a meal containing viscous polysaccharides to rats, more fat was absorbed from the ileum (Imaizumi et al., 1982). Since nutrients have a trophic effect on the small intestine, a downward shift in the site of absorption would explain the observations that the ileal epithelium tends to hypertrophy after chronic administration of guar gum (Imaizumi and Sugaro, 1986). We have suggested that a greater exposure of the ileum to fat could explain the second meal phenomenon, in which administration of viscous polysaccharides does not only reduce the postprandial glycaemia of the test meal but also the meal afterwards. The reason for this is that the presence of a significant amount of fat in the ileum, such as might occur at the time of the second meal, can cause substantial suppression of the motility of the stomach and proximal intestine and also induce sensations of satiety to occur with ingestion of smaller amounts of food (Read et al., 1984).

Do Viscous Polysaccharides Affect the Degree of Absorption?

The important question regarding the action of viscous polysaccharides in the small intestine is: does this lead to any change in the degree of absorption of nutrients from a meal? Higham and Read (1992) attempted an answer by incorporating guar gum into the diet of patients with ileostomies fashioned from the terminal few centimetres of ileum. Guar gum was administered with every meal for a period of seven days and care was taken to keep the nutrient intake constant. The results showed that the volume of ileostomy effluent was increased by ingestion of guar gum and increased amounts of fat and protein, water and electrolytes. Carbohydrate output was not significantly influenced by addition of guar gum. Surprisingly, mouth to caecum transit time was unchanged under the conditions of these experiments and the viscosity of the ileal effluent was not increased, but was lower than the control studies in which guar was not given. Patients reported that their ileal effluent was much more runny during ingestion of guar gum. These unexpected results could be explained by dilution caused by, for example, increased pancreatic secretions. An alternative explanation is the degradation of the polysaccharide by contaminant bacteria in the ileum, though the absence of an increase in breath hydrogen response to the meal did not support this possibility. Similar effects on protein and fat excretion from the ileum have been observed in the rat (Isaksson et al., 1983a).

Unresolved Issues

Can the Effect of Supplementing the Diet with Non-starch Polysaccharides on Gastro-intestinal Viscosity be Predicted from Measurements of Viscosity in Vitro?

The answer to this question is either, "No" or "Not necessarily". There are several reasons for this.

1. Dilution with digestive juices can produce marked reductions in viscosity and this effect can be much greater with some polysaccharides than with others (Morris, 1986; Edwards et al., 1987). This effect has been confirmed using pigs fitted with intestinal cannulae, in which direct measurements of duodenal viscosity have been carried out in response to dietary supplementation with samples of guar gum of differing molecular sizes and physical properties (F.G. Roberts, unpublished data).

2. Different sources of the same polysaccharide can show great variation in their physical properties in solution and this is directly related to their molecular weights (Morris, 1986; Ellis et al., 1986).

3. Non-starch polysaccharides form non-Newtonian solutions. That is to say that their viscosity varies according to the force or shear rate to which they are subjected. Agitation or stirring at rapid rates causes a relative reduction in viscosity as the polysaccharide chains disentangle and the rate of disentanglement exceeds the rate of re-entanglement. This phenomenon is known as shear-thinning. Thus in order to predict the effect of a polysaccharide in the gut, it is necessary to know the forces to which that solution is subjected by gastro-intestinal contraction and the geometry of the system (see Chap. 3).

Morris has shown that for a given polysaccharide, there is a linear relationship between viscosity and the product of viscosity with a fixed power of the shear rate and this slope and intercept of this relationship varies with different polysaccharides (Morris, 1990). This not only provides a means of describing the behaviour of a polysaccharide over the whole range of shear conditions, but it may also provide the possibility of deriving a value for the predominant shear conditions that may exist in the intestine by comparing the relative effects of two or more polysaccharides that differ widely in the slopes of their viscosity/shear rate relationship. Although theoretically possible, this approach would require a knowledge of the concentration of the polysaccharide in the operationally dominant region of the gut.

4. Another consideration is the difficulty in measuring the viscosity of gastro-intestinal contents – or what to do with the lumps? As anybody who has examined the composition of vomitus knows, gastric contents are not homogeneous; the solids, liquids and the oils separate out and there is often an unusually high proportion of tomato skins, pieces of carrot and maize husks. Since the stomach functions as a blender or homogeniser, the material that enters the small intestine is much more homogeneous, but lumps can still be present, particularly after administration of viscous polysaccharides.

Most methods that are currently used to measure viscosity require samples to be small and reasonably homogeneous. Lumps can produce considerable distortion, but removal of the lumps by sieving could also produce an unacceptable bias in the data, since the lumps must exert a major influence on rheological behaviour. There is, we believe, a need to develop and validate a method for measuring the rheological properties of gastro-intestinal contents, "lumps and all". Perhaps the answer is to use sufficiently large viscometers.

How Can the Rheological Properties of Whole Foods be Studied?

The development of an acceptable method for measuring the viscosity of gastro-intestinal contents would also facilitate measurements of the rheological properties of whole foods and their fate in the gut. There is very little insight into the effects on rheology in vitro and in the gut of different food combinations, such as proteins and polysaccharides, starch and non-starch polysaccharides, carbohydrate and fat in pastries or cakes and the availability of nutrients from these combinations. Starch granules are intimately associated with a protein matrix that may impair digestion. The glycaemic response to gluten-free flour is greater than to gluten containing flour indicating more complete absorption of carbohydrate (Jenkins et al., 1987).

Most of our food is subjected to physical forces, such as heat, pressure, microwaving, and cold before we eat it. We need more insight into the effects of food preparation on rheological properties of digesta. Recent studies in the pig have shown that incorporating guar gum into bread still causes an increase in the viscosity of intestinal contents and a reduction in postprandial glucose concentrations (Roberts et al., 1990).

What is the Effect of Long-term Supplementation with Viscous Polysaccharides?

There is evidence that the ileal epithelium hypertrophies in response to chronic ingestion of viscous polysaccharides and as suggested above, this may be related to a change in the site of absorption. Is there any evidence for functional or physiological adaptation?

Chronic ingestion of vegetarian or high-fibre diets may sensitise the gastro-intestinal chemoreceptors that control gastro-intestinal transit and eating behaviour to the action of nutrients. We have previously observed that the infusion of lipids into the duodenum produced a much more marked inhibition of gastric emptying in vegetarians than in subjects on a normal mixed diet. Furthermore the gastric emptying of a high fat meal became much slower after two weeks habituation of normal volunteers to a low fat diet (Cunningham et al., 1991). By diluting intestinal contents and impairing the access of nutrients to the intestinal epithelium, there is a possibility that non-starch polysaccharides could sensitise nutrient receptors. This could produce an adaptive inhibition of food intake, gastric emptying and intestinal transit from foods of higher nutrient density.

Can Non-starch Polysaccharides Reduce Absorption by Mechanisms Other than Increasing the Viscosity of Gastro-intestinal Contents?

Displacement of Nutrients?

Not all the non-starch polysaccharides that may reduce postprandial glycaemia or cholesterolaemia produce viscous solutions. Diets high in beans or wheat bran or beet fibre can be very helpful, but this could have more to do with what is displaced from the diet than what is added (for references, see Chap. 16). We designed a study to ask the question, "Does the addition of either soluble or insoluble fibre to a sensible diabetic diet confer any special benefit in terms of diabetic control?". Type II diabetic patients were randomised to one of three diets, a sensible high carbohydrate, low fat diet with minimal fibre, and the same diet supplemented with 15g guar gum or wheat bran (Beattie et al., 1988). Care was taken to ensure that the nutrient intake was kept constant with all three diets. At the end of 20 weeks, the patients on all three diets had similar reductions in fasting plasma glucose and glycosylated haemoglobin and had lost equivalent amounts of weight. Our conclusion was that the long-term supplementation of normal diets with high-fibre foods improved diabetic control because it worked as a device to assist patients to achieve a more healthy diet. This conclusion is in the spirit of the British Diabetic Association, which recommends a diet rich in complex polysaccharide and low in fat without specifying whether the carbohydrate be available or not.

Sequestration

In plants, polysaccharides either form part of the skeleton or they are an energy store or they are secreted as gums or mucilages for protection against microorganisms. Many of the storage or skeletal forms may be sequestered inside rigid waxy or lignified cell walls, which need to be broken open by milling, grinding or chewing before the carbohydrate is released (O'Dea et al., 1980; Southgate, 1986). The important function of chewing in releasing starch for digestion was emphasised by a study that compared the low postprandial plasma glucose levels when meals of apple, potato, maize and rice were served in large particles and not chewed compared with the marked postprandial glycaemia when these foods were chewed thoroughly (Read et al., 1986). The importance of sequestration or particle size is also implicit in the much higher plasma insulin responses to apple juice compared with whole apples (Haber et al., 1977), and in the plasma insulin and glucose responses to isocaloric wheat-based meals that varied according to the degree of milling of the wheat (Jenkins et al., 1986; Heaton et al., 1988; O'Donnell et al., 1989). All of these studies showed that the smaller the particles, the greater the metabolic responses (Heaton et al., 1988).

Jenkins has popularised the glycaemic index, the ratio of the glycaemic response to 50 g of test carbohydrate to the glycaemic response to 50 g glucose as a means of measuring the metabolic responses of a variety of carbohydrate foods (Jenkins et al., 1981). Bread and potatoes have a high glycaemic index whereas legumes have low glycaemic indices. The implication is that it is more healthy for diabetics and even healthy people to eat foods of low glycaemic indices because this avoids the harmful effects of high plasma glucose and high insulin secretion. This theory breaks down in the context of mixed meals, when other components of the meal may influence the way in which carbohydrate is digested. For example, putting a lump of butter on a potato is a very effective way to reduce the glycaemic index, probably because the fat interacts with duodenal receptors to delay the delivery of the carbohydrate from the stomach and hence limit digestion (Cunningham and Read, 1989).

Food Preparation

Cooking as well as chewing releases polysaccharides and may be necessary for the rapid development of viscous properties. Heating in the presence of water bursts open starch grains; the glycaemic responses to uncooked potato or wheat starch are minimal (Collings et al., 1981). It is likely that some non-starch polysaccharides require heat treatment before they are released from the cell wall. Pectins in uncooked vegetables show much less adhesion and are much more soluble in intestinal fluids than those in uncooked vegetables (Selvendran, 1985). Cooking may also reduce the availability of starch. Englyst and

Cummings (1987) have shown that the cooking, cooling and reheating of starch foods can result in the production of a form of retrograded starch that is resistant to digestion by pancreatic amylase.

The current enthusiasm for high-fibre diets and eating vegetables in their raw state may mean that large amounts of polysaccharide remain sequestered within rigid cell walls and are not released into the intestinal lumen. Under these conditions, the fibre influences gastro-intestinal physiology by displacing or diluting nutrients or by acting as a non-specific "irritant" (see later).

Cooking or other forms of preparation of plant foods often denatures the natural toxins. It is possible that some of the effects attributed to "fibre" in uncooked vegetables and fruits could be signs of intoxication.

Fermentation

When non-starch polysaccharides reach the colon, they are fermented by the vast numbers of anaerobic bacteria to release short chain or volatile fatty acids, predominantly acetic acid, butyric acid and propionic acid with smaller concentrations of lactic acid and branched chain acids. It has been suggested that propionic acid reduces postprandial glycaemia by actions on hepatic metabolism (Jenkins, 1979; see also Chaps. 7 and 10). This factor may be crucial to the long-term effects of fibre in diabetic control. Propionic acid also reduces cholesterol synthesis in isolated rat hepatocytes (Chen et al., 1984), but this observation appears not to be relevant to the reduction in plasma cholesterol by viscous polysaccharides in vivo (see Chap. 17).

Villous Atrophy

Although diets rich in non-starch polysaccharides can be associated with a relative hypertrophy of the epithelium of the distal intestine, the major absorptive site in the proximal small intestine often shows atrophic changes. Villi are stunted, disaccharidase production is reduced, and there are compensatory increases in crypt cell production rate and cell turnover (Johnson and Gee, 1986; Roberts, 1991). These features are similar to those found in coeliac disease and therefore suggest epithelial toxicity. By the use of specific lectins to stain for specific sugar residues, Roberts (1991) has shown intense galactose and mannose staining in the small intestinal glycocalyx and even in the lymphatics, suggesting incorporation of the polysaccharide into the epithelium. The intriguing question from these observations is: "Does dietary fibre damage the epithelium?".

Binding of Bile Acids

One of the most popular theories for the hypocholesteraemic action of fibre is that it may sequester and even chemically bind bile acids. This may then limit fat absorption by bile acid depletion and impaired micellisation (see Chap. 17). Bile acids bind with phenolic and uronic residues on the polysaccharide matrix, particularly when the pH in the intestinal lumen is low (Eastwood and Hamilton, 1968).

Effects on the Colon

The addition of non-starch polysaccharides to the diet can increase stool output, accelerate colonic transit time and increase the expulsion of colonic gases. Not all polysaccharides produce all of these effects; some have little effect on any of them, others produce some effects but not others, and the effects may vary with time. In other words, the colon appears to be able to adapt to the continued presence of a non-starch polysaccharide by varying its function.

The physical properties of polysaccharides may change significantly in the colon. Some are immediately fermented and removed from the lumen. Others may be chemically modified by the bacteria in a way that changes their physical properties; very little is known about the impact of bacterial metabolism on these plant materials. The more acidic colonic environment will reduce the ionisation of uronic and phenolic acid radicals present on some polysaccharides and on lignin, increasing the binding of bile acids and reducing the binding of minerals. The bacterial mass itself will be altered by the presence of polysaccharides; fermentable substrates will increase bacterial numbers and alter types of bacteria present and it is probable that some of the properties, such as cation exchange, acceleration of transit time and stool bulking, may in fact be properties of the bacterial cell mass.

Increased Stool Output

The increased stool output is most commonly thought to be related to the water-holding capacity of the polysaccharide, but it is not the water-holding capacity of the polysaccharide as ingested that is most important; studies have shown that substances with the highest water-holding capacity in vitro, such as guar gum or pectin, are often the poorest laxatives (Eastwood et al., 1983). The key factor is the water-holding capacity after exposure to colonic bacteria (McBurney et al., 1985; Adiotomre et al., 1990). Many non-starch polysaccharides are rapidly broken down by colonic bacteria to small molecular weight units that have no ability to sequester or retain water. These have little laxative action. The substances that appear to have the greatest effects on stool weight are the polysaccharides such as carboxymethylcellulose, xanthan gum, ispaghula that resist breakdown or wheat bran which contains highly lignified material which is virtually non-biodegradable in the human colon. The water-holding capacity of bran even before exposure to colonic bacteria is very low. Is the bulk of the bran itself without any associated water sufficient to increase stool output or does its laxative action depend on another mechanism? And how does cooking wheat bran to form Kellogg's All-Bran yield a product that is a less effective stool bulker than whole bran (Wyman et al., 1976)?

Transit Time

The inverse relationship between stool weight and whole gut transit time implies a causal relationship; either the increase in colonic bulk stimulates propulsion or the acceleration of colonic transit reduces the contact time for absorption. Supplementing the diet with non-starch polysaccharides does not support a causal relationship because this often stimulates colonic propulsion without affecting stool bulk or increases stool output without affecting transit time (Tomlin and Read, 1988a). By examining the effects of a number of non-starch polysaccharides, Tomlin and Read (1988b) have proposed that non-starch polysaccharides that retain at least some of their complex structure retain water and increase stool bulk while fermentation of non-starch polysaccharides is associated with an acceleration of transit time. They have further suggested that the best laxatives are those that undergo some fermentation but retain sufficient of their complex structure to retain fluid and bulk the stool.

If fermentation is associated with acceleration of transit time, which of the fermentation products are responsible? The strongest candidates would appear to be short chain fatty acids, but current data from our laboratory (unpublished data) suggest that in the concentration range normally found in the colonic lumen, acetic acid, propionic acid and butyric acid and a cocktail of all three acids inhibit colonic motility. The effect of luminal lactic acid on colonic motility has not been investigated. The other fermentation products are the gases. Perhaps gaseous distension of the caecum induces colonic propulsion. Certainly there is evidence that fluid distension of the right colon causes regular propulsive colonic pressure waves (Chauve et al., 1986).

Laxative Action of Sequestered Bile Acids and Fatty Acids

Laxatives stimulate colonic secretion and colonic propulsion and it seems likely that they act on mucosal receptors to stimulate a neural programme for colonic clearance. It is possible that fibre may have the same effect. Wheat bran binds bile acids causing increased delivery into the colon and bile acids have been termed nature's laxative because they stimulate colonic propulsion and secretion (Read, 1988). Small concentrations of bile acids also increase rectal sensitivity, lowering the distension threshold required to cause a desire to defecate (Edwards et al., 1989). Similarly the ingestion of non-starch polysaccharides may cause impaired absorption of long chain fatty acids and bile acids in the small intestine and increased delivery to the colon. Long chain fatty acids also induce colonic propulsion and secretion (Read, 1988).

Direct Irritant Effect of Particles

It is well known that coarse particles of bran have a greater laxative action than the same amount of bran that has been ground up into much finer particles (Brodribb and Groves, 1978; Heller et al., 1980; Smith et al., 1981). This result has been explained simply on the basis of the greater water retention within the fibre matrix of the larger particles, but water-holding capacity of bran is less impressive than other "fibres".

Tomlin and Read (1988b) have suggested an alternative mechanism: the edges of large particles may induce secretion and propulsive motor activity in the colon by stimulating mucosal mechano-receptors. This mechanism was proposed as a result of observations that pieces of polyvinyl tubing cut up to the same dimensions as coarse bran particles increased stool output, accelerated transit time and made the stool consistency more watery. Polyvinyl has negligible water-holding capacity and yet the effects of plastic fibre were indistinguishable from coarse wheat bran. As there were no plasticisers present these chemicals could not have leaked out to induce a chemical laxation. Other studies have demonstrated similar laxative properties after administration of polystyrene particles to dogs (Cherbut and Ruckebusch, 1985).

Gas Formation

Fermentation of unabsorbed carbohydrate in the colon produces short chain or volatile fatty acids and gases, carbon dioxide, hydrogen and methane. Hydrogen and methane cannot be produced by mammalian cells and are an important means of disposal of the hydrogen ions produced during bacterial fermentation (Bond and Levitt, 1978).

It is likely that several litres of gas are produced in the colon every day. Most of this gas is absorbed across the colonic epithelium and excreted in the breath, but between about half a litre and 2 litres can be evacuated as flatus (Tomlin et al., 1991). The ingestion of an elemental diet containing no polysaccharides reduces flatus production to about 200 ml, whereas it is well established that the administration of non-starch polysaccharides increases flatus production (Calloway and Burroughs, 1969). The relationship between the entry of carbohydrate into the colon and gas production is unlikely to be a simple one. It depends on the source of carbohydrate; not all carbohydrates can be fermented in the colon and different carbohydrates may be fermented in different ways yielding different amounts of products (Eastwood et al., 1986). It is misleading to use breath hydrogen excretion after administration of a non-absorbable carbohydrate such as lactulose to test the degree of absorption of another carbohydrate such as starch (Levitt and Donaldson, 1970). Different carbohydrates are fermented by different strains of bacteria. Fermentation characteristics are, after all, the current basis of bacterial taxonomy. The rate of delivery of carbohydrate also influences gas production. Some bacteria can utilise hydrogen and there is a balance between hydrogen production and hydrogen utilisation. Slowing the delivery of substrate may reduce hydrogen production to such an extent that it is barely detectable (Read et al., 1985).

Not all the population can produce methane, but those that do tend to live in the same communities (Tadesse et al., 1980; McKay et al., 1985). Among animal species, methane tends to be produced by herbivores and not by carnivores (McKay and Eastwood, 1984). Gibson et al. (1990) have suggested that methane production only occurs in the absence of sulphate-reducing bacteria.

How Does the Colon Adapt to Fibre?

"It worked for the first week, then I started to get bunged up again and I haven't been since." How many times have constipated patients said that to their doctors after they have been prescribed non-starch polysaccharides such as ispaghula? Why should the colon adapt to the fibre? It seems likely that it is the colonic bacteria that have modified their function. There is certainly evidence that colonic bacteria may acquire the ability to break down a polysaccharide after exposure. Xanthan gum is very poorly broken down by colonic bacteria, but after feeding normal volunteers xanthan for a week, most of them had acquired the ability to degrade xanthan in the colon (J. Daly, J. Tomlin, N. W. Read, unpublished data).

"Just keep taking the medicine and the discomfort will go away." Is this just wishful thinking on the part of the doctor or is there any evidence that gas production and distension will diminish as patients continue to take ispaghula for their constipation? After a few days the volume of hydrogen expelled by fermentation of lactulose decreases (McLean Ross et al., 1983; Florent et al., 1985). The phenomenon of long-term adaptation to the ingestion of complex polysaccharides requires much more study.

References

Adiotomre J, Eastwood MA, Edwards CA, Brydon WG (1990) Dietary fibre: in vitro methods that anticipate nutrition and metabolic activity in humans. Am J Clin Nutr 52:123–134

Beattie VA, Edwards CA, Hosker JP et al. (1988) Comparison of guar gum, a fibre rich diet and a low fat sugar diet in the management of newly diagnosed Type 2 diabetes. Br Med J 296:1147–1149

Blackburn NA, Redfern JS, Jarjis M et al. (1984a) The mechanism of action of guar gum in improving glucose tolerance in man. Clin Sci 66:329–336

Blackburn NA, Holgate AM, Read NW (1984b) Does guar gum improve postprandial hyperglycaemia in humans by reducing small intestinal contact area? Br J Nutr 52:197–204

Bond JH, Levitt MD (1978) Effect of dietary fibre on intestinal gas production and small bowel transit time in man. Am J Clin 31:S169–S174

Brodribb AJM, Groves C (1978) Effect of bran particle size in stool weight. Gut 19:60–63

Brown NJ, Worlding J, Rumsey RDE, Read NW (1988) The effect of guar gum on the distribution of a radiolabelled meal in the gastrointestinal tract of the rat. Br J Nutr 59:223–231

Bueno L, Praddaude F, Fioramonti J, Ruckebusch Y (1981) Effect of dietary fibre on gastrointestinal motility and jejunal transit time. Gastroenterology 80:701–707

Calloway DH, Burroughs SE (1969) Effect of dried beans and silicone on intestinal hydrogen and methane production in man. Gut 10:180–184

Chauve A, Devroede G, Bastin E (1986) Intraluminal pressure during perfusion of the human colon in situ. Gastroenterology 70:336–345

Chen W-J, Anderson JW, Jennings D (1984) Propionate may mediate the hypocholesterolemic effects of certain soluble plant fibres in cholesterol fed rats. Proc Soc Exp Biol Med 175:215–218

Cherbut C, Ruckebusch Y (1985) The effect of indigestible particles on digestive transit time and colonic motility in dogs and pigs. Br J Nutr 53:549–557

Collings P, Williams C, MacDonald I (1981) Effect of cooking on serum glucose and insulin responses to starch. Br Med J 282:1032

Cunningham K, Read NW (1989) Effect of incorporating lipid in different compounds of a standard meal on gastric emptying and postprandial plasma glucose and insulin levels. Br J Nutr 61:285–290

Cunningham KM, Daly J, Horowitz M, Read NW (1991) Gastrointestinal adaptation to diets of differing fat composition in human volunteers. Gut 32:483–486

Dunaiff G, Schneeman BO (1981) The effect of dietary fibre on human pancreatic enzyme activity in vitro. Am J Clin Nutr 34:1034–1035

Eastwood MA, Hamilton D (1968) Fatty acids in the lumen of the small intestine of man following a lipid containing meal. Scand J Gastroenterol 5:225–230

Eastwood MA, Robertson JA, Brydon WG, Macdonald D (1983) Measurement of water-holding properties of fibre and their faecal bulking ability in man. Br J Nutr 50:539–547

Eastwood MA, Brydon WG, Anderson DMW (1986) The effect of the polysaccharide composition and structure of dietary fibres on caecal fermentation and faecal excretion. Am J Clin Nutr 44:51–55

Edwards CA, Blackburn NA, Craigen L et al. (1987) Viscosity of food gums determined in vitro related to their hypoglycaemic actions. Am J Clin Nutr 46:72–77

Edwards CA, Johnson IT, Read NW (1988) Do viscous polysaccharides slow absorption by inhibition diffusion or convection? Eur J Clin Nutr 42:307–312

Edwards CA, Baxter J, Brown S, Bannister JJ, Read NW (1989) Effect of bile acids on anorectal functions in humans. Gut 30:383–386

Ellis PR, Morris ER, Low AG (1986) Guar gum: the importance of reporting data on its physicochemical properties. Diabetic Med 3:490–491

Elsenhans B, Zenker D, Caspary WF (1981) Long-term feeding of unavailable carbohydrate gelling agents. Influence of dietary concentration and microbial degradation on adaptive responses in the rat. Am J Clin Nutr 34:1836–1844

Englyst HN, Cummings JH (1987) Resistant starch, a 'new' food component: a classification of starch for nutritional purposes. In: Morton ID (ed) Cereals in a European context. Ellis Horwood, Chichester, pp 221–233

Florent C, Florie B, Lebland A et al. (1985) Influence of chronic lactulose ingestion on the colonic metabolism of lactulose in man (an in vivo study). J Clin Inv 75:608–613

Gibson GR, Cummings JH, MacFarlane GT et al. (1990) Alternative pathways for hydrogen disposal during fermentation in the human colon. Gut 31:679–683

Haber GB, Heaton KW, Murphy D, Burroughs LF (1977) Depletion and disruption of dietary fibre, effect on satiety, plasma glucose and serum insulin. Lancet ii:679–682

Heaton KW, Marcus SN, Emmett PM, Bolton CH (1988) Particle size of wheat maize, oat test meals; effects on plasma glucose and insulin responses and rate of starch digestion in vitro. Am J Clin Nutr 47:675–682

Heller SN, Hackler LR, Rivers JM et al. (1980) Dietary fiber: the effect of particle size of wheat bran on colonic function in young adult men. Am J Clin Nutr 33:1734–1744

Higham SE, Read NW (1992) The effects of ingestion of guar gum on ileostomy effluent. Br J Nutr 67:115–122

Holt S, Heading RC, Cater DC, Prescott LF, Tothill P (1979) Effect of gel-forming fibre on gastric emptying and absorption of glucose and paracetamol. Lancet i:636–639

Imaizumi K, Sugaro M (1986) Dietary fibre and intestinal lipoprotein secretion. In: Vahouny GV, Kritchevsky D (eds) Dietary fibre: basic and clinical aspects. Plenum Press, New York, pp 287–308

Imaizumi K, Tominaga A, Maivatari K, Sugaro M (1982) Effect of cellulose and guar gum on the secretion of mysenteric lymph chylomicrons in meal-fed rats. Nutr Rep Int 26:263–269

Isaksson G, Lundquist I, Ihse I (1982) Effect of dietary fibre on pancreatic enzyme activity in vitro. Gastroenterology 82:918–924

Isaksson G, Asp N-G, Ihse I (1983a) Effect of dietary fibre on pancreatic enzyme activities of ileostomy evacuates and on excretion of fat and nitrogen in the rat. Scand J Gastroenterol 18:417–423

Isaksson G, Lilja P, Lundquist I, Ihse I (1983b) Influence of dietary fibre on exocrine pancreatic function in the rat. Digestion 27:57–62

Jenkins DJA (1979) Dietary fibre, diabetes and hyperlipidaemia. Lancet ii:1287–1290

Jenkins DJA, Wolever TMS, Taylor RH et al. (1981) Glycaemic index of foods: a physiological basis for carbohydrate exchange. Am J Clin Nutr 34:362–366

Jenkins DJA, Wolever TMS, Jenkins AL et al. (1986) Low glycaemic response to traditionally produced wheat and rye products, bulgar and pumpernickel bread. Am J Clin Nutr 43:516–520

Jenkins DJA, Thorne MJ, Wolever TM (1987) The effect of starch protein interaction in wheat on the glycaemic response and rate of in vitro digestion. Am J Clin Nutr 45:946–951

Johnson IT, Gee JM (1981) Effect of gel forming food gums on the intestinal unstirred layer and sugar transport in vitro. Gut 22:398–403

Johnson IT, Gee JM (1986) Gastrointestinal adaptation in response to soluble non-available polysaccharides in the rat. Br J Nutr 55: 497–505

Levitt MD, Donaldson RM (1970) The use of respiratory hydrogen excretion to detect carbohydrate malabsorption. J Lab Clin Med 75:937–945

McBurney MI, Horvath PJ, Jeraci JL, Van Soest PJ (1985) Effect of in vitro fermentation using faecal inoculum on the water-holding capacity of dietary fibre. Br J Nutr 53:17–24

McKay LF, Eastwood MA (1984) A comparison of bacterial fermentation end products in carnivores, herbivores and primates including man. Proc Nutr Soc 43:35A

McKay LF, Eastwood MA, Brydon WG (1985) Methane excretion in man – a study of breath, flatus and faeces. Gut 26:69–74

McLean Ross AH, Eastwood MA, Brydon WG et al. (1983) A study of the effects of dietary gum arabic in humans. Am J Clin Nutr 37:368–375

Meyer JH, Elashoff YGJ, Reedy T, Fressman J, Amidon G (1986) Effects of viscosity and fluid outflow on postcibal gastric emptying of solids. Am J Physiol 250:G161–G164

Morris ER (1986) Molecular origin of hydrocolloid functionally. In: Phillips GO et al. (eds) Gums and stabilisers for the food industry, vol 3. Elsevier Applied Science, London, pp 3–16

Morris ER (1990) Shear thinning of random coil polysaccharides: characterisation by two parameters from a simple linear plot. Carbohydr Polym 13:85–96

O'Dea K, Nestle PJ, Anatoff L (1980) Physical factors influencing postprandial glucose and insulin responses to starch. Am J Clin Nutr 33:760–765

O'Donnell JD, Emmett PM, Heaton KW (1989) Size of flour particles and its relation to glycaemia, insulinaemia and colonic disease. Br Med J 298:1616–1617

Phillips DR (1986) The effect of guar gum in solution on diffusion of cholesterol mixed micelles. J Sci Food Agri 37:548–552

Prove J, Ehrlein HJ (1982) Motor function of gastric antrum and pylorus for evacuation of low and high viscosity meals in dogs. Gut 23:150–156

Rainbird AL, Low AG (1986) Effect of guar gum on gastric emptying in growing pigs. Br J Nutr 55:87–98

Read NW (1988) Relationship between colonic transport and motility. Pharmacology 36:S1:119–124

Read NW, Davies RJ, Holdsworth CD, Levin RJ (1977) Electrical assessment of functional lactase activity in conscious man. Gut 18:640–643

Read NW, MacFarlane A, Kinsman R et al. (1984) Effect of infusion of nutrient solutions into the ileum on gastric transit and plasma levels of neurotensin and enteroglucagon in man. Gastroenterology 86:274–280

Read NW, Bates TE, Al-Janabi MN, Cann PA (1985) The interpretation of the breath hydrogen profile after a solid meal containing unabsorbable carbohydrate. Gut 26:834–842

Read NW, Welch IMcL, Austen CJ et al. (1986) Swallowing food without chewing; a simple way to reduce postprandial glycaemia. Br J Nutr 55:43–47

Roberts FG (1991) PhD Thesis. University of London

Roberts FG, Smith HA, Low AG, Ellis PR (1990) Influence of wheat breads containing guar flour supplements of high and low molecular weights on viscosity of jejunal digesta in the pig. In: Southgate DAT, Waldron K, Johnson IT, Fenwick GR (eds) Dietary fibre: chemical and biological aspects. Royal Society of Chemistry, London, pp 164–168

Scarpello J, Vinik A, Owyang C (1982) The intestinal phase of pancreatic polypeptide release. Gastroenterology 82:406–412

Schwartz SE, Levine GD (1980) Effect of dietary fibre on intestinal glucose absorption and glucose tolerance in rats. Gastroenterology 79:833–836

Selvendran RR (1985) Developments in the chemistry and biochemistry of pectin and hemicellulosic polymers. J Cell Sci (Suppl)2:51–88

Smith AN, Drummond E, Eastwood MA (1981) The effect of coarse and fine Canadian red spring wheat and French soft wheat bran on colonic motility in patients with diverticular disease. Am J Clin Nutr 34:2460–2463

Southgate DAT (1986) The relation between composition and properties of dietary fibre and physiological effects. In: Vahouny GV, Kritchevsky D (eds) Dietary fibre: basic and clinical aspects. Plenum Press, New York, pp 35–48

Tadesse K, Smith D, Eastwood MA (1980) Breath hydrogen and methane excretion patterns in normal man and in clinical practice. Q J Exp Pysiol 65:85–97

Tomlin J, Read NW (1988a) The relation between bacterial degradation of viscous polysaccharides and stool output in human beings. Br J Nutr 60:467–475

Tomlin J, Read NW (1988b) Laxative properties of indigestible plastic particles. Br Med J 297:1175–1176

Tomlin J, Lewis C, Read NW (1991) Investigation of normal flatus production in healthy individuals. Gut 32:665–669

Wyman JB, Heaton KW, Manning AP, Wicks ACB (1976) The effect on intestinal transit and the faeces of raw and cooked bran in different doses. Am J Clin Nutr 29:1474–1479

Chapter 6

Bacterial Fermentation in the Colon and Its Measurement

C.A. Edwards and I.R. Rowland

Introduction

The colonic microflora is of crucial importance to any consideration of the role of dietary fibre in health and disease since many of the physiological effects of fibre on the gut are dependent on, or are influenced by, the activities of the colonic bacteria. This area of interaction between bacteriology and gut physiology is still poorly understood, mainly because of the inaccessibility of the proximal colon.

Fermentation

In the human colon, fermentation generally involves the anaerobic degradation by the colonic microflora of oligosaccharides and polysaccharides from the diet or mucins derived from host secretions.

The factors which determine whether a particular polysaccharide is fermented include the carbohydrate chemistry and structure, the presence of bacterial enzymes (these may be inducible), the environment (pH, bile acids, mixing rate) and the gut transit time (a long transit time provides more opportunity for slowly fermentable sources to be degraded (Van Soest et al., 1982).

Colonic Bacteria

The microbial population that inhabits the human colon is a large (about 10^{11} organisms/g contents) and highly complex community comprising 400–500 bacterial species (Moore et al., 1978). The predominant organisms of this ecosystem are non-sporing, obligate anaerobes from the genera *Bacteroides*, *Fusobacterium* (Gram negative rods), *Eubacterium* and *Bifidobacterium* (Gram positive rods). Gram positive anaerobic cocci are also present in large numbers (Drasar, 1988).

It has been calculated that the daily amount of carbohydrate needed to sustain the colonic microflora is 60–70 g (Wolin, 1981; Cummings et al., 1970). This is considerably more than the quantity entering the colon from undigested dietary carbohydrates (non-starch polysaccharides and "resistant" starch) which has been estimated, in studies with ileostomy patients, to be 25–35 g (Schweizer et al., 1990). The large discrepancy between the two values suggests that host secretions are important as substrates for bacterial fermentation in the colon.

Carbohydrate Fermentation by Gut Bacteria

Despite the evidence from human and animal studies that the colonic flora is the agent responsible for breakdown of dietary fibre, identification of the main organisms responsible is difficult and the results of such studies need to be interpreted with caution for the following reasons:

1. The demonstration of carbohydrate fermentation by a pure culture in vitro does not prove that the same organism performs the reaction in the colon since other, more easily utilised substrates may be available.

2. Incubations of pure cultures of anaerobes with polysaccharides do not take into account the complexities of the colonic environment which may markedly influence polysaccharide fermentation (Salyers et al., 1977a; Roberton and Stanley, 1982).

3. Purified forms of dietary fibre may be more, or less, susceptible to bacterial attack than when in their natural, plant cell wall complexes (as discussed for cellulose below).

4. Degradation of some polysaccharides may require two, or more, bacteria acting in a "consortium", so fermentation would not be apparent in the presence of just one of the organisms.

Dietary Fibre

The major contributors to undigested dietary carbohydrates are the poly-saccharides that compose the plant cell wall. The plant cell wall is a very complex structure containing a variety of polysaccharides with varying degrees of fermentability.

On the basis of in vitro incubations, several species of colonic bacteria can utilise polysaccharides found in plant cell walls (Table 6.1). Hemicelluloses, pectins and plant gums appear to be the most readily utilised as substrates by pure cultures of gut organisms (Salyers et al., 1977b). This in vitro data is supported by some elegant in vivo experiments by Salyers and Pajeau (1989) in which mutants deficient in their capacity to utilise specific carbohydrates were tested for ability to compete with wild type strains for colonisation of germfree mouse gut. These studies indicate that *Bacteroides thetaiotaomicron* is a scavenger, able to utilise small amounts of different carbohydrates available in vivo.

Table 6.1. Fermentation of carbohydrates by gut anaerobes

Group	Cellulose	Hemicellulose	Pectin	Gums[a]	Starch	Mono/disaccharides
Bacteriodes						
fragilis	−	−	−	(+)	+	+
thetaiotaomicron	−	+	+	−	+	+
ovatus	−	+	+	(+)	+	+
vulgatus	−	+	(+)	−	+	+
distasonis	−	−	−	−	−	+
3452	−	+	+	−	−	+
0061-1	−	+	−	+	+	+
sp	+	NT	NT	NT	NT	+
uniformis	NT	NT	NT	(+)	NT	NT
varibilis	NT	NT	NT	(+)	NT	NT
Bifidobacterium						
adolescentis	−	+	−	−	+	+
breve	−	−	−	−	+	+
infantis	−	+	−	−	−	+
longum	−	+	−	(+)	−	+
Eubacterium						
aerofaciens	−	−	−	−	−	+
elegans	−	−	+	−	−	+
rectale	−	−	−	−	+	+
Fusobacterium						
prauznitzii	−	−	−	−	+	+
Peptostreptococcus						
productus	−	−	−	−	−	+

−   not fermented
+   fermented
(+) fermented by some strains
NT, Not tested
[a] Gum arabic, guar, tragacanth
Data from Salyers et al., 1977a, b; McCarthy and Salyers, 1988; Betian et al., 1977; Tomlin et al., 1988.

In contrast, none of the predominant species of gut bacteria has been shown to degrade cellulose, although cellulolytic bacteria have been isolated from faeces sporadically and in low numbers by enrichment culture (Betian et al., 1977). In vivo however, cellulose particularly in the form of bran and cabbage fibre can be degraded (Ehle et al., 1982) suggesting that a consortium of organisms is required or that the forms of cellulose used in the in vitro studies, usually microcrystalline in structure, cannot be utilised as easily as the hydrated cellulose and hemicellulose/cellulose complexes present naturally in foods.

Other plant polysaccharides such as mucilages and indigestible storage polysaccharides are also included in dietary fibre as are some bacterially produced polysaccharides such as xanthan and gellan. The latter are used in small amounts as food stabilisers and thickeners but are often included in fermentation experiments amongst dietary fibre polysaccharides.

Plant polysaccharides which are readily fermented when fed in a pure or semi-isolated form include guar gum, pectin and gum arabic. The less fermentable include cellulose and ispaghula.

Oligosaccharides

Many carbohydrate-requiring bacteria cannot utilise polysaccharides and presumably subsist on dietary sugars and oligosaccharides which escape digestion in the small intestine. These include stachyose and raffinose in plants such as leguminous seeds. Lactulose which is often used as a marker of small bowel transit time is also readily fermented. Polydextrose and polyfructose structures are now being used as soluble food ingredients. The former appears to be partially digested in the small intestine and partially fermented in the colon. In contrast, polyfructose escapes digestion in the small intestine and is fermented by the colonic flora (Figdor and Rennhard, 1981; Hosoya et al., 1988). Other small molecules which may be fermented and which have been little studied include the sugar alcohols such as sorbitol, which are often used in manufactured food (Würsch et al. 1990).

Low molecular weight carbohydrates can be generated in the colon by the activities of the polysaccharide degraders and then scavenged by those organisms unable to utilise polysaccharides (Salyers et al., 1981). Such cross-feeding has been widely reported in rumen cultures. Thus the polysaccharide degraders play a crucial role in metabolism in the colon since they convert macromolecular diet components to simpler substances which can then be utilised by other groups in the ecosystem.

Resistant Starch

Many of the anaerobes in the gut are starch fermenters (Table 6.1) and it seems likely that starch which escapes digestion in the small intestine (Englyst and Cummings, 1986), provides a source of carbon and energy for the colonic flora.

Mucins and Mucopolysaccharide

In vivo studies in man and rats provide strong evidence that mucins, produced in the intestine by the host, are utilised by the colonic microflora (Vercellotti et al., 1977; Gustafsson and Carlstedt-Duke, 1984; Midtvedt et al., 1986). Indeed, the fact that people ingesting a completely absorbable diet can support a complex gut microflora suggests that mucins and other host secretions are important sources of nutrients for gut bacteria as reviewed by Rowland et al. (1985).

Despite the above evidence for mucin breakdown in the gut, and by faeces in vitro (Hoskins and Boulding, 1981; Perman and Modler, 1982; Hill, 1986) it has proved difficult to isolate mucin-degrading bacteria from faeces (Roberton and Stanley, 1982). There is, however, evidence that certain strains of *Bifidobacterium bifidum, Bacteroides fragilis* and *Ruminococcus* torques have some mucin-degrading activity (Salyers et al., 1977b; Roberton and Stanley, 1982).

Mucopolysaccharides (glycosaminoglycans) can be fermented by several *Bacteroides* spp although since the amounts entering the colon are small by comparison to mucin, mucopolysaccharides are probably not a major source of nutrients for the microflora (McCarthy and Salyers, 1988).

Enzymes Involved in Polysaccharide Degradation

Even relatively simple polysaccharide structures require several enzymes for their degradation. Usually the degradation proceeds stepwise with the breakdown of the polysaccharide into oligosaccharides, which are then hydrolysed by glycosidases into their component monomers. Further enzymes may be required to cleave sidechains and substituent groups such as sulphate residues (Salyers and O'Brien, 1980).

Most of the polysaccharide fermenting organisms possess a broad spectrum of enzyme activities. For examples, *Bacteroides thetaiotaomicron* produces β-glucanase, polygalacturonase and chondroitin lyase (Salyers and Leedle, 1983).

In general, the polysaccharidases and glycosidases of *Bacteroides* spp are cell-associated rather than extracelluar (Salyers and Leedle, 1983; Berg, 1981) with some being membrane bound (Salyers and O'Brien, 1980). Despite the cellular location of the enzymes, small amounts of disaccharides and oligosaccharides appear to "leak" from the cells allowing the possibility of cross-feeding of non-polysaccharide degraders in the colon. Such cross-feeding may be more common during fermentation of viscous polysaccharides such as guar gum for which there is some evidence for involvement of extracelluar enzymes (Tomlin et al., 1988).

The polysaccharidases of human colonic bacteria appear to be subject to regulation. Their activities are induced by exposure to substrate and there is evidence for repression of enzyme synthesis by products of the reaction (Salyers and Leedle, 1983).

Fermentation Products

Carbohydrates and oligosaccharides are degraded by the Embden–Meyerhof pathway to short chain fatty acids (SCFA), carbon dioxide, hydrogen and methane.

Short Chain Fatty Acids

The SCFA produced from polysaccharide fermentation will depend on the substrates supplied and the bacteria which ferment them. The bacterial flora is

Table 6.2. The patterns of SCFA production from the fermentation of various complex carbohydrates by human faecal bacteria in vitro

Carbohydrate	% Acetate	% Propionate	% Butyrate	Reference
Starch	50	22	29	Englyst et al., 1987
Resistant starch	41	21	38	Englyst and MacFarlane, 1986
Wheat bran	52	11.4	19.2	Adiotomre et al., 1990
	61.4	19.1	19.5	McBurney and Thompson, 1987
Pectin	84	14	2	Englyst et al., 1987
	71	14.8	8.5	Adiotomre et al., 1990
	69	13	17	Vince et al., 1990
Cellulose	61	20	19	Vince et al., 1990
Gum arabic	68.2	19.6	8.2	Adiotomre et al., 1990
Guar gum	57.7	27.2	8.0	Adiotomre et al., 1990
	61.4	24.7	13.7	McBurney and Thompson, 1987
Tragacanth	67	18.5	8.2	Adiotomre et al., 1990
Xanthan	71	18.6	3.2	Adiotomre et al., 1990
Gellan	62.2	19.6	7.0	Adiotomre et al., 1990
Karaya	63	9.9	9.5	Adiotomre et al., 1990
Xylan	82	15	3	Englyst et al., 1987
Arabinogalactan	50	42	8	Englyst et al., 1987
	60	22.4	17.3	Vince et al., 1990
Ispaghula	56.3	26.3	9.5	C.A. Edwards unpublished data
Oat bran	57	20.8	22.5	McBurney and Thompson, 1987
Lactulose	67	13	20	Vince et al., 1990

extremely complex and is usually examined as a complete ecosystem. However, it is important to note that particular SCFA are produced by different groups of bacteria and are not all produced by each species (Macy and Probst, 1979; Mandelstam et al., 1982). Thus the combination of diverse substrates and the variability of the flora composition produces large variations in the proportion of SCFA in human faeces. The patterns of SCFA produced by the fermentation of a range of polysaccharides by mixed human faecal bacteria in vitro are shown in Table 6.2. Although there is some variation in the percentage of the individual SCFA produced from a single polysaccharide between laboratories (this is due mainly to different donors, different background media and culture methods), distinct patterns can be seen. Acetic acid is invariably the major SCFA produced from all fermentable polysaccharides. Starch, wheat bran and oat bran are associated with large proportions of butyric acid, while arabinogalactan, ispaghula (an arabinoxylan), guar gum and starch are associated with large proportions of propionic acid.

Products of Protein and Amino Acid Degradation

The catabolism of protein and amino acids by the colonic bacteria has been studied very little. In the rumen it has been shown that the bacteria convert casein to CO_2, NH_3 and branched SCFA (Hespell and Smith, 1983). In vitro fermentation of albumin and casein by human faecal flora has shown production of branched chain SCFA and ammonia (MacFarlane et al., 1986; Mortenson et al., 1988) which are also found throughout the human colon and in faeces (MacFarlane et al., 1986; Zarling and Ruchim, 1987). These branched chain fatty acids may have important roles in the colon; they have been shown to stimulate bacterial growth (Hespell and Smith, 1983).

Gaseous Products

Hydrogen is the most studied of the gaseous products of fermentation. Breath hydrogen is easy to measure and its use as a marker of fermentation is discussed below. Breath hydrogen rises rapidly when a fermentable substrate reaches the colon. In contrast, methane levels are constant throughout the day (Tadesse and Eastwood, 1978). The colonic production of methane is not so well studied. It is reported that only 33% of some populations produce methane (Haines et al., 1977) in the breath. However, most faecal incubations produce methane readily, indicating the importance of environment on methane production. In the rumen there is virtually no hydrogen but mainly methane. Methanogenic bacteria act as hydrogen acceptors using hydrogen and carbon dioxide to produce methane.

The most detectable result of gas production must be distension which may lead to colonic propulsion and the production of flatus, a somewhat undesirable effect of a sudden increase in the intake of fermentable non-starch polysaccharides.

Measurement of Colonic Fermentation In Vivo

The major obstacle in measuring fermentation of carbohydrate in vivo is the inaccessibility of the proximal colon where the majority of fermentation is thought to occur. The most direct way to measure fermentation is to sample from the colon itself but this is very difficult and only possible in a few laboratories. Alternatives are to look at fermentation indirectly by measuring products of fermentation that are excreted in the faeces, breath or urine. These studies are very restricted in the information they can provide. Animal studies provide an alternative way of gaining access to the colon but the problem of finding a suitable animal model then arises.

Human Models

Intubation of the human colon is difficult and involves substantial interference with the normal physiology of the subject. Studies of colonic motility and absorption have often concentrated on the rectum and sigmoid colon because of the problems of intubating the more proximal colon (Snape et al., 1978; NcNeil et al., 1978) though some reach the transverse colon (Narducci et al., 1987). A few laboratories have managed successfully to intubate the proximal colon. This is usually performed by passing a tube by mouth down the gut either completely through the colon (Fink and Friedman, 1960) or to the proximal colon alone or in association with a tube passed rectally (Ruppin et al., 1980). The normal physiology of the gut may be severely disturbed by intubation both by the presence of the tube which may alter transit time (Read et al., 1983) and also by any wash out or bowel preparation carried out before the study. This interference of normal luminal contents limits the usefulness of intubation studies to measure normal fermentation but they can be used to measure the fermentation of specific substrates. Florent et al. (1985) reported some impressive studies of the fermentation of lactulose. They sampled from the ileum and caecum to monitor fermentation in detail following the appearance and disappearance of the intermediates and correlated their results with breath hydrogen measurements. However, as this study was carried out using lactulose, the contents may have been more liquid than if a polysaccharide had been used when aspiration of caecal contents up a narrow tube may be more difficult.

An alternative method of sampling colonic contents is in vivo dialysis (Wrong et al., 1965) where subjects swallow a dialysis bag. The contents of the gut equilibrate with the contents of the dialysis bag and small molecules such as SCFA can be measured after the bag is egested from the body. This however will provide only a single measure of material sampled throughout the colon and delivered some unknown time after it reached the caecum and therefore can give only an indirect impression of events occurring in the proximal colon.

A more direct method is the use of radio telemetric pills (Bown et al., 1974; Evans et al., 1988). These are usually pH electrodes that are swallowed and transmit measurements of luminal pH as they pass down the gut. This technique has been used by several laboratories to study the normal pH of different parts of the colon and the effects of lactulose (Bown et al., 1974) and bran (Evans et al., 1988). However, fermentation of many polysaccharides may not decrease colonic pH and transit through the colon cannot be controlled unless the pill is tethered at the mouth resulting in some of the problems of colonic intubation.

Plasma SCFA in man can be measured only in peripheral blood and unfortunately acetate is the only SCFA in man which remains in blood after passage through the liver (Pomare et al., 1985). Since acetate is also produced by human cells, plasma levels are difficult to interpret. Breath hydrogen measurements are often used to give an indication of fermentation occurring in the colon, but cannot really be used quantitatively. There may be a large baseline variation in breath hydrogen depending on background diet and antibiotic use (Gilat et al., 1978). It was originally suggested that the hydrogen produced from a known dose of lactulose could be used as a standard to indicate the amount of carbohydrate fermented in the colon by breath hydrogen measurement (Bond and Levitt, 1972; Thornton et al., 1986). However, even the amount of hydrogen produced with lactulose is variable and may be affected by prolonged intake. Indeed, a smaller postprandial rise in breath hydrogen may not mean less fermentation. Florent et al. (1985) showed that fermentation of lactulose may become more efficient on repeated dosing but with a reduction in the amount of breath hydrogen produced. The amount of hydrogen detected in the breath depends not only on the fermentation of substrate but also on the activity of hydrogen utilising bacteria and perhaps colonic blood flow. Mouth to caecum transit time may affect breath hydrogen profiles, but significant differences in transit time did not have significant effects on the area under the hydrogen curve (Rumessen et al., 1989).

Patients with Colostomies

The use of ileostomy patients has supplied much useful information about the amount of nutrients escaping absorption in the small bowel. The use of patients with stomas giving access to colonic lumen would, in theory, enable direct studies of colonic function. However, the flora of the colon in these individuals may not be representative of that of intact subjects and in practice the recruitment of such patients in sufficient numbers to allow controlled and interpretable studies is very difficult. Colonic SCFA have been measured in such patients (Mitchell et al., 1985).

Faecal Analysis

Many studies of the fermentation of dietary fibre rely on measurements of faecal constituents. The ease of faecal collection makes this an easy if unpleasant option. Faecal samples must be processed very carefully as fermentation may continue after stool passage. During and after feeding trials faecal samples may be analysed for such as residual fibre, SCFA, bile acids and pH. Residual fibre measurements can certainly reveal the human fermentability of particular carbohydrate, but measurements of faecal SCFA and pH may not give any information about fermentation patterns in the proximal colon as some or most of the SCFA may be absorbed before the distal colon. This is particularly important for fibres which are rapidly fermented. The relationship of faecal to proximal colonic SCFA will thus depend on the type of dietary fibre consumed. Faecal samples can also be analysed for bacteria and bacterial enzymes.

Animal Models

The use of animal models allows controlled diet studies as well as access to the colonic lumen. It is very difficult to assess and ensure compliance of human subjects to a test diet especially over long time periods. The background diet in many studies is uncontrolled and may be responsible for the large inter-individual variation often seen. In contrast, the dietary intake of animals can be controlled and monitored. However, there is little standardisation of conditions for animal feeding trials and each laboratory has its own favourite basal diet, the details of which are not always described in the resulting paper. Some studies use low fibre semi-synthetic diets of varied recipe for their basal diet period (Nyman and Asp, 1988) others use elemental liquid diets (Walter et al., 1988). Animals may have been previously on a stock diet (Illman et al., 1982) which is usually high in dietary fibre, or may have been acclimatised to the test diet for any time between three days (Nyman et al., 1986) or four weeks (Walter et al., 1986). Other laboratories use a run-in period of varying length on the basal or control diet before including the test fibre. Thus results may reflect the effects of refeeding a substrate deprived flora or the effects of reducing overall fibre intake. The duration of the feeding trial may vary from 3 days to 18 months. Walter et al. (1986) showed that the stability of fermentative capacity of the rat is still changing four weeks after inclusion of a new substrate and that dietary trials of less than this may not measure the true fermentative capacity. The amount of fibre fed also varies. Many laboratories use 10% fibre supplementation. This may be excessively high when a fibre with large water-holding capacity is used. Fermentability may be affected by the dose administered especially if transit time is accelerated due to colonic distension.

The question with any animal model is whether the fermentation of the animals' colonic flora is representative of that in man. The colonic fermentation of each species is dependent on its diet, the transit time of food through the colon and the presence, size or absence of a caecum. The comparative physiology and anatomy of the colon of man and other non-ruminant species have been well documented (Argenzio and Stevens, 1984; Von Englehardt et al., 1989). The most frequently used species for fermentation studies as a model for man are the rat and the pig. The rat has a large caecum but probably a shorter colonic transit time than man (Van Soest et al., 1982). They may be described on the whole as caecal fermenters. Rats are also coprophagic. The effects of dietary fibre on stool output of the rat, however, are well correlated with their effects in man (Nyman et al., 1986).

The use of the pig as an animal model is limited to those laboratories with suitable facilities. The pig is an omnivore like man but some ileal fermentation does occur in the pig (Graham and Aman, 1987). Although the pig has a larger caecum and a greater capacity for fibre fermentation than man, the pig has similar faecal and blood SCFA (Graham and Aman, 1987) and as it is a larger animal than the rat or rabbit, it may provide larger samples of colonic contents and allow easier surgery for direct sampling from the colon or portal blood vessels.

Although the use of an animal model should allow detailed in vivo studies of colonic fermentation most laboratories working on dietary fibre still concentrate on stool characteristics and only some measure events occurring in the caecum. Very few studies investigate ongoing fermentation by sampling from the colon in the live animal although the measurement of portal and peripheral blood SCFA concentrations is providing much useful information (Illman et al., 1982; Demigné and Rémésy, 1985).

Measurement of Colonic Fermentation In Vitro

The difficulties encountered in human and, to a lesser extent, in animal in vivo studies of fibre fermentation outlined above, (namely, sampling the colon contents, dietary control, measurement of SCFA and gaseous reaction products) can be partially overcome or at least circumvented in in vitro studies. In particular, the lack of intestinal absorption of products in vitro facilitates the measurement of rates of formation and the relative proportions of the various gases and SCFA produced.

However the limitations of in vitro studies should be kept in mind. Firstly, the source of the inoculum for in vitro cultures is usually faeces – how representative the faecal flora is of that in the colon has been the subject of debate (Fernandez et al., 1985; Drasar, 1988). In most instances, however, it is the only practical means of obtaining a sample of the lower gut flora from the healthy human. Alternative methods, of varying degrees of complexity and unpleasantness for the subject, have several disadvantages and do not necessarily provide samples representative of the gut region under study (Drasar and Barrow, 1985). A second more serious limitation of in vitro studies is the virtual impossibility of mimicking ex vivo the biotic and physico-chemical conditions of the human colon. Consequently, as soon as a faecal sample is transferred to culture medium its bacterial composition and metabolic activity starts to change. Furthermore in static cultures, it continues to do so throughout the period of incubation and end products of metabolism can build up to bacteriostatic concentrations.

Some of these limitations can be partially overcome, at the expense of increased complexity by the use of continuous and semi-continuous models of the human colonic flora.

Static In Vitro Systems

The usual procedure for studying carbohydrate fermentation in vitro is similar to that used extensively for investigating gut microflora metabolism of foreign compounds, for which the methodology and conditions have been discussed critically by Coates et al. (1988). Briefly a freshly collected faecal sample is diluted in buffer or culture medium and incubated under anaerobic conditions at 37 °C with the carbohydrate under investigation (McBurney and Thompson, 1987; Goering and Van Soest, 1970; Tomlin et al., 1988; Mortensen et al., 1988; Jeraci and Horvath, 1989). The head space can be sampled for gases and the incubation mixture for SCFA and residual fibre analyses and also for monitoring changes in physico-chemical characteristics of fibre during fermentation.

Despite the simplicity of the method, it can supply useful information on the degree of fermentability of a fibre source and on any changes in physico-chemical characteristics, such as water-holding capacity, likely to be engendered by bacterial degradation (McBurney et al., 1985). Where more sophisticated measurements are undertaken such as rates of gas production and SCFA formation, the limitations of the method become apparent (McBurney and Thompson, 1990). The relative amounts of the different SCFA and gases, hydrogen and methane produced from vegetable and cereal fibres varies with the time of incubation over 4 to 24 hours. The authors conclude that the in vitro system underestimates H_2 production and overestimates CH_4 production due to an increase in H_2 partial pressure stimulating CH_4 production in the closed system. It would seem advisable to use short incubation periods (4 hours) rather than extended ones (24 hours) to minimise the above problem, since this would also have the effect of minimising changes in the balance of the flora and in the build up of SCFA which would lower the culture pH and possibly inhibit bacterial metabolism. It should be noted however that fermentation of slowly fermentable substrates may not be detectable with short incubation times and a combination of in vitro and in vivo studies may be needed.

A further problem that may be encountered in static culture incubations is the presence of fermentable material in the faecal inocula themselves. This can result in two- to three-fold increases in SCFA concentration in the incubations over 24 hours (Mortensen et al., 1988). The inclusion of control incubations without added fibre (Mortensen et al., 1988) would also seem prudent. McBurney and Thompson (1990) point out that some fibre preparations (e.g wheat bran) contain carbohydrate and protein fractions which in vivo may be digested and absorbed, but in vitro are available for fermentation, thus affecting SCFA and gas production. It is important, therefore, to pre-digest such fibre preparations with pancreatic enzymes.

Despite these limitations, the method can provide useful information on the extent and products of fermentation and provides a rapid means of comparing a large number of fibres. In addition, the effect of source of faecal sample on fermentation of fibre can be studied. For example, although the fermentation capacity of faecal samples collected from a single individual on several occasions was similar, that of faecal samples from six different individuals varied considerably (McBurney and Thompson, 1987, 1989). Inter-individual variation has also been noted by Mortensen et al. (1988). The finding that ingestion of Solka floc modifies pectin fermentation in man suggests that diet may be one cause of inter-individual variation (Jeraci and Horvath, 1989).

Continuous and Semi-continuous Culture Systems

The aim of these various models is to establish in vitro, a mixed population of bacteria, similar to that of the colon, in a near steady state or equilibrium, so that studies of metabolism and microbial ecology can be performed over long periods (up to several weeks or months). Although offering a number of advantages over batch cultures, these more complex systems are considerably more expensive and time consuming to use.

The essential difference between continuous and semi-continuous methodologies lies in the maintenance in the former system of a bacterial population near to a steady state by the continuous addition of fresh growth medium and the continuous removal, at the same rate, of spent culture (Veilleux and Rowland, 1981). In contrast, in semi-continuous systems, culture is removed and replenished at intervals during the day to mimic the periodic entry of ileal chyme into the colon (Miller and Wolin, 1981). The systems vary in complexity from those using single culture vessels (Miller and Wolin, 1981; Edwards et al., 1985) to those in which two or more vessels (sometimes poised at different pH values) placed in series are used to provide more heterogeneity of physico-chemical conditions and to mimic pH gradients in the colon (Veilleux and Rowland, 1981; Gibson et al., 1988).

Both continuous and semi-continuous systems use freshly collected human faeces from a single donor as the source of inoculum, so results may be generated which are peculiar to that person and not applicable to a wider population. On the basis of the production, or equilibrium concentrations, of SCFA these models appear to mimic bacterial fermentation in the human gut quite closely. The total SCFA concentration ranged from about 35 to 135 mmol/litre (with acetate usually comprising the highest proportion and propionate and butyrate contributing about 5% to 20% each (Miller and Wolin, 1981; MacFarlane et al., 1989; Edwards et al., 1985; Bearne et al., 1990; Duncan and Henderson, 1990). Levels of SCFA in human faeces are reported to be 66–163 mmol/litre with acetate predominating. In some of the culture systems the production of hydrogen and methane has been demonstrated (Miller and Wolin, 1981; Duncan and Henderson, 1990).

Despite the progress that has been made with the design of continuous and semi-continuous culture systems, further work is clearly needed to improve their similarity to the colon and in particular to overcome the practical problems of delivering and emptying fibrous and viscous materials without blocking the tubes and ports of the system.

Studies of Carbohydrate Fermentation

The SCFA concentration in the continuous and semi-continuous culture models of the human colon have been shown to alter in response to changes both in the amount (Edwards et al., 1985, 1986; Duncan and Henderson, 1990) and type (Miller and Wolin, 1981) of carbohydrate provided in the growth medium. Recently such models have been used to compare the fermentability and fermentation products of different types of dietary fibre. For example, Rumney (1989) compared wheat bran and sugar beet fibre in a semi-continuous culture system. Total SCFA production was higher with sugar beet fibre and this correlated with a higher rate of non-starch polysaccharide utilisation from this substrate.

In addition to facilitating studies of fermentation products, continuous flow cultures can provide information on the consequences of alterations in transit time, which can be simulated by altering the dilution rate or the number of feeds per day. Furthermore the influence of amount or type of carbohydrate on bacterial types and their metabolic activities can be studied over extended periods. For example, the effect of the endogenously produced glycoprotein mucin on activity of bacterial glycosidases and proteases and on sulphate reduction and methanogenesis has been investigated (Gibson et al., 1988; MacFarlane et al., 1989). Similarly, the influence of wheat bran and sugar beet fibre on bacterial nitrate reduction and ammonia production have been studied (Rumney, 1989). A useful feature of continuous and semi-continuous cultures is that the cultures can act as their own controls giving more meaningful results than with batch cultures.

The ability of the gut flora maintained in continuous culture to adapt metabolically over a long period to a novel substrate (Mallett et al., 1985) could be of great potential use in the study of fermentation of novel fibres, which may require the induction of enzymes or selection of normally rare bacterial types for their breakdown in the gut. Conversely, suppression, in vivo, of the fermentative capacity of the microflora by, for example, ingestion of Solka floc has been shown to be reproduced in a continuous culture model (Jeraci and Horvath, 1989).

Conclusions

The methods used to study fermentation of carbohydrate by the human colon flora vary enormously in complexity and in the type of information that they provide. The particular method used will depend on the question being asked. For example, is a fibre fermentable? Is it fermented in vivo? Does it stimulate epithelial cell turnover? In some cases, no single method will provide the answer and a combination of approaches must be used.

Despite the difficulties involved, it is clearly important to study colonic fermentation not only because of its impact on physico-chemical properties and physiological action of dietary fibre (e.g. reduction in stool bulking effects) but also because the products of fermentation can be of benefit and detriment to man. Many of the beneficial consequences of fibre fermentation centre on the production of SCFA. These can provide energy, not only for the colonic mucosa (Roedigger, 1980) but also for the body as a whole. The SCFA may also have effects on liver metabolism, particularly propionic acid which may affect gluconeogenesis (Anderson and Bridges, 1984) and cholesterol synthesis (Chen et al., 1984), and their contribution to the lowering of gut luminal pH may reduce tumorigenesis in the colon (Jacobs, 1990).

The increased growth of bacteria in the presence of fermentable carbohydrate may reduce ammonia production (Vince et al., 1990) but can also raise the activity of potentially undesirable enzymes such as β-glucuronidase and glycosidase thus increasing the generation of toxic or carcinogenic metabolites in the colon (Rowland and Mallett, 1990).

It is clear from this review that a number of methodological problems need to be addressed, in particular the difficulties in sampling from the proximal colon, but it is hoped that with the development of present methods our knowledge of fermentation in the colon will soon match the current level of understanding of rumen fermentation.

References

Adiotomre J, Eastwood MA, Edwards CA, Brydon WG (1990) Dietary fiber: in vitro methods that anticipate nutrition and metabolic activity in humans. Am J Clin Nutr 52:128–134

Anderson JW, Bridges SR (1984) Short chain fatty acid fermentation products of plant fibre affect glucose metabolism of isolated rat hepatocytes. Proc Soc Exp Biol Med 177:372–376

Argenzio RA, Stevens CE (1984) The large bowel – a supplementary rumen. Proc Nutr Soc 43:13–23

Bearne CA, Mallett AK, Rowland IR, Brennan-Craddock WE (1990) Continuous culture of human faecal bacteria as an in vitro model for the colonic flora. Toxicol In Vitro 4:522–525

Berg J-O (1981) Cellular localization of glycoside hydrolases in *Bacteroides fragilis*. Curr Microbiol 5:13–17

Betian HG, Lineham BA, Bryant MP, Holdeman LV (1977) Isolation of a cellulolytic *Bacteroides* sp. from human feces. Appl Environ Microbiol 33:1009–1010

Bond JH, Levitt MD (1972) Use of pulmonary (H_2) measurements to quantitate carbohydrate absorption. J Clin Invest 51:1219–1225

Bown ML, Gibson JA, Sladen GE, Hicks B, Dawson AM (1974) Effect of lactulose and other laxatives on ileal and colonic pH as measured by a radiotelemetric device. Gut 15:999–1004

Chen W-J, Anderson JW, Jennings D (1984) Propionate may mediate the hypocholesterolaemic effects of certain soluble plant fibres in cholesterol fed rats. Proc Soc Exp Med 175:215–218

Coates ME, Drasar BS, Mallett AK, Rowland IR (1988) Methodological considerations for the study of bacterial metabolism. In: Rowland IR (ed) Role of the gut flora in toxicity and cancer. Academic Press, London, pp 1–21

Cummings JH, Southgate DAT, Branch W, Houston H, Jenkins DJA, James WPT (1970) Colonic response to dietary fibre from carrot, cabbage, apple, bran and guar gum. Lancet i:5–8

Demigné C, Rémésy C (1985) Stimulation of absorption of volatile fatty acids and minerals in the caecum of rats adapted to a very high fibre diet. J Nutr 115:53–60

Drasar BS (1988) The bacterial flora of the intestine. In: Rowland IR (ed) The role of the gut flora in toxicity and cancer. Academic Press, London, pp 23–38

Drasar BS, Barrow PA (1985) Intestinal microbiology. American Society for Microbiology, Washington (Aspects of microbiology 10)

Duncan A, Henderson C (1990) A study of the fermentation of dietary fibre by human colonic bacteria grown in vitro in semi-continuous culture. Microb Ecol Health Dis 3:87–98.

Edwards CA, Duerden BI, Read NW (1985) Metabolism of mixed human colonic bacteria in a continuous culture mimicking the human caecal contents. Gastroenterology 88:1903–1909

Edwards CA, Duerden BI, Read NW (1986) Effect of clindamycin on the ability of a continuous culture of colonic bacteria to ferment carbohydrate. Gut 27:411–417

Ehle FR, Robertson JB, Van Soest PJ (1982) Influence of dietary fibres on fermentation in the human large intestine. J Nutr 112:158–166

Englyst HN, Cummings JH (1986) Digestion of the carbohydrates of banana, in the human small intestine. Am J Clin Nutr 44:42–50

Englyst HN, MacFarlane GT (1986) Breakdown of resistant and readily digestible starch by human gut bacteria. J Sci Food Agric 37:699–706

Englyst HN, Hay S, MacFarlane GT (1987) Polysaccharide breakdown by mixed populations of human faecal bacteria. Microbiol Ecol 95:163–171

Evans DF, Crompton J, Pye G, Hardcastle D (1988) The role of dietary fibre on acidification of the colon in man. Gastroenterology 94:118 (abstract)

Fernandez F, Kennedy H, Hill M, Truelove S (1985) The effect of diet on the bacterial flora of ileostomy fluid. Microbiol Aliment Nutr 3:47–52

Figdor SK, Rennhard HH (1981) Caloric utilisation and deposition of [^{14}C] polydextrose in the rat. J Agric Food Chem 29:1181–1189

Fink S, Friedman S (1960) The differential effects of drugs on the proximal and distal colon. Am J Med 534–540

Florent C, Flourié B, Leblond A, Raurureau M, Bernier JJ, Rambaud JC (1985) Influence of chronic lactulose ingestion on the colonic metabolism of lactulose in man (in vivo study). J Clin Invest 75:608–613

Gibson GR, MacFarlane GT, Cummings JH (1988) Occurrence of sulphate-reducing bacteria in human faeces and the relationship of dissimilatory sulphate reduction to methanogenesis in the large gut. J Appl Bacteriol 65:103–111

Gilat T, Benhur H, Gelman Malachi E, Terdiman R, Peled Y (1978) Alterations of the colonic flora and their effect on the hydrogen breath test. Gut 19:602–605

Goering HK, Van Soest PJ (1970) Forage fiber analysis. Apparatus, reagents, procedures and some applications. US Dept. Agriculture, Washington (Agriculture handbook no. 379)

Graham H, Aman P (1987) The pig as a model in dietary fibre digestion studies. Scand J Gastroenterol 22 (Suppl 129):55–61

Gustafsson BE, Carlstedt-Duke B (1984) Intestinal water soluble mucins in germfree, ex-germfree and conventional animals. Acta Pathol Microbiol Immunol Scand (B) 92:247–252

Haines A, Metz G, Dilawari J, Blendis L, Wiggins HS (1977) Breath methane in patients with cancer of the large bowel. Lancet ii:481–483

Hespell RB, Smith CJ (1983) Utilisation of nitrogen sources by gastrointestinal tract bacteria. In: Hentges DJ (ed) Human intestinal flora in health and disease. Academic Press, London, pp 167–187

Hill RRH (1986) Digestion of mucin polysaccharides in vitro by bacteria isolated from the rabbit cecum. Curr Microbiol 14:117–120

Hoskins LC, Boulding ET (1981) Mucin degradation in human colon ecosystems. J Clin Invest 67:163–172

Hosoya N, Dhorranintra D, Hikada H (1988) Utilisation of ^{14}C oligofructo-oligosaccharides in man as energy resources. J Clin Biochem 5:67–74

Illman RJ, Trimble RP, Snoswell AM, Topping DL (1982) Daily variation in concentrations of volatile fatty acids in the splanchnic blood vessels of rats fed diets high in pectin and bran. Nutr Rep Intern 26:439–446

Jacobs LR (1990) Influence of soluble fibres on Experimental Colon Carcinogenesis. In: Kritchevsky D et al. (eds) Dietary fiber: chemistry, physiology and health effects. Plenum Press, New York, pp 399–402

Jeraci JL, Horvath PJ (1989) In vitro fermentation of dietary fiber by human fecal microorganisms. Anim Feed Sci Technol 23:121–140

MacFarlane GT, Cummings JH, Allison C (1986) Protein degradation by human intestinal bacteria. J Gen Microbiol 132:1647–1656

MacFarlane GT, Hay S, Gibson GR (1989) Influence of mucin on glycosidase, protease and arylamidase activities of human gut bacteria grown in a 3-stage continuous culture system. J Appl Bacteriol 66:407–417

Macy JM, Probst I (1979) The biology of gastrointestinal bacteroides. Ann Rev Microbiol 33:561–594

Mallett AK, Rowland IR, Bearne CA, Purchase R, Gangolli SD (1985) Metabolic adaptation of rat faecal microflora to cyclamate in vitro. Food Chem Toxicol 23:1029–1034

Mandelstam J, McQuillen K, Dawes I (eds) (1982) Biochemistry of bacterial growth, 3rd edn. Blackwell Scientific, Oxford

McBurney MI, Thompson LU (1987) Effect of human faecal inoculum on in vitro fermentation variables. Br J Nutr 58:233–243

McBurney MI, Thompson LU (1989) Effect of human faecal donor on in vitro fermentation variables. Scand J Gastroenterol 24:359–367

McBurney MI, Thompson LU (1990) Fermentative characteristics of cereal brans and vegetable fibres. Nutr Cancer 13:271–280

McBurney MI, Horvath PJ, Jeraci JL, Van Soest PJ (1985) Effect of in vitro fermentation using human faecal inoculum on the water-holding capacity of dietary fibre. Br J Nutr 53:17–24

McBurney MI, Thompson LU, Cuff DJ, Jenkins DJA (1988) Comparison of ileal effluents, dietary fibers and whole foods in predicting the physiological importance of colonic fermentation. Am J Gastroenterol 83:536–540

McCarthy RE, Salyers AA (1988) The effects of dietary fibre utilisation on the colonic microflora. In: Rowland IR (ed) Role of the gut flora in toxicity and cancer. Academic Press, London, pp 295–313

McNeil NI, Cummings JH, James WPT (1978) Short chain fatty acid absorption by the human large intestine. Gut 19:819–822

Midtvedt T, Carlstedt-Duke B, Höverstad T et al. (1986) Influence of peroral antibiotics upon the biotransformatory activity of the intestinal microflora in healthy subjects. Eur J Clin Invest 16:11–17

Miller TL, Wolin MJ (1981) Fermentation by the human large intestine microbial community in an in vitro semi-continuous culture system. Appl Environ Microbiol 42:400–407

Mitchell BL, Lawson MJ, Davies M et al. (1985) Volatile fatty acids in the human intestine: studies in surgical patients. Nutr Res 5:1089–1092

Moore WEC, Cato EP, Holdeman LV (1978) Some current concepts in intestinal bacteriology. Am J Clin Nutr 31:533–542

Mortensen PB, Holtug K, Ramussen HS (1988) Short chain fatty acid production from mono-disaccharides in a fecal incubation system: implications for colonic fermentation of dietary fiber in humans. J Nutr 118:321–325

Narducci F, Basotti G, Gabburi M, Morelli A (1987) Twenty-four-hour manometric recording of colonic motor activity in healthy man. Gut 28:17–25

Nyman MG, Asp N-G (1988) Fermentation of oat fibre in the rat intestinal tract. A study of different cellular areas. Am J Clin Nutr 48:274–279

Nyman MG, Asp N-G, Cummings J, Wiggins H (1986) Fermentation of dietary fibre in the intestinal tract comparison between man and rat. Br J Nutr 55:487–496

Perman JA, Modler S (1982) Glycoproteins as substrates for production of hydrogen and methane by colonic bacterial flora. Gastroenterology 83:388–393

Pomare EW, Branch WJ, Cummings JH (1985) Carbohydrate fermentation in the human colon and its relationship to acetate concentrations in venous blood. J Clin Invest 75:1448–1454

Read NW, Al-Janabi MN, Bates TE, Barber DC (1983) Effect of gastrointestinal intubation on the passage of a solid meal through the stomach and small intestine in humans. Gastroenterology 84:1568–1572

Roberton AM, Stanley RA (1982) In vitro utilization of mucin by *Bacteroides fragilis*. Appl Environ Microbiol 43:325–330

Roedigger WEW (1980) Role of anaerobic bacteria in the metabolic welfare of the colonic mucosa in man. Gut 21:793–798

Rowland IR and Mallett AK (1990) The influence of dietary fibre on microbial enzyme activity in the gut. In: Kritchevsky D et al. (eds) Dietary fibre: Chemistry, physiology and health effects. Plenum Press, New York, pp 195–206

Rowland IR, Mallett AK, Wise A (1985) The effect of diet on the mammalian gut microflora and its metabolic activities. CRC Crit Rev Toxicol 16:31–103

Rumessen JJ, Hamberg O, Gudmand-Hoyer E (1989) Influence of orocaecal transit time on hydrogen excretion after carbohydrate malabsorption. Gut 30:811–814

Rumney CJ (1989) In vitro study of the metabolic activities of bacteria from the human colon. PhD thesis, Robert Gordon's Institute for Technology, Aberdeen

Ruppin H, Bar-Meir S, Soergel KH, Wood CM, Schmitt MG (1980) Absorption of short chain fatty acids by the colon. Gastroenterology 78:1500–1507

Salyers AA, Leedle JAZ (1983) Carbohydrate metabolism in the human colon. In: Hentges D (ed) Microflora in health and disease. Academic Press, New York, pp 129–146

Salyers AA, O'Brien M (1980) Cellular location of enzymes involved in chondroitin sulfate breakdown by *Bacteroides thetaiotaomicron*. J Bacteriol 143:772–780

Salyers AA, Pajeau M (1989) Competitiveness of different polysaccharide utilization mutants of *Bacteroides thetaiotaomicron* in the intestinal tracts of germfree mice. Appl Environ Microbiol 55:2572–2578

Salyers AA, Vercellotti JR, West SEH, Wilkins TD (1977a) Fermentation of mucin and plant polysaccharide by strains of *Bacteroides* from the human colon. Appl Environ Microbiol 33:319–322

Salyers AA, West SEH, Vercellotti JR, Wilkins TD (1977b) Fermentation of mucins and plant polysaccharides by anaerobic bacteria from the human colon. Appl Environ Microbiol 34:529–533

Salyers AA, Gherardini F, O'Brien M (1981) Utilization of xylan by two species of human colonic *Bacteroides*. Appl Environ Microbiol 41:1065–1068

Schweizer TF, Anderson H, Langkilde AM, Reimann S, Torsdottir I (1990) Nutrients excreted in ileostomy effluents after consumption of mixed diets with beans or potatoes. II. Starch, dietary fibre and sugars. Eur J Clin Nutr 44:567–575

Snape WJ, Matarazzo SA, Cohen S (1978) Effect of eating and gastrointestinal hormones on colonic myoelectric and motor activity. Gastroenterology 75:373–378

Southgate DAT, Houston H, James WPT, Cummings JH, Branch W, Jenkins DJA (1978) Colonic response to dietary fibre from carrot, cabbage, apple, bran and guar gum. Lancet i:5–8

Tadesse K, Eastwood MA (1978) Metabolism of dietary fibre components in man assessed by breath hydrogen and methane. Br J Nutr 30:393–396

Thornton JR, Dryden A, Kelleher J, Losowsky MS (1986) Does super-efficient starch absorption promote diverticular disease? Br Med J 292:1708–1710

Tomlin J, Read NW, Edwards CA, Duerden BI (1988) The degradation of guar gum by individual strains of colonic bacteria in vivo. Microb Ecol Health Dis 1:163–167

Van Soest PJ, Jeraci J, Fosse T, Wrick K, Ehle F (1982) Comparative fermentation of fibre in man and other animals. In: Wallace CR, Bells L (eds) Fibre in human and animal nutrition. The Royal Society of New Zealand, Wellington, pp 75–80 (Bulletin 20)

Veilleux BG, Rowland I (1981) Simulation of the rat intestinal ecosystem using a two stage continuous culture system. J Gen Microbiol 123:103–115

Vercellotti JR, Salyers AA, Bullard WS, Wilkins TD (1977) Breakdown of mucin and plant polysaccharides in the human colon. Can J Biochem 55:1190–1196

Vince AJ, McNeil NI, Wager JD, Wrong DM (1990) The effect of lactulose, pectin, arabinogalactan and cellulose on the production of organic acids and metabolism of ammonia by intestinal bacteria in a faecal incubation system. Br J Nutr 63:17–26

Von Engelhardt W, Ronnau K, Rechkermanes G, Sakata T (1989) Absorption of short chain fatty acids and their role in the hindgut of monogastric animals. Anim Feed Sci Technol 23:43–53

Walter DJ, Eastwood MA, Brydon WG (1986) An experimental design to study colonic fibre fermentation in the rat: the duration of feeding. Br J Nutr 55:465–479

Walter DJ, Eastwood MA, Brydon WG, Elton RA (1988) Fermentation of wheat bran and gum arabic in rats fed an elemental diet. Br J Nutr 60:225–232

Wolin MJ (1981) Fermentation in the rumen and human large intestine. Science 213:1463–1468

Wrong O, Metcalfe-Gibson A, Morrison BI, Ing ST, Howard AV (1965) In vivo dialysis of faeces as a method of stool analysis. I. Technique and results in normal subjects. Clin Sci 28:357–375

Würsch P, Koellreutter B, Getaz F, Arnaud MJ (1990) Metabolism on maltitol by conventional rats and mice and germfree mice and comparative digestibility between maltitol and sorbitol in germ-free mice. Br J Nutr 63:7–15

Zarling EJ, Ruchim MA (1987) Protein origin of the volatile fatty acids isobutyrate and isovalerate in human stool. J Lab Clin Med 109:566–570

Commentary

Cummings: Methane is the major route for disposing of gaseous hydrogen (H_2) in fermentation. However in man not everyone excretes methane. In rural Africans about 80% to 90% of the population excrete methane, while this figure may be as low as 30% to 40% in some western adult groups. Methane is produced by methano-bacteria which are acquired in early life (usually after the age of two). Environmental influences are important. If neither parent produces methane then only 6% of children will do so. If one parent is a methane excretor, 50% of the children will be, whilst if both parents are excretors then 90% of the children will do so (Bond et al., 1971; Peled et al., 1985). Studies of identical twins however show that they may be discordant for methane. Furthermore, institutionalised people tend to have similar methane production status, thus suggesting an environmental rather than a genetic determinant. Non-methane excretors are likely to be carriers of sulphate reducing bacteria (SRB) in the bowel (Gibson et al., 1988, 1990). In marine sediments SRB outcompete methano-bacteria for H_2 and thus reduce methane excretion. In man, feeding sulphate by mouth will stop methane excretion in 50% of methanogenic subjects, and stimulate growth of SRB (Christl et al., 1990).

References

Bond JH, Engel RR, Levitt MD (1971) Factors influencing pulmonary methane excretion in man. J Exp Med 133:572–588

Christl SU, Gibson GR, Florin THJ, Cummings JH (1990) The role of dietary sulfate in the regulation of methanogenesis in the human large intestine. Gastroenterology 98:A164

Gibson GR, MacFarlane GT, Cummings JH (1988) Occurrence of sulphate-reducing bacteria in human faeces and the relationship of dissimilatory sulphate reduction to methanogenesis in the large gut. J Appl Bacteriol 65:103–111

Gibson GR, Cummings JH, MacFarlane GT et al. (1990) Alternative pathways for hydrogen disposal during fermentation in the human colon. Gut 31:679–683

Peled Y, Gilat T, Liberman E, Bujanover Y (1985) The development of methane production in childhood and adolescence. J Pediatr Gastroenterol Nutr 4:575–579

Chapter 7

Metabolism and Utilisation of Short Chain Fatty Acids Produced by Colonic Fermentation

C. Rémésy, C. Demigné and C. Morand

Background

Most of the carbohydrates of the fibre fraction are extensively broken down by the microflora when they reach the large intestine; this metabolic process results in the production of gas and short chain fatty acids (SCFA; essentially acetic, propionic and butyric acids). In non-ruminant mammals, including humans, the large intestine is the major site of SCFA production and they are extensively absorbed. The mechanisms for SCFA absorption depend on conditions prevailing in the intestinal lumen; basically, the SCFA always diffuse along the concentration gradient, mainly the non-ionised (protonated) form. However, SCFA absorption may involve facilitated transfers: when the lumen pH is close to neutral, SCFA absorption is parallel to a net secretion of bicarbonate (Hoverstad, 1986). This process contributes to water and mineral recovery from the large intestine. Absorption capacity from the human colon has been estimated at 200 to 700 mmol/24 hours (Cummings, 1984), which is in accordance with an estimated breakdown of 30 to 60 g carbohydrates in the colon. There is also a minor production of some other SCFA (isobutyrate, *n*-valerate, isovalerate), the iso C4 and C5 monocarboxylates chiefly arise from the de-amination of branched chain amino acids.

Other minor sources of SCFA in humans are SCFA consumed with fermented products (vinegar, sauerkraut) or butyrate from milk triglycerides. These SCFA are mainly absorbed in the upper part of the digestive tract, especially the stomach. In addition, the hepatic metabolism of ethanol may lead to a substantial production of acetate.

Metabolism of SCFA by the Digestive Tract

The SCFA absorbed from the large intestine are partly metabolised by the mucosa, directly during absorption itself by the colonic mucosa, or indirectly (SCFA present in the systemic blood) by the small intestine mucosa. Theoretically, the rate of absorption of aliphatic monocarboxylates increases in parallel to the chain length; yet, butyrate is found in a lower proportion in the blood draining the large intestine (the caecum, for example) than in the lumen (Rémésy and Demigné, 1976). It has been shown that butyrate is metabolised to CO_2 and ketone bodies by colonocytes; according to Roediger (1982), butyrate could be the major energetic fuel for colonocytes, in preference to glucose or glutamine. In the rat, ketogenesis from butyrate by the caecal wall is low, much lower than ketogenesis in the rumen wall or in the caecum of herbivorous species such as rabbits (Henning and Hird, 1972). In humans, ketone bodies production could be higher in the proximal than in the distal colon (Roediger, 1980). The hierarchy for energetic fuels for isolated colonocytes in vitro seems to be butyrate → acetoacetate → glutamine → glucose (Roediger, 1982; Ardawi and Newsholme, 1985), in contrast to the small intestine where 3-hydroxybutyrate is an important fuel. The metabolism of the other SCFA seems quite limited: propionate utilisation is very low (in the rumen there is a substantial capacity for propionate metabolism – to lactate essentially – but activation to propionyl-CoA is inhibited by butyrate). Acetate is also a minor substrate for the metabolism of the large intestine, however a noticeable utilisation has been reported in the distal colon of rabbit (Marty and Vernay, 1984) and in rat colonocytes (Fleming et al., 1991).

Besides their role as energetic fuels, SCFA affect various cellular processes in the large intestine. SCFA can stimulate proliferation of the colonic mucosa (Sakata and Yajima, 1984; Kripke et al., 1989) and SCFA infusion in the large intestine accelerates healing of colonic anastomosis in the rat, butyrate being the most effective (Rolandelli et al., 1986). Accordingly, germ-free animals exhibit atrophy of the large intestinal mucosa, together with altered capacities of absorption. It has also been shown, with cultures of carcinoma cells, that 1 mmol/l butyrate enhanced the doubling time from 26 to 72 hours and increased the proportion of cells expressing alkaline phosphatase (Whitehead et al., 1986). Insofar as butyrate is permanently present in the large intestine, its protective role against colon cancer is still questionable; nevertheless, it has been recently observed that subjects with adenomatous polyps or colon cancer have a significantly higher incidence of low butyrate fermentation (Weaver et al., 1988). The effect of SCFA on the digestive mucosa could be reinforced by the presence of fibres themselves, as illustrated by the effects of pectin on cell proliferation in the small intestine and the colon (Rombeau et al., 1989). Besides their direct effects, SCFA could also affect the development of intestinal mucosa via nervous or systemic humoral pathways (Sakata, 1986). It has been shown that butyrate may affect the expression of some oncogenes (Bahn et al., 1988; Herold and Rothenberg, 1988). The role of butyrate is nevertheless equivocal since it has been argued that sodium butyrate may act as a tumour promoter in the human colon by selecting for epithelial cells which have acquired a reduced response to terminal differentiation signals (Berry and Paraskeva, 1988).

The epithelial cells of the large intestine are exposed to very high concentrations of SCFA, up to 150 mmol/l (Rémésy and Demigné, 1976; Cummings, 1981; Bugaut, 1987). Due to their high diffusibility, these anions are potentially toxic for a great variety of cell types. In the colon, the rate of transfer from the lumen to the blood plasma is very high, which may hinder any accumulation in the colonocytes; another possibility is that the K_m of enzymes for activation of SCFA could be higher than in other tissues, to limit their metabolisation in the mucosa.

Comparison of SCFA and Glucose Absorption

Most of the data in the field have been collected on animal models, due to difficulties in sampling blood from portal-drained viscera in humans. In contrast to glucose, SCFA absorption is relatively continuous during the 24 hour light/dark cycle. SCFA absorption is minimum 2–3 hours after the beginning of food intake, during the dark period in the rat (Demigné and Rémésy, 1982). Even with a standard diet, there is a noticeable absorption of SCFA in the rat, all the more since glucose absorption is low under such conditions. Diets containing resistant starch are a useful model to study the replacement of glucose by SCFA. We have observed, by replacing 50% of wheat starch by amylomaize starch, that glucose absorption was 63% depressed whilst SCFA absorption was enhanced nine-fold. Furthermore, SCFA absorption was markedly higher than in control rats during the post-absorptive period. Comparable studies have been carried out in pigs (Rérat al., 1987) showing that, after a single meal containing 6% fibre, the 12-hour absorption of SCFA may range from 400 to 450 mmoles.

Hepatic Metabolism of SCFA

SCFA concentrations in the portal vein are closely dependent on the dietary fibre level (Fig. 7.1). In pigs, SCFA range from 0.5 to 1.0 mmol/l for acetate, from 0.15 to 0.30 mmol/l for propionate and are generally less than 0.10 mmol/l for butyrate (Rérat et al., 1987). In humans, data are still scarce: post mortem values have been presented by Cummings et al. (1987), namely acetate 0.26 mmol/l, propionate 0.09 mmol/l and butyrate 0.03 mmol/l. This probably

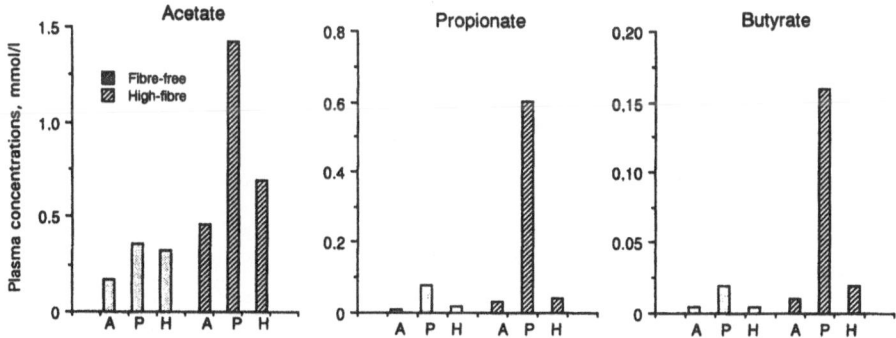

Fig. 7.1. Plasma concentrations of SCFA in the artery (A), portal vein (P) and hepatic vein (H). The rats were fed semi-purified diets containing basically 18% casein, 5% ground nut oil and 70% carbohydrate (with adequate mineral and vitamin supply, making up to 7% of the diet). The carbohydrate supply was either 70% wheat starch (fibre-free group) or 30% resistant starch (amylomaize starch), beet fibre (chiefly hemicellulose) 20%, wheat bran 15% and pectin 5%. The animals were sampled during the digestive period, namely 8 hours after the beginning of food intake.

reflects the fact that current occidental diets are rather poor in fibres; conceivably, higher values could be found in populations consuming high-fibre diets.

When present in physiological concentrations in the portal vein (max. 0.5 mmol/l) propionate and butyrate are almost completely taken up by the liver (hence, observed only in trace amounts in extrasplanchnic blood). In contrast, acetate is only partly taken up and this process is affected by the portal concentrations (in the physiological range, the higher the portal acetate the higher the hepatic uptake) and by physiological conditions (fed state, starvation, diabetes, etc.).

SCFA are activated to acyl-CoA with a concomitant production of adenosine monophosphate (AMP) and of pyrophosphate (PPi), by various short chain acyl-CoA synthetases. Acetyl-CoA synthetase activity has been described in liver cytosol ($K_m \approx 0.1$ mmol/l) and mitochondria ($K_m \approx 10$ mmol/l). Activation of propionate and butyrate takes place almost exclusively in the mitochondrial matrix. A propionyl-CoA synthetase (K_m 0.2 mmol/l) has been identified, but there is no specific butyryl-CoA synthetase in the liver (although butyrate is readily activated in liver mitochondria) and butyrate activation is probably mediated by medium chain acyl-CoA synthetase(s) (Groot et al., 1974; Scholte and Groot, 1975).

SCFA uptake by liver cells is very different under in vivo and in vitro conditions. In vitro, the plot of the rate of utilisation against medium concentration (Fig. 7.2) shows that acetate uptake is very low for concentrations lower than 1 mmol/l, whereas propionate or butyrate are readily metabolised (in

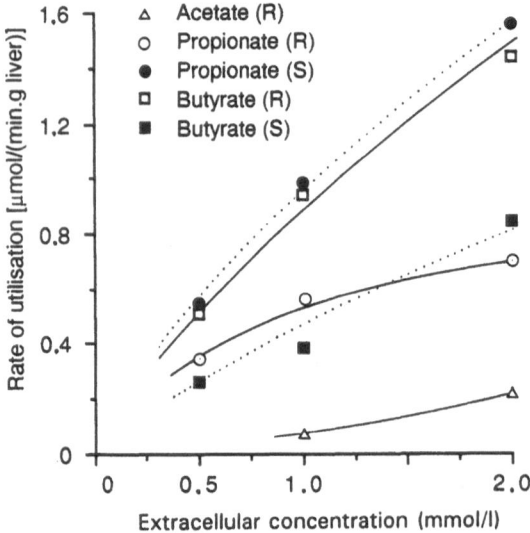

Fig. 7.2. Rates of propionate and butyrate utilisation by rat (R) or sheep (S) hepatocytes. The data represent measurements on six batches of cells for each species. The rate of SCFA utilisation was determined by sequential measurement of substrate disappearance from the medium over the initial period of linear uptake (See Demigné et al., 1986b). Acetate utilisation was hardly detectable at concentrations lower than 1.0 mmol/l and only data for rat hepatocytes are presented. Regressions are given as continuous lines for rat hepatocytes and as dotted lines for sheep hepatocytes.

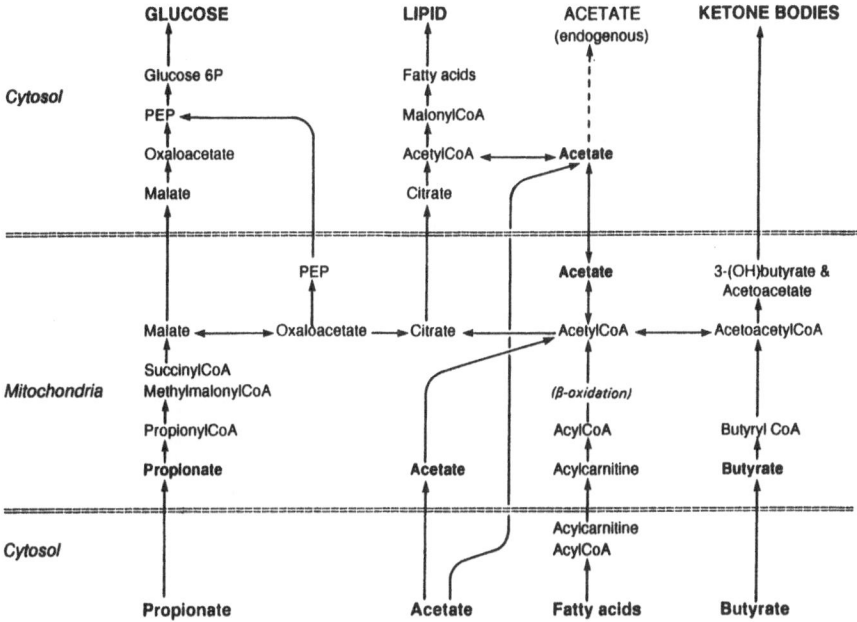

Fig. 7.3. General aspects of the metabolism of SCFA in the liver. PEP, phosphoenolpyruvate.

rat, butyrate → propionate; in sheep, propionate → butyrate; Demigné et al., 1986a). In vivo, the rate of acetate uptake is quite measurable in the rat (Buckley and Williamson, 1977), up to 0.5 μmol/(min. g liver) for 1 mmol/l acetate in afferent plasma (Demigné et al., 1986b). Furthermore, it is difficult to detect any difference in the uptake percentage of propionate and butyrate in vivo, close to 100%, in physiological conditions. However, when their concentrations are experimentally enhanced by SCFA infusion, it appears that the capacity for hepatic uptake saturates for higher concentrations of butyrate than of propionate (Rémésy et al., 1980).

A scheme summarising the hepatic metabolism of SCFA is shown in Fig. 7.3 and the metabolism of acetate, propionate and butyrate outlined below in more detail.

Acetate Metabolism

There is a relatively high capacity for acetate activation in the liver, and it has been long disputed as to whether acetate activation is predominantly cytosolic or mitochondrial (Snoswell et al., 1982; Söling and Rescher, 1985; Jessop et al., 1986; Crabtree et al., 1990). Theoretically, the low K_m (0.1 mmol/l) of the cytosolic isoenzyme supports the view that acetate activation is chiefly cytosolic. However, the pH conditions in the subcellular compartments should favour SCFA accumulation in the mitochondrial matrix ([mito]/[external] gradient ≈ 3) rather than in cytosol ([cytosol]/[external] gradient ≈ 0.6). Crabtree et al. (1990)

have proposed that most of acetyl-CoA synthesis from acetate occurs in the mitochondria and that the substrate cycling between acetate and acetyl-CoA in this compartment is very low, due to the fact that acetyl-CoA hydrolysis is chiefly cytosolic (see also Baranyai and Blum, 1989). This is consistent with the data of Inoue et al. (1989) showing that acetate leads to a dramatic accumulation of PPi in liver mitochondria, especially in the presence of noradrenaline and glucagon. In turn, in the presence of Ca^{++}, PPi accumulation can inhibit acetate metabolism (Inoue et al., 1989).

As for glucose, activated by a high-K_m kinase in the liver, high concentrations of acetate in portal blood are required for an effective utilisation of acetate. This is illustrated by the fact that, paradoxically, exogenous acetate utilisation is increased by ethanol, merely due to the rise in acetate and acetyl-CoA levels in hepatocytes (Baranyai and Blum, 1989). However, additional factors may play a role in the control of the hepatic metabolism of acetate: the cytosolic acetyl-CoA synthetase is inducible by insulin (like glucokinase) and it could account for most of acetate metabolism in situations of active lipogenesis (Del Boca and Flatt, 1969; Knowles et al., 1974). It is noteworthy that, in vitro in isolated hepatocytes, in parallel to glucose cycling, there is a high rate of acetyl-CoA hydrolysis which masks the effective activation of acetate in cytosol and mitochondria. Acetate may be released by the liver in vivo, provided that portal acetate concentration is low and that β-oxidation is activated (Buckley and Williamson, 1977) but this process is seldom observed in vivo, except in diabetics. Endogenous acetate constitutes a minor vehicle for the release of C2 units by the liver, compared to ketone bodies. High rates of acetate production are observed with ethanol only, and not from acetyl-CoA arising from β-oxidation of long chain fatty acids.

The metabolic effects of acetate will depend on its site of activation. When activated in the cytosol, acetate should constitute an effective precursor for lipogenesis (acetyl-CoA has been proposed as an inhibitor of carnitine acyltransferase, hence fatty oxidation; MacCormick et al., 1983). When activated in mitochondria, acetate can also contribute to lipogenesis: Des Rosiers et al. (1991) have shown that the pool of mitochondrial acetyl-CoA is not isotopically homogeneous and acetyl-CoA produced from acetate is preferentially used for citrate synthesis. Acetate activation in mitochondria could be inhibited by propionate and butyrate (Lumeng and Davis, 1973) which are activated by low-K_m acyl-CoA synthetases (which depletes the free CoA pool and enhances matrix PPi). If such an inhibition is effective with high-fibre diets, the cytosolic pathway should account for a substantial part of acetate metabolism. It seems that long chain fatty acids have priority for energy supply in the liver and acetate utilisation is rather channelled towards lipogenesis, this is illustrated by the observation that, in ruminants, the liver is a minor site for acetate utilisation and for lipogenesis (Pethick et al., 1981).

Propionate Metabolism

The hepatic uptake of propionate is mediated by a system (facilitated transfer) with a relatively low apparent K_m, about 0.15 mmol/l (Fafournoux et al., 1985). Once propionate has been activated in the mitochondria, propionyl-CoA is transformed into methylmalonyl-CoA (propionyl-CoA carboxylase, ATP dependent); the subsequent conversion to succinyl-CoA is mediated by a methylmalonyl-CoA mutase with vitamin B_{12} as a cofactor. The catabolism of certain amino acids also yields propionyl-CoA or succinyl-CoA (valine, isoleucine, methionine, threonine).

Propionate is an excellent precursor for gluconeogenesis since it is readily taken up and activated in the liver, and it does not depend on the rate-controlling step of pyruvate carboxylase. The net adenosine triphosphate (ATP) requirement for the conversion of 2 propionate into a glucose molecule is particularly low: 4 ATP, versus 6 ATP for {2 lactate → 1 glucose} or 10 ATP for {2 alanine → 1 glucose}. In rats fed a very high-fibre diet, propionate may be the major glucogenic substrate removed by the liver (Demigné et al., 1986a), all the more since propionate can inhibit the utilisation of the other glucogenic substrates, such as lactate (Blair et al., 1973; Anderson and Bridges, 1984). The various CoA intermediates of propionate metabolism may affect the activity of pyruvate carboxylase but this effect is complex since propionyl-CoA could be an activator whereas succinyl-CoA or methylmalonyl-CoA are inhibitors (Barritt et al., 1976). When there are large amounts of propionate, methylmalonyl-CoA accumulates (Corkey et al., 1982) because the methylmalonyl-CoA mutase is the rate-limiting enzyme of the pathway. A deficiency in vitamin B_{12} or in methylmalonyl-CoA mutase may lead to the accumulation of methylmalonate which is itself an inhibitor of gluconeogenesis (Arinze et al., 1979).

In herbivorous species, gluconeogenesis and glycogen synthesis are tightly dependent on the availability of propionate. In ruminant hepatocytes, it has been shown that propionate is a potent activator of glycogen synthetase, but in omnivorous species, lactate is a more efficient activator than propionate (Morand et al., 1990, 1991). In rats fed high-fibre diets, it appears that the average concentration of glycogen is lower than with a high-carbohydrate diet, but with limited fluctuations during the dark/light cycle owing to the continuous supply of SCFA from the digestive fermentations. It is still uncertain whether propionate is quantitatively utilised for gluconeogenesis in any circumstances. In monogastric species, gluconeogenesis is very low after a high-carbohydrate meal, yet propionate is completely metabolised by the liver. It is conceivable that propionate can provide acetyl-CoA, via the citrate cycle, like pyruvate or lactate. Even in ruminants, which have a permanently active gluconeogenesis in the liver, the yield of the conversion of propionate to glucose is lower than 100% (Bergman, 1990). In fact, the mitochondrial metabolism of propionate results in a rise in the redox state which limits gluconeogenesis from oxaloacetate. In this view, ethanol (which enhances both cytosolic and mitochondrial redox state) is a potent inhibitor of gluconeogenesis from propionate in ruminants and to a lesser extent in the rat (Demigné et al., 1991). The higher sensitivity to ethanol inhibition in the ruminant may reflect the fact that phosphoenolpyruvate carboxykinase (PEPCK) is present in the cytosol and in mitochondria (only cytosolic in the rat), as in humans. In fact, precise data are still lacking for humans. Insofar as a high rate of propionate utilisation might be connected to the presence of an active mitochondrial PEPCK, it is conceivable that the rate of propionate utilisation could be higher in humans than in rats.

Propionate may affect the rate of ureogenesis. This has been ascribed to the inhibition by propionyl-CoA of the synthesis of N-acetylglutamate, which activates the carbamoylphosphate synthase (CPS) (Coudé et al., 1979).

However, such an inhibition requires high concentrations of propionate since, at 0.5 mmol/l, the reaction with propionyl-CoA represents only 4% of that with acetyl-CoA (Sonoda and Tatibana, 1983). In turn, ammonia could affect propionate metabolism. There is an enhanced absorption of ammonia from the large intestine with high-fibre diets, in spite of an extensive utilisation of ammonia for bacterial proteosynthesis. SCFA are likely to provide energy for ureogenesis, together with acetyl-CoA for CPS activation. However, excess ammonia may inhibit propionate metabolism, or channel it towards the synthesis of amino acids rather than glucose. In the post-absorptive period, there is a progressive mobilisation of protein amino acids for gluconeogenesis and it would be interesting to assess whether propionate may contribute to spare protein during that period.

Several sites of impact on liver lipid metabolism have been reported for propionate. Propionate could inhibit the β-oxidation of fatty acids since propionyl-CoA leads to a "suicide-inactivation" of the FAD dehydrogenase of the even short chain acyl-CoA (Shaw and Engel, 1985). This inhibition should concern long chain fatty acids rather than butyrate. A part of the antiketogenic effects of propionate, besides an enhanced supply of oxaloacetate in mitochondria, could be ascribed to succinylation (using succinyl-CoA) of hydroxymethyl-glutaryl-CoA synthase (Lowe and Tubbs, 1985), a rate-limiting enzyme of the ketogenesis pathway. An inhibition of the acylcarnitine transferase I (hence of fatty acid transfer into mitochondria) by methylmalonyl-CoA has been observed in liver mitochondria from sheep (Brindle et al., 1985); however, the physiological relevance of this observation remains to be established (especially as to the existence of a cytosol pool of methylmalonyl-CoA).

Butyrate Metabolism

In contrast to acetate and propionate, there is a noticeable binding of butyrate to plasma albumin, from 10% in rat to 30% in sheep (Rémésy and Demigné, 1974); the capacity for hepatic uptake of butyrate is nevertheless very high, resulting in a quantitative uptake under any physiological conditions. Butyrate uptake could also be facilitated by the presence of a butyrate-binding protein in the cytosol (Marioka and Ono, 1978). Butyrate is a carnitine-independent source of acetyl-CoA in mitochondria and it is a ketogenic substrate during the post-absorptive period. In fed subjects, butyrate is certainly an excellent precursor for lipogenesis; furthermore, high concentrations of butyrate inhibit propionate utilisation (Demigné et al., 1986a). Due to the provision of acetyl-CoA in mitochondria, butyrate is an effective activator of gluconeogenesis from lactate and of ureogenesis; thus, butyrate probably thwarts some of the inhibitory effects of propionate on gluconeogenesis.

Butyrate has very specific effects on cellular metabolism, but studies on the relationship between butyrate and the orientations of hepatic metabolism are still scarce. It has been shown that the activation of butyrate leads to a dramatic accumulation of PPi which can trap the mitochondrial Ca^{2+}, especially after addition of calcium-dependent hormones (Davidson and Halestrap, 1988).

Butyrate also affects cell division and differentiation processes. One mechanism involves hyperacetylation of histones resulting from inhibition of histone deacylase, leading to arrest of cell proliferation (Kruh, 1982). More specifically, it has been shown that butyrate can modulate the expression of tyrosine aminotransferase, a highly inducible enzyme (Plesko et al., 1983; Staecker and Pitot, 1988). Like colonocytes, hepatocytes are probably adapted to a permanent supply of butyrate and other cell types might be more responsive to butyrate effects. This awaits further investigations on butyrate effects on hepatomas, especially secondary hepatomas.

Extrasplanchnic Metabolism of Acetate

A large portion of acetate arising from digestive fermentation escapes hepatic uptake (from 30% to 80%) and the splanchnic balance of acetate is always positive, even during fasting periods (Rémésy and Demigné, 1983). Most of the peripheral tissues can metabolise acetate: adipose tissue and mammary gland contain a cytosolic acetyl-CoA synthetase, and muscles, kidneys and the heart contain a mitochondrial enzyme (Groot et al., 1974). The cytosolic localisation should channel acetate towards lipogenesis whereas the mitochondrial localisation favours its utilisation for energy supply in the Krebs cycle.

The turnover of acetate is particularly rapid ($T\frac{1}{2} \approx 2$–4 min) and there are noticeable arteriovenous differences in muscles ($\approx 30\%$) (Rémésy, 1973). Acetate uptake by muscles is, to a large extent, dependent on its arterial concentration; this process has been extensively investigated since there are large changes in blood acetate after ethanol ingestion or during haemodialysis (Crouse et al., 1968; Desch et al., 1982). Acetate apparently fails to alter energy consumption by muscles and this suggests that it may replace long chain fatty acids as a fuel (Karlsson, 1976), all the more since acetate is antilipolytic (Abramson and Arky, 1968; Akanji et al., 1989). The utilisation of glucose by muscles is not affected by acetate, but glucose – probably via insulin secretion – enhances acetate utilisation. In consequence, there is a severe reduction in the peripheral utilisation of acetate and a considerable increase in systemic concentrations in diabetic animals (Knowles et al., 1974; Akanji and Hokaday, 1990). Most of the above data have been obtained with resting muscles; since acetate has vasodilator effects (Liang and Lowenstein, 1978), there is a possible role of acetate in exercise hyperaemia (Steffen et al., 1982).

SCFA and Lipid Metabolism

Dietary fibres have been reported to depress plasma lipids (Story, 1985; Vahouny, 1985; Mazur et al., 1990a). However, not all fibres display the same potency; generally, the soluble fibres are the most effective. Since these fibres are extensively broken down by the microflora, it is conceivable that their effects could be chiefly ascribed to SCFA. In this view, Chen et al. (1984) have suggested that propionate may have an hypocholesterolaemic effect. Such an effect has been experimentally observed in rats or pigs (Thacker and Bowland, 1981; Illman et al., 1988). It has been proposed that propionate decreases cholesterolaemia by shifting circulating cholesterol from serum to the tissue pool. However, this is not consistent with the fact that propionate is present only in trace amounts in peripheral blood.

The estimation of lipogenesis or cholesterogenesis rate using acetate as a precursor may be misleading in the presence of propionate, since propionate may inhibit acetate activation itself. In addition, propionate affects the availability of acetyl-CoA for lipid synthesis, by channelling it towards complete oxidation. More direct effects of propionate on the microsomal HMG-CoA reductase are still speculative, all the more since the various CoA esters of propionate metabolism are sequestered into mitochondria. Furthermore, it turns out that high concentrations of propionate in portal vein are unable to counteract the rise of the activity of HMG-CoA reductase observed in rats fed low-fat, high-fibre diets. The replacement of a part of dietary glucose by SCFA may considerably alter liver and peripheral metabolism as well as the hormonal status. For example, a high-fibre diet has been reported to normalise the insulin/glucagon ratio in obese Zucker rats (Mazur et al., 1990b). The suppressive effect of food intake on gluconeogenesis with a high-fibre diet is certainly less than with a high-carbohydrate diet; this should have repercussions on lipid metabolism since gluconeogenesis and lipogenesis are strongly antagonistic. In the liver, the general orientation of metabolism rather than SCFA themselves may condition the impact of fibre diets on lipid metabolism, all the more since SCFA provide C_2 units for lipogenesis. In adipose tissue, the supply of acetyl-CoA is frequently limiting for lipogenesis (Del Boca and Flatt, 1969) and acetate is an excellent substrate for acetyl-CoA synthesis; furthermore acetate and glucose synergistically stimulate lipogenesis.

Energy Aspects

The energy value of most fibres is not negligible: it has been estimated in the range of 2 kcal/g (Livesey, 1990) and this value essentially reflects the contribution of SCFA. Even with fibres that are completely broken down by the microflora, the energy losses (for the host) during digestion in the large intestine are substantial: gas production, utilisation of fuels for anabolic and energetic requirements of the microflora. Furthermore, once absorbed, SCFA have a relatively low calorie value per gram (acetate 3.49, propionate 4.96 and butyrate 6.16), and it must be kept in mind that acetate is the major SCFA absorbed. The yield of the metabolisable energy is lower for SCFA than for glucose (reference value: 100): from 84% for acetate to 87% for butyrate (Blaxter, 1971). This reflects the high cost of the energy of activation of SCFA, compared with the energy recovered. As a result, even with diets containing substantial amounts of fibre, the energy contribution of SCFA is probably limited (seldom higher than 5%) in humans; however, it is noteworthy that a large part (generally >50%) is metabolised in the liver, and it is conceivable that SCFA may have a noticeable impact on splanchnic tissues.

The specificities of the different SCFA have to be considered. Fermentation of fibre carbohydrates results in a considerable loss of glucogenic substrates, since only propionate is glucogenic (the contribution of *n*-valerate, isobutyrate and isovalerate is very low). As a result, fibres enhance the contribution of non-glucogenic substrates to energy metabolism. In peripheral tissues, acetate metabolism is tightly dependent on glycaemia and, in ruminant species acetate infusion alone leads to an increment of heat production, but glucose or propionate abolish this heat increment (Lobley and McRae, 1985). In humans, the contribution of acetate to energy metabolism is lower but heat increment has been shown upon ethanol administration and concomitant hypoglycaemia (Akanji et al., 1989).

Conclusion

In conclusion, dietary fibres affect metabolism in different ways: indirectly, on digestion (by delaying and decreasing glucose and lipid absorption), or directly by provision of SCFA. In the digestive tract various processes may result in enhanced losses of energy for the host; hypertrophy of some parts, increase in cell turnover, modification of peristalsis and irrigation. It must be noted that a part of this energy may be provided by SCFA themselves. In the liver, the hepatic lipogenesis is generally lower with high-fibre diets, but whether this is specifically due to SCFA or to an overall shift of hepatic metabolism is still uncertain. The substitution of glucose by SCFA probably leads to a lower efficiency of energy utilisation, but to an improved nitrogen retention (Vermorel, 1968). In this view, the utilisation of relatively high-fibre diets could be advocated for slimming treatments: the slower absorption of nutrients together with an almost continuous absorption of SCFA probably limits the periods of intensive storage of energy (as glycogen and lipids) and the concomitant episodes of hyperinsulinaemia. It appears that, quantitatively, the metabolic aspects of SCFA are now taken into account, but some other more qualitative effects on cell division and differentiation are becoming of increasing interest.

References

Abramson EA, Arky RA (1968) Acute antilipolytic effects of ethyl alcohol and acetate in man. J Lab Clin Med 72:105–118

Akanji AO, Hockaday TD (1990) Acetate tolerance and the kinetics of acetate utilization in diabetic and nondiabetic subjects. Am J Clin Nutr 51:112–118

Akanji AO, Bruce MA, Frayn KN (1989) Effect of acetate infusion on energy expenditure and substrate oxidation rates in non-diabetic and diabetic subjects. Eur J Clin Nutr 43:107–115

Anderson JW, Bridges SR (1984) Short chain fatty acid fermentation products of plant fiber affect glucose metabolism of isolated rat hepatocytes. Proc Soc Expt Biol Med 177:372–376

Ardawi MSM, Newsholme EA (1985) Fuel utilization on colonocytes of the rat. Biochem J 231:713–719

Arinze IJ, Waters D, Donaldson MK (1979) Effect of methylmalonic acid on gluconeogenesis in isolated rat and guinea-pig hepatocytes. Biochem J 184:717–719

Bahn RS, Zeller JC, Smith TJ (1988) Butyrate increases *c-erb* A oncogene expression in human colon fibroblasts. Biochem Biophys Res Comm 150:259–262

Baranyai JM, Blum JJ (1989) Quantitative analysis of intermediary metabolism in rat hepatocytes incubated in the presence and absence of ethanol with a substrate mixture including ketoleucine. Biochem J 258:121–140

Barritt GJ, Zander GL, Utter MF (1976) The regulation of pyruvate carboxylase activity in glucogenic tissues. In: Hanson RW, Mehiman MA (eds) Gluconeogenesis: its regulation in mammalian species. Wiley, New York, pp 3–46

Bergman EN (1990) Energy contribution of volatile fatty acids from the gastrointestinal tract in various species. Physiol Rev 70:567–590

Berry RD, Paraskeva C (1988) Expression of carcinoembryonic antigen by adenoma and carcinoma derived epithelial cell lines: possible marker of tumour progression and modulation of expression by sodium butyrate. Carcinogenesis 9:447–450

Blair JB, Cook DE, Lardy HA (1973) Interaction of propionate and lactate in the perfused rat liver. J Biol Chem 248:3608–3614

Blaxter KL (1971) Methods of measuring the energy metabolism of animals and the interpretation of the results obtained. Fed Proc 30:1436–1443

Brindle NPJ, Zammit VA, Pogson CI (1985) Inhibition of sheep liver carnitine palmitoyltransferase by methylmalonyl-CoA. Biochem Soc Trans 33:880–881

Buckley BM, Williamson DH (1977) Origin of blood acetate in the rat. Biochem J 166:539–545

Bugaut M (1987) Occurrence, absorption and metabolism of short chain fatty acids in the digestive tract of mammals. Comp Biochem Physiol 86B:439–472

Chen W-JL, Anderson JW, Jennings D (1984) Propionate may mediate the hypocholesterolemic effects of certain soluble plant fibers in cholesterol-fed rats. Proc Soc Exp Biol Med 175:215–218

Corkey BE, Martin-Requero A, Walajtys-Rode E, Williams RJ, Williamson JR (1982) Regulation of the branched chain α-ketoacid pathway in liver. J Biol Chem 257:9668–9676

Coudé FX, Sweetman L, Nyhan WL (1979) Inhibition by propionyl-coenzyme A of N-acetylglutamate synthetase in rat liver mitochondria. J Clin Invest 64:1544–1551

Crabtree B, Gordon M-J, Christie SL (1990) Measurement of the rates of acetyl-CoA hydrolysis and synthesis from acetate in rat hepatocytes and the role of these fluxes in substrate cycling. Biochem J 270:219–225

Crouse JR, Gerson CD, DeCarli LM, Lieber CS (1968) Role of acetate in the reduction of plasma free fatty acids produced by ethanol in man. J Lipid Res 9:509–512

Cummings JH (1981) Short chain fatty acids in the human colon. Gut 22:763–779

Cummings JH (1984) Colonic absorption: the importance of short chain fatty acids in man. Scand J Gastroenterol 20:88–99

Cummings JH, Pomare EW, Branch WJ, Naylor CPE, MacFarlane GT (1987) Short chain fatty acids in human large intestine, portal, hepatic and venous blood. Gut 28:1221–1227

Davidson AM, Halestrap AP (1988) Inorganic pyrophosphate is located primarily in the mitochondria of the hepatocyte and increases in parallel with the decrease in light-scattering induced by gluconeogenic hormones, butyrate and ionophore A23187. Biochem J 254:379–384

Del Boca J, Flatt JP (1969) Fatty acid synthesis from glucose and acetate and the control of lipogenesis in adipose tissue. Eur J Biochem 11:127–134

Demigné C, Rémésy C (1982) Influence of unrefined potato starch on cecal fermentations and volatile fatty acid absorption in rats. J Nutr 112:2227–2234

Demigné C, Yacoub C, Rémésy C (1986a) Effects of absorption of large amounts of volatile fatty acids on rat liver metabolism. J Nutr 116:77–86

Demigné C, Yacoub C, Rémésy C, Fafournoux P (1986b) Propionate and butyrate metabolism in rats or sheep hepatocytes. Biochim Biophys Acta 875:535–545

Demigné C, Yacoub C, Morand C, Rémésy C (1991) Interactions between propionate and aminoacid metabolism in sheep hepatocytes. Br J Nutr 65:301–317

Desch G, Polito C, Descomps B et al. (1982) Effect of acetate on ketogenesis during haemodialysis. J Lab Clin Med 99:98–106

Des Rosiers C, David F, Garneau M, Brunengraber H (1991) Nonhomogeneous labeling of liver mitochondrial acetyl-CoA. J Biol Chem 266:1574–1578

Fafournoux P, Rémésy C, Demigné C (1985) Propionate transport in rat liver cells. Biochim Biophys Acta 818:73–80

Fleming SE, Fitch MD, De Vries S, Knight C (1991) Nutrient utilization by cells isolated from rat jejunum, cecum and colon. J Nutr 121:869–878

Groot PHE, Scholte HR, Hülsmann WC (1974) Fatty acid activation: specificity, localization, and function. In: Paoletti R, Kritchevsky D (eds) Advances in lipid research. Academic Press, New York, pp 75–126

Henning SJ, Hird FJR (1972) Ketogenesis from butyrate and acetate by the caecum and the colon of rabbits. Biochem J 130:785–790

Herold KM, Rothenberg PG (1988) Evidence for a labile intermediate in the butyrate reduction of the level of c-myc RNA in SW837 rectal carcinoma cells. Oncogene 3:423–428

Hoverstad T (1986) Studies of short chain fatty acid absorption in man. Scand J Gastroenterol 21:257–260

Illman RJ, Topping DL, McIntosh GH et al. (1988) Hypocholesterolaemic effects of dietary propionate: studies in whole animals and perfused rat liver. Ann Nutr Metab 32:97–107

Inoue T, Yamada T, Furuya E, Tagawa K (1989) Ca^{2+}-induced accumulation of pyrophosphate in mitochondria during acetate metabolism. Biochem J 262:965–970

Jessop NS, Smith GH, Crabtree B (1986) Measurement of substrate cycle between acetate and acetyl-CoA in rat hepatocytes. Biochem Soc Trans 14:146–147

Karlsson N (1976) Acetate metabolism in skeletal muscle. Thesis, in: Acta Universitatis Upsaliensis, Uppsala

Knowles SE, Jarrett IG, Filsell OH, Ballard FJ (1974) Production and utilization of acetate in mammals. Biochem J 142:401–411

Kripke SA, Fox AD, Berman JM, Settle RG, Rombeau JL (1989) Stimulation of intestinal mucosal growth with intracolonic infusion of short chain fatty acids. J Parenteral Enteral Nutr 13:109–116

Kruh J (1982) Effects of sodium butyrate, a new pharmacological agent, on cells in culture. Molec Cell Biochem 42:65–82

Liang C-S, Lowenstein JM (1978) Metabolic control of the circulation. Effects of acetate and pyruvate. J Clin Invest 62:1029–1038

Livesey G (1990) Energy values of unavailable carbohydrate and diets: an inquiry and analysis. Am J Clin Nutr 51:617–637

Lobley GE, McRae JC (1985) Acetate utilization in sheep. In: Moe PW, Tyrrell HF, Reynolds PJ (eds) Energy metabolism of farm animals. Rowman & Littlefield, Beltsville, MD, pp 38–41

Lowe DM, Tubbs PK (1985) Succinylation and inactivation of 3-hydroxy-3-methylglutaryl-CoA synthase by succinyl-CoA and its possible relevance for the control of ketogenesis. Biochem J 232:37–42

Lumeng L, Davis J (1973) The oxidation of acetate by liver mitochondria. FEBS Lett 79:124–126

MacCormick K, Notar-Francesco VJ, Sriwatannakul K (1983) Inhibition by acetyl-CoA of hepatic carnitine acyltransferase and fatty acid oxidation. Biochem J 216:499–502

Marioka K, Ono T (1978) Butyrate-binding protein from rat and mouse liver. J Biochem 83:349–356

Marty J, Vernay M (1984) Absorption and metabolism of volatile fatty acids in the hind-gut of the rabbit. Br J Nutr 51:265–277

Mazur A, Rémésy C, Gueux E, Levrat M-A, Demigné C (1990a) Effects of diets rich in fermentable carbohydrates on plasma lipoprotein levels and on lipoprotein catabolism in rats. J Nutr 120:1037–1045

Mazur A, Rémésy C, Demigné C (1990b) The effect of high fibre diet on plasma lipoprotein and hormones in genetically obese Zucker rats. Eur J Clin Nutr 20:600–606

Morand C, Redon C, Rémésy C, Demigné C (1990) Non-hormonal and hormonal control of glycogen metabolism in isolated sheep liver cells. Int J Biochem 22:873–881

Morand C, Rémésy C, Demigné C (1991) Contrôle du métabolisme du glycogène au niveau du foie. Diabète Métabolisme (in press)

Pethick DW, Lindsay DB, Barker PJ, Northrop AJ (1981) Acetate supply and utilization by the tissues of the sheep in vivo. Br J Nutr 46:97–110

Plesko MM, Hargroves JL, Granner DK, Chalkley R (1983) Inhibition by sodium butyrate of enzyme induction by glucocorticoids and dibutyryl cyclic AMP. J Biol Chem 258:13738–13744

Rémésy C (1973) Contribution à l'étude de la production et du métabolisme des acides gras volatils chez le rat. Thèse, Université Clermont-Ferrand

Rémésy C, Demigné C (1974) Determination of volatile fatty acids in plasma after ethanolic extraction. Biochem J 141:86–91

Rémésy C, Demigné C (1976) Partition and absorption of volatile fatty acids in the alimentary canal of the rat. Ann Rech Vétér 7:39–55

Rémésy C, Demigné C (1983) Changes in availability of glucogenic and ketogenic substrates and liver metabolism in fed or starved rats. Ann Nutr Metab 27:57–70

Rémésy C, Demigné C, Chartier F (1980) Origin and utilization of volatile fatty acids in the rat. Reprod Nutr Develop 20:1339–1349

Rérat A, Fiszlewicz M, Giusi A, Vaugelade P (1987) Influence of meal frequency on postprandial variations in the production and absorption of volatile fatty acids in the digestive tract of the conscious pigs. J Anim Sci 64:448–456

Roediger WE (1980) Role of anaerobic bacteria in the welfare of the colonic mucosa in man. Gut 21:793–798

Roediger WE (1982) Utilization of nutrients by isolated epithelial cells of rat colon. Gastroenterology 83:424–429

Rolandelli RH, Koruda MJ, Settle RG, Rombeau JL (1986) Effects of intraluminal infusion of short chain fatty acids in the healing of colonic anastomosis in the rat. Surgery 100:198–200

Rombeau JL, Rolandelli RH, Kripke SA, Settle RG (1989) Citrus pectin and short chain fatty acids in intestinal dysfunction. In: Cummings JH (ed) The role of dietary fiber in enteral nutrition. Abbott International, Abbott Park, IL, pp 75–84

Sakata T (1986) Effects of indigestible dietary bulk and short chain fatty acids on the tissue weight and epithelial cell proliferation rate of the digestive tract in rats. J Nutr Sci Vitaminol 32:355–362

Sakata T, Yajima T (1984) Influence of short chain fatty acids on the epithelial cell division of digestive tract. Q J Exp Physiol 69:639–648

Scholte HR, Groot PHE (1975) Organ and intracellular localization of short-chain acyl-CoA synthetases in rat and guinea-pig. Biochim Biophys Acta 409:283–296

Shaw L, Engel PC (1985) The suicide inactivation of ox liver short chain acyl-CoA dehydrogenase by propionyl-CoA. Biochem J 230:723–731

Snoswell AM, Trimble RP, Fishlock RC, Storer GB, Topping DL (1982) Metabolic effects of acetate in perfused rat liver. Studies on ketogenesis, glucose output, lactate uptake and lipogenesis. Biochim Biophys Acta 716:290–297

Söling H-D, Rescher C (1985) On the regulation of cold-labile cytosolic and of mitochondrial acetyl-CoA hydrolase in rat liver. Eur J Biochem 147:111–117

Sonoda T, Tatibana M (1983) Purification of N-acetyl-L-glutamate synthetase from rat liver mitochondria and substrate and activator specificity of the enzyme. J Biol Chem 258:9839–9844

Staecker JL, Pitot HC (1988) The effect of sodium butyrate on tyrosine aminotransferase induction in primary cultures of normal adult rat hepatocytes. Arch Biochem Biophys 261:291–298

Steffen RP, McKenzie JE, Haddy FJ (1982) The possible role of acetate in exercise hyperemia in dog skeletal muscle. Pflügers Arch 392:315–321

Story JA (1985) Dietary fiber and lipid metabolism. Proc Soc Exp Biol Med 180:447–452

Thacker PA, Bowland JP (1981) Effects of dietary propionic acid on serum lipids and lipoproteins of pigs fed diets supplemented soybean meal or canula meal. Can J Anim Sci 61:439–448

Vahouny GV (1985) Dietary fiber and lipid metabolism. Fed Proc 41:2801–2806

Vermorel M (1968) Utilisation énergétique de la triacétine par le rat en croissance. Ann Biol Anim Bioch Biophys 8:453–455

Weaver GA, Krause JA, Miller TL, Wolin MJ (1988) Short chain fatty acid distributions of enema samples from a sigmoidoscopy population: an association of high acetate and low butyrate ratios with adenomatous polyps and colon cancer. Gut 29:1539–1542

Whitehead RH, Young GP, Bhatal PS (1986) Effects of short chain fatty acids on a new human colon carcinoma cell line (LIM1215). Gut 27:1457–1463

Commentary

Kritchevsky: Could you comment on the inhibition of cholesterol synthesis by propionate?

Authors' reply: The estimation of lipogenesis or cholesterogenesis rate in the presence of propionate is difficult, since propionate may inhibit acetate activation itself. In addition, propionate affects the availability of acetyl-CoA for lipid synthesis, by channelling it towards complete oxidation. More direct effects of propionate on microsomal HMG-CoA reductase are still speculative, all the more since the various CoA esters of propionate metabolism are confined in mitochondria. In fact high concentrations of propionate are unable to counteract the paradoxical induction of HMG-CoA reductase observed in rats fed low-fat, high-fibre diets.

Section II
Physiological Effects

Chapter 8

The Influence of Dietary Fibre on Protein Digestion and Utilisation

B.O. Eggum

Introduction

Dietary fibre (DF), an index mainly for plant cell wall materials, has recently received considerable attention with regard to its effect on protein digestion and utilisation. Not only has the number of studies and publications in the area increased exponentially but so has the number of high fibre food products available for the consumers.

Dietary fibre affects many processes along the entire gastro-intestinal tract from ingestion to excretion (Heaton, 1980). In the small intestine, however, the effect of DF depends on the chemical and structural composition of the plant cell wall. In general, purified viscous polysaccharides such as gums and pectin substances reduce the rate of nutrient absorption, whereas insoluble DF sources (e.g. wheat bran) will have only little effect on nutrient absorption in the small intestine. Consequently, DF may modify and usually decrease digestibility of proteins, along with lipids and certain minerals (Kritchevsky, 1988).

In the hind-gut DF profoundly alters the metabolism of the bacteria and as a consequence nitrogen metabolism is changed (Mason, 1984). The effect of fibre on nitrogen (N) balance and N excretory patterns is influenced by many factors, including its chemical composition and degradability (Eggum et al., 1984). The effect of fibre on the apparent digestibility of nitrogen depends on the nature of the DF, digestibility of dietary carbohydrates and the digestibility and level of dietary protein (Beames and Eggum, 1981). Furthermore, fibre reduces the transit time significantly (Raczynski et al., 1982), and thus leaves less time for microbial fermentation.

The proteins (or rather amino acids) not absorbed from the small intestine, including those of endogenous origin, will sustain the microbial population in the hind-gut with nitrogen (Beames and Eggum, 1981; Mason, 1984; MacFarlane et al., 1986). Together with the undigested carbohydrates that act as energy sources, nitrogen will stimulate microbial activity leading to substantial increases of bacterial nitrogen in the faecal matter.

Numerous studies have been carried out to study the effect of fibre on protein utilisation (as was reviewed by e.g. Eggum, 1973; Gallaher and Schneeman, 1986). Results obtained by different groups have been contradictory in that some found a decrease in protein utilisation with increasing fibre levels and others found no differences. Some of the contradictions may have been due to the type of fibre source that was included in the diets. For example, Eggum (1973) in work with rats found no effect of including cellulose powder up to a level of 30% in the diet on true protein digestibility, biological value and net protein utilisation of casein in rats. On the other hand, Breite (1973) and Meier and Poppe (1977) found a decrease in protein digestibility as well as amino acid availabilities when including increasing amounts of natural DF sources to rats. Hulls from faba beans, peas and sunflower seed were included at increasing levels in diets for rats containing 20% casein. No differences were found if sawdust or cellulose powder were used. Bergner et al. (1975) in work with labelled amino acids and wheat straw as a dietary fibre source presumed that native fibre influences the process of intestinal sloughing and in addition is able to adsorb amino acids, peptides or proteins.

However, the validity of the faecal analysis methods for determination of the apparent digestibility of protein and amino acids is often questioned partly because of endogenous protein secretions into the digestive tract and partly because of the effects of micro-organisms in the hind-gut. The micro-organisms may influence protein metabolism and thereby confound the determination of protein and amino acid digestibilities. Bacterial enzymes in the large intestine could bring about hydrolysis of undigested protein through peptides of decreasing length to free amino acids. These free amino acids may either be absorbed as such or broken down further to yield ammonia and carbon skeletons. The latter compounds, in turn, may be absorbed by the individual or be used for de novo bacterial protein synthesis (Mason, 1984). It is also demonstrated that amino acids infused into the caecum of pigs rather than fed orally led to almost complete and rapid excretion of their N into the urine and no improvement in N balance (Zebrowska, 1973, 1975; Just et al., 1981).

An additional problem would be to separate the influence of anti-nutritional factors associated to the fibres (Liener and Kakade, 1980; Bach Knudsen and Eggum, 1984; Vandergrift et al., 1983). It is also difficult to separate the nitrogen associated to the fibre having a low availability (Donangelo and Eggum, 1985) from other nitrogen containing material in faeces.

It appears from the discussion above that many factors can be of great importance when determining the influence of DF on protein digestion and utilisation in vivo. The present work will be discussing several of these aspects based on experiments with rats, pigs and humans.

Experiments with Rats

In balance studies with natural protein foods and feeds Eggum (1973) showed that there exists a strict negative relationship ($P<0.001$) between true protein digestibility (TD) and the fibre level in various protein sources. However, when replacing starch with pure cellulose powder in the diets from 0% to 30% of dry matter no relationship between the fibre level and TD or protein utilisation was found. These two studies indicate that fibre in natural food sources affects protein utilisation differently compared with purified fibre sources. However, in the review of Gallaher and Schneeman (1986) it could be seen also that purified fibres could have a negative effect on protein digestibility in studies on rats while the two human studies reported showed no effect of purified fibre on protein digestibility.

Many fibre-rich sources contain significant quantities of cell wall bound protein which can influence the digestibility data since part of this protein is indigestible (Donangelo and Eggum, 1985). This points out a potential difference in the source of faecal nitrogen between purified fibres and natural fibre-rich sources. For the purified fibres containing no cell wall bound protein, the source of faecal protein must derive from incomplete digestion of the dietary protein, secreted digestive enzymes, sloughed mucosal cells, and microbial protein. In the case of natural fibre sources, cell wall bound proteins will contribute to the faecal nitrogen. Thus, a low protein digestibility may be due in part to the presence of undigestible cell wall protein (Gallaher and Schneeman, 1986).

Agarwal and Chauhan (1989) found in experiments with Indian plant foods, high in dietary fibre, that the various food sources affected TD significantly and more than pure cellulose. TD of the cellulose group was thus significantly higher than any of the other food groups. It was also demonstrated in the same material that lignin had a much stronger negative effect on TD than hemicellulose, cellulose and pectin. In studies with 15 natural food sources Mongeau et al. (1989) showed that several food fibre fractions, and possibly associated substances, influenced protein digestibility. Purified cellulose did not have the same physiological behaviour as food cellulose from the viewpoint of protein digestibility and fibre fermentability which is in agreement with the studies of Agarwal and Chauhan (1989).

Radha and Geervani (1985) studied the influence of neutral detergent fibre from Bengal gram on the utilisation of protein in rats. Four market samples of Bengal gram varieties harvested at three different stages of maturity were used for the study. TD of Bengal gram ranged between 45% and 87% and net protein utilisation between 33.9% and 79.9%. It could be observed that digestibility decreased with maturity which probably is due to an increase in the neutral detergent fibre (NDF) content. The authors concluded from their study that it was evident that factors such as varietal differences, in the content of tannins, cellulose, hemicellulose and lignin have to be considered in accounting for low protein digestibility and utilisation. Storage changes might also be different from one variety to another.

Bach Knudsen and Eggum (1984) showed in balance experiments with rats – given botanically defined mill fractions of barley – that TD and digestible energy were negatively correlated to insoluble dietary fibre, acid detergent fibre (ADF), and tannin. The fibres of endosperm – soluble dietary fibre and β-glucans – did not contribute to any negative effect on digestibility. Insoluble fibre was more closely associated to TD than was ADF.

In a further study with the same botanical fractions of barley Bach Knudsen et al. (1984) showed that the microbial activity in the hind-gut was strongly influenced by the amount and type of nutrients reaching the lower gut. It was demonstrated that the aleuron fractions having a low digestibility in the small intestine, contributed significant amounts of easily fermentable energy and protein to the microflora in the hind-gut. In work with cereals Heger et al. (1990) found in balance experiments with rats a strict negative relationship between TD, soluble and insoluble fibre respectively, while the biological value was positively correlated with both fibre fractions. These works prove that DF in natural food sources affect nitrogen excretion patterns in rats significantly.

Increased loss of endogenous faecal nitrogen when fibre is added to the diet may be due to a number of factors. Increased secretion of digestive enzymes (trypsin, chymotrypsin, lipase and amylase) has been shown to occur when pectin is added to diets of rats (Foreman and Schneeman, 1980). The possibility that fibre might increase the sloughing of intestinal mucosal cells has been suggested (Bergner et al., 1975; Sheard and Schneeman, 1980). A lowering of intestinal reabsorption of endogenous amino acids secreted into the gut has been observed with a fibre-supplemented diet (Bergner et al., 1975). Any reduction in intestinal transit time associated with fibre-containing diets could also leave less time for digestion and absorption of dietary protein.

To understand the mechanisms by which fibre affects the utilisation of protein, the physico-chemical nature of the fibre material in conjunction with the observed effect on nitrogen digestibility, faecal nitrogen excretion and growth should be considered. Cellulose is a linear polymer of high molecular weight of glucose that has a very low solubility and no functional moieties other than the hydroxyl group. Pectin is a hydrophillic polymer that contains ionisable carboxylic groups of galacturonic acid (Shah et al., 1982). Depending on ionic conditions, and its degree of methyl esterifications, pectin may form either viscous solutions or a gel matrix (or indeed, both). This viscous property may decrease accessibility of protein molecules held in the matrix to the digestive enzymes and of the products of digestion to the absorptive sites. Further, it can inhibit enzyme activity and thereby increase proteolytic enzyme secretion. Pectin may also coat the absorptive lining of the gut thereby interfering with the absorption of the products of digestion.

Guar gum, a galactomannan contains only two sugars, galactose and mannose and produces solutions of very high viscosity. It shows physico-chemical properties similar to pectin, except that it lacks a uronic acid moiety. Unlike pectin, increasing levels of guar gum caused increased excretion of both dietary and endogenous faecal nitrogen per gram of food intake (Shah et al., 1982). As discussed by the authors the reason might possibly be that guar gum does not have acidic functional groups.

Lignin, a polymer of phenyl propyl alcohols and acids, is insoluble and hydrophobic in nature. The percentage of lignin in foods is lower than that of the other fibre components. The effect of lignin, while qualitatively similar to those of other fibres, must reflect in some way its unique structure, due, for example, to hydrophobic binding of essential amino acids (Shah et al., 1982).

Wheat bran contains protein, fat, starch, cellulose, pectin, lignin and uronic acid-containing hemicellulose (Anderson and Clydesdale, 1980). It may also contain protease inhibitors (Mistunaga, 1974). Therefore, wheat bran can be expected to affect protein utilisation via all the mechanisms discussed above as well as by direct inhibition of proteolysis. As shown by Kies and Fox (1978) increasing the level of wheat bran lowers apparent and true nitrogen digestibility by increasing the excretion of both endogenous and dietary faecal nitrogen per gram of food intake.

Rémésy and Demigné (1989) measured the specific effects of fermentable carbohydrates on blood urea flux and ammonia absorption in the rat caecum. Caecal weight and pH values were not different among rats fed diets containing 10% lactulose, pectin or guar gum, or 25% amylomaize starch. However, the caecal wall weight was markedly higher with lactulose feeding than with the other polysaccharides, whereas volatile fatty acid concentrations were lower with lactulose. The fibre diets depressed caecal ammonia, particularly in the case of the amylomaize starch diet, whereas the lactulose diet enhanced the concentration of ammonia. Owing to caecal enlargement and enhanced blood flow, the diets containing fermentable carbohydrates promoted a higher flux of urea to the caecum and also higher ammonia absorption in spite of low concentration of ammonia in the caecum. The study of Rémésy and Demigné (1989) suggests that fermentable fibre will affect protein metabolism in the rat significantly.

Conclusion from Experiments with Rats

From experiments with rats it can be concluded that fibre in general has a negative influence on protein digestibility and utilisation. However, purified fibre sources seem to have a lesser and often insignificant negative effect while fibre in natural food sources has a much more pronounced effect. The reason for this is certainly that nitrogen/protein associated with cell wall material is less digestible than regular storage plant proteins. Furthermore, anti-nutritional factors are often associated with the fibre-rich parts of plant foods and thus have a negative effect on protein utilisation. The influence of fibre is strongly determined by the chemical composition of the DF fraction. Fermentable fibre in the digestive tract will be a better energy source for the microflora than less fermentable DF – and thus more nitrogen will be built into microbial protein and thus escape absorption.

Experiments with Pigs

The fistulated pig is a frequently used animal model when studying the significance of the microflora in the digestive tract on the utilisation of various nutrients. Since the fistulation technique on pigs became routine more detailed information can be obtained as sampling of digesta can be performed at various sites of the digestive tract (Low and Zebrowska, 1989). As the microbial activity primarily is located to the hind-gut (Bach Knudsen et al., 1990) it is convenient to be able to sample digesta prior to this organ. By comparing values obtained on digesta collected at the terminal ileum with values obtained on faecal material a good estimate of the influence of the microbial activity on various nutrients can be obtained. Since dietary fibre can be metabolised only through microbial fermentation, under the use of nitrogen, this model will give detailed information concerning the influence of dietary fibre on protein digestion and utilisation.

The catabolic activities of the bacteria in the large intestine are closely related to the inflow of nitrogenous compounds which leave the ileum. These consist partly of undigested dietary residues but also substantial amounts of endogenous proteins from epithelial cells, mucus, as well as urea and bacteria (Zebrowska et al., 1977; Low, 1979).

The anabolic processes of the microflora are as dependent on available substrates as are the catabolic processes. The bacterial requirements for their own cell components and secretions are largely met by urea, ammonia, amino acids, and peptides, together with a suitable energy source – usually carbohydrate and mostly in the form of non-starch polysaccharides. The quantitative importance of this activity is indicated by the observation that 60%–80% of faecal nitrogen in pigs appears to be bacterial (Mason et al., 1976; Low et al., 1978; Meinl and Kreienbring, 1985). More recently, Mason et al. (1982) found that substitution of one-third of the cereal in a high-barley diet with grass meal increased faecal and bacterial N output by 60% and 63% respectively, resulting in a low protein digestibility.

Infusion of starch into the caecum of pigs given a barley-meal and bone meal diet (Zebrowska et al., 1980) depressed faecal apparent digestibility of nitrogen by 3–4 percentage units, and of amino acids by 4–7 percentage units, compared with the control group. N excretion in the urine was reduced, and N balance was unaffected, indicating that the route of nitrogen excretion was modified by starch and that microbial growth and metabolism was limited by the available energy supply. Similar conclusions have been drawn from studies by Just et al. (1981), Misir and Sauer (1982), and Zebrowska et al. (1984). When cellulose rather than starch was infused into the caecum of pigs, however, little effect on digestibility of N was observed by Zebrowska et al. (1978) because of its low fermentability. Mosenthin and Henkel (1983) and Mosenthin (1984) compared a basal diet with a diet supplemented with pure straw cellulose (120 g/kg) and pectin 80 g/kg in pigs fitted with ear-vein catheters. Urea labelled with ^{15}N was infused and faecal (^{15}N) ammonia and ^{15}N in bacteria were measured, as well as ^{15}N in urine. The supplemented diet led to increased faecal weight, bacteria, and N (^{15}N and unlabelled) and decreased urinary N (of both types), with no change in N balance. Ammonia labelled with ^{15}N appeared in faeces at the highest level after only 6 hours, while faecal output of bacterial ^{15}N was highest after 24 to 48 hours. It was concluded that blood urea served as a N source for bacteria in the gut: the rapid appearance of faecal (^{15}N) ammonia suggested that secretion of urea into the large intestine had occurred, while the delayed increase in incorporation into bacteria implied that the secretion was mainly into the small intestine.

It can be concluded that the large intestinal microflora has a significance for measurements of protein digestibility but the microflora of the stomach and small intestine are of importance. Dierick et al. (1990) could thus demonstrate that in ileum, 25% and in faecal digesta 45% of the total N was of bacterial origin.

Den Hartog et al. (1988) compared the effects of different carbohydrate sources on amino acid digestibility. They substituted 50 g/kg of a basal diet containing corn, barley, soybean meal, and meat meal with either pectin, cellulose, or ground straw (as a lignin-rich source). All amino acids (except arginine) were digested to a lower extent when straw meal was incorporated in the diet. There was no statistically significant effect of either pectin or cellulose inclusion on ileal amino acid digestibility. However, Dierick et al. (1983) found that the addition of pectin and sugar beet pulp had a much larger effect on ileal digestibility of essential and non-essential amino acids than addition of cellulose. There was a considerable reduction in digestion of the nutrients at the ileal level dependent on source and level of fibre. The influence of pectin and dried sugar beet pulp was much more pronounced than cellulose. The significant reduction in digestion of dry matter, protein and amino acids amounted to 10 to 15 units at the ileal level. The effect in the faeces was greatly reduced, illustrating the importance of hind-gut fermentation.

The referred works with fistulated pigs demonstrate an excellent model for studying the fate of undigested protein in the large bowel of monogastric animals and man and the importance of DF.

Conclusion from Experiments with Pigs

The referred experiments with pigs demonstrate a similar negative influence of dietary fibre on protein digestibility and utilisation as in rats. Purified fibre sources of low fermentability have a much lower negative effect than more fermentable fibres and fibres in natural foods. This is probably due to associated factors as anti-nutritional components in common feed and foodstuffs.

Experiments with Humans

As for the rat and pig, dietary fibre, more than any other dietary component affects the large bowel function of humans, causing an increase in stool output, dilution of colonic contents, a faster rate of passage through the gut and changes in the colonic metabolism of dietary fractions (Stephen and Cummings, 1980). It is thought that these changes are brought about by fibre passing through the gut undigested and holding water within its cellular structure. The way in which contrasting types of DF act in the large bowel depends on the extent to which they are digested.

In most studies of the effects of fibre on humans, cereal fibres were fed (Gallaher and Schneeman, 1986). However, Stephen and Cummings (1980) showed that cabbage fibre, which is extensively broken down, provides a readily usable substrate for the stimulation of microbial growth, whereas wheat fibre remains largely undigested and retains water in the gut lumen. These authors compared the effect of 18 g fibre given as wheat bran or as cabbage to a control diet. The changes seen with cabbage fibre were quite different: stool output increased by 54.3 g per day (69%), a smaller increase than with wheat fibre but nevertheless highly significant, transit time fell by 15.8 hours and nitrogen excretion increased from 1.5 g to 2.1 g per day.

Cabbage fibre influences colonic function through its stimulation of microbial growth. Analysis of the bacterial fraction for nitrogen in the study of Stephen and Cummings (1980) showed that 0.42 g of the 0.67 g per day (63%) increase in nitrogen excretion is associated with this fraction, whereas with wheat fibre only 0.18 g of the 0.53 g (34%) increase is in the bacteria. Two distinct mechanisms thus emerge whereby fibre affects the human colon. Stephen and Cummings (1980) assume that the stimulation of microbial growth is the more usual one in man because very little fibre survives digestion by the bacteria when sources such as apple, carrot, guar, pectin or mixed diets are fed. Wheat fibre, and most cereals in general, may prove to be the exception as they have small cells with highly lignified cell walls which resist digestion. The rest of the nitrogen is presumably present in the undigested cell wall material.

Kelsay et al. (1981) studied the effects of diets containing fruits and vegetables as sources of DF. A low-DF diet was compared with three diets containing increasing levels of fibre in fruits and vegetables. Mean NDF intakes on the four diets were 1.9, 10.1, 19.4 and 25.6 g/day for diets 1, 2, 3 and 4, respectively. Energy, nitrogen, and faecal fat excretions increased and apparent digestibilities decreased as the fibre content of the diet increased. Nitrogen digestibilities decreased from 89.9% on diet 1 (low in fibre) to 81.2% on diet 4 containing the highest amount of fruits and vegetables. Apparent digestibility of NDF was in the range of 30% to 40% for all diets and did not differ significantly. This indicates an active microbial protein fermentation which can explain the decreasing nitrogen digestibility with increasing fibre in the diets.

In a study with ileostomy patients receiving 15 g citrus pectin per day Sandberg et al. (1983) found only a slight increase in ileal output of nitrogen. It was concluded that this may either be due to decreased digestion and absorption of protein or increased endogenous losses of nitrogen.

Legumes in general have a low protein digestibility (Beames and Eggum, 1981). This was also confirmed in studies on man by Radha and Geervani (1984). They gave three cereal legume diets differing in NDF content to women in a balance study. The three groups were given either a low-fibre diet, a normal diet or a high-fibre diet. In this study the mean faecal excretion of nitrogen on a low-fibre diet was 2.13 g/day, while it was 2.50 g/day on a normal diet and 4.21 g/day on a high-fibre diet. The apparent protein digestibility of a high-fibre diet was significantly ($P < 0.01$) lower than on low-fibre diet. The percentage nitrogen retained expressed on the basis of intake in normal (19.6%), low-fibre (35.5%) and high-fibre (9.52%) diets were also proportional to the fibre content of the diet. The results indicate strict adverse influence of fibre on nitrogen utilisation. The study of Radha and Geervani (1984) demonstrates that dietary fibre might adversely affect the protein situation of a population when protein supply is marginal.

Kaneko et al. (1986) gave five female subjects four types of test diets (white or brown rice) containing various levels of protein and fibre for four consecutive 5-day periods. It was shown that apparent digestibility of protein was significantly depressed with an increasing fibre level from 0, 12, 16 to 18 g/day. The high-fibre diet (18 g/day) was based on brown rice and apparent protein digestibility was only 55.5% vs. 81.2% in a zero-fibre diet based on sugar and starch and soyprotein isolates. It could also be seen that the negative effect of fibre on apparent protein digestibility was more pronounced on a low-protein diet (27 g/day) compared to a high-protein diet (67 g/day).

In a study by Wisker et al. (1988) where the fibres almost exclusively originated from cereals, a low-fibre diet (19.7 g/day) and a high-fibre diet (48.3 g/day) were given and the digestibility of various dietary components measured. The main fibre constituents in both diets were polymers containing glucose, xylose and arabinose. Apparent digestibility of N was 87.4% in the low-fibre diet and 79.6% in the high-fibre diet. The corresponding digestibility for DF was 70.5% and 46.6% respectively. The authors concluded from their study that the reason for the lower digestibility of N in the high-fibre diet probably was due to a higher microbial protein synthesis and/or a higher proportion of dietary N associated with the fibre having a low digestibility.

The fate of undigested protein in the colon of man is not so intensively studied as in pigs although this topic has attracted special interest. Only few data are available concerning the physiological mechanisms which control protein breakdown or amino acid fermentation in vivo. About 50% of normal adults harbour methanogenic bacteria in their large intestine (Miller et al., 1984). The presence of methane-producing bacteria would probably alter the end-products formed during protein breakdown.

Protease activities in human ileal effluent are approximately 20 times greater than in normal faeces of man (MacFarlane et al., 1988). Substantial quantities of proteinaceous material enter the human large intestine (approx. 12 g/day) in the form of a complex mixture of proteins and peptides, that are of both endogenous and dietary origin. In the large gut, these substances are metabolised by the microflora to produce organic acids, toxic metabolites such as ammonia, phenols and indoles, and the gases hydrogen, carbon dioxide and methane (MacFarlane and Allison, 1986). The initial step in protein degradation by bacteria involves hydrolysis of the polypeptides and amino acids that are produced and then become available for assimilation.

MacFarlane et al. (1986) showed that human colonic contents are strongly proteolytic and it seems probable that this activity results from the continued actions of both bacterial and host-produced proteases (Bohe et al., 1983). However, the nature of the bacterial contribution to the large gut proteolysis is far from clear. MacFarlane et al. (1988) have shown that high levels of proteolytic activity occur in human faeces and that a large proportion of this activity is of microbial origin. Proteolysis is the first step in the utilisation of protein by bacteria and the large oligopeptides which are initially formed are subsequently degraded into smaller peptides and amino acids (Hespell and Smith, 1983) which can be either assimilated directly into microbial protein or fermented with the production of ammonia and volatile fatty acids (Allison, 1978). At present, few data are available concerning the extent and nature of protein degradation in the human colon, or of the proteolytic bacteria which may take part in this process, although it appears likely that a combination of microbial and pancreas derived proteolytic enzymes (trypsin, chymotrypsin and elastase) may be involved (Prins, 1977).

Conclusion from Experiments with Humans

Although less detailed information is available from studies on humans compared with rats and pigs concerning the influence of fibre on protein digestion and utilisation, very similar conclusions can be drawn. Fibre, especially fibre associated with natural food sources, has a negative influence on protein utilisation. The influence depends greatly on the structure and composition of the dietary fibre. Soluble dietary fibre found primarily in fruits and vegetables is more fermentable than insoluble fibre, mainly found in cereals, and will as such stimulate microbial growth resulting in a relatively high excretion of microbial proteins together with undigested protein.

General Conclusion

In this review the current knowledge of the effects of dietary fibre and associated components on protein digestibility and utilisation are discussed. Results from rats, pigs and humans are included. Although it is not fully understood how DF affects the utilisation of various nutrients, it can be concluded that the implications and the mechanisms behind the effect of soluble and insoluble DF on protein digestibility and utilisation are quite different. Hence, insoluble DF, because of its low degradability by the microflora will effect increased faecal bulk and faecal nitrogen excretion primary due to an increased excretion of cell wall bound protein. Contrary to this, soluble DF increases faecal bulk and faecal nitrogen due to an increased excretion of microbial nitrogen. The overall effect of both mechanisms is a decrease in apparent protein digestibility. Furthermore anti-nutritional factors are often associated with the fibrous parts of plant foods, which can have an additional negative effect on protein digestibility and utilisation.

A number of studies suggest that fibrous products and leguminous foods in particular, will have an adverse effect on protein utilisation. People in the Western World in general consume excess amounts of protein from animal sources, hence, the risk of developing protein deficiencies due to increased fibre consumption is very low indeed. However, as a general rule, when major dietary changes are recommended for any population group (as is the case for dietary fibre) the overall nutritional effects should be considered. The situation for the people in the Third World countries, however, is somewhat different. People consuming the highest amounts of dietary fibre are often the same people who are marginal in dietary protein. A reduced protein utilisation due to fibre might make the difference between protein adequacy and inadequacy under these conditions.

A matter of controversy is the influence of DF on endogenous nitrogen excretion and factors affecting the losses of nitrogen in this way. Although it is now widely recognised that very substantial amounts of protein are secreted into the digestive tract, it is not known if fibre as a dietary component acts as a secretogogue. Such information could lead to methods of reducing endogenous losses with consequent improved metabolic efficiency of dietary protein. It is still extremely hazardous to distinguish with confidence between dietary and endogenous proteins within the digestive tract, although knowledge of such partition would be helpful in interpreting data on digestibility of dietary proteins. Fundamental studies on the hormonal regulation of endogenous secretions are clearly worthwhile from both fundamental and practical viewpoints.

References

Agarwal V, Chauhan BM (1989) Effect of feeding some plant foods as source of dietary fibre on biological utilization of diet in rats. Plant Foods Hum Nutr 39:161–167

Allison MJ (1978) Production of branched chain volatile fatty acids by certain anaerobic bacteria. Appl Environ Microbiol 35:872–877

Anderson NE, Clydesdale FM (1980) An analysis of the dietary fiber content of a standard wheat bran. J Food Sci 45:336–340

Bach Knudsen KE, Eggum BO (1984) The nutritive value of botanically defined mill fractions of barley. 3. The protein and energy value of pericarp, testa, germ, aleuron, and endosperm-rich decortication fractions of the variety Bomi. Z Tierphysiol Tierernährg u Futtermittelkde 51:130–148

Bach Knudsen KE, Wolstrup J, Eggum BO (1984) The nutritive value of botanically defined mill fractions of barley. 4. The influence of hindgut microflora in rats on digestibility of protein and energy of pericarp, testa, germ, aleuron and endosperm-rich decortication fractions of the variety Bomi. Z Tierphysiol Tierernährg u Futtermittelkde 52:182–193

Bach Knudsen KE, Borg Jensen B, Andersen JO, Hansen I (1990) Gastrointestinal implications in pigs of wheat and oat fractions. 2. Microbial activity in the gastrointestinal tract. Br J Nutr 65:233–248

Beames RM, Eggum BO (1981) The effect of type and level of protein, fibre and starch on nitrogen excretion patterns in rats. Br J Nutr 46:301–313

Bergner H, Simon O, Zimmer M (1975) Contents of crude fiber in the diet as affecting the process of amino acid resorption in rats. Arch Tierernährg 25:95–104

Bohe M, Borgstrom S, Ohlsson GK (1983) Determination of immunoreactive trypsin, pancreatic elastase and chymotrypsin in extracts of human feces and ileostomy drainage. Digestion 27:8–15

Breite S (1973) Modelluntersuchungen zum Einfluss exogener Faktoren auf die Aminosäuren-resorbierbarkeit. Dissertation (Promotion A), University of Rostock

Den Hartog KA, Huisman J, Thielen WJG, Van Schayk GHA, Boer H, Van Weerden EJ (1988) The effect of including various structural polysaccharides in pig diets on ileal and faecal digestibility of amino acids and minerals. Livestock Prod Sci 18:157–170

Dierick N, Vervaeke I, Decuypere J, Henderickx HK (1983) Influence de la nature et du niveau des fibres brutes sur la digestibilité iléale et fécale apparente de la matiére séche, des proteines et des acides aminée et sur la rétention azotée chez les porcs. Revue de l'agriculture 36:1691–1712

Dierick NA, Vervaeke IJ, Decuypere JA, Henderickx HK (1990) Bacterial protein synthesis in relation to organic matter digestion in the hindgut of growing pigs; contribution of hindgut fermentation to total energy supply and growth performances. J Anim Physiol Anim Nutr 63:220–235

Donangelo CM, Eggum BO (1985) Comparative effects of wheat bran and barley husk on nutrient utilization in rats 1. Protein and energy. Br J Nutr 54:741–751

Eggum BO (1973) A study of ceratin factors influencing protein utilization in rats and pigs. Rep. No 406, Nat Inst Anim Sci, Copenhagen, pp 1–173

Eggum BO, Beames RM, Wolstrup J, Bach Knudsen KE (1984) The effect of protein quality and fibre level in the diet and microbial activity in the digestive tract on protein utilization and energy digestibility in rats. Br J Nutr 51:305–314

Foreman LP, Schneeman BO (1980) Effects of dietary pectin and fat on the small intestinal contents and exocrine pancreas of rats. J Nutr 110:1992–1999

Gallaher D, Schneeman (1986) Effect of dietary fiber on protein digestibility and utilization. In: Spiller GA (ed) Handbook of dietary fiber in human nutrition. CRC Press, Boca Raton, pp 143–164

Heaton KW (1980) Dietary fibre in perspective. Hum Nutr Clin Nutr 37C:151–170

Heger J, Salek M, Eggum BO (1990) Nutritional value of some Czechoslovak varieties of wheat, triticale and rye. Anim Feed Sci Technol 29:89–100

Hespell RB, Smith CJ (1983) Utilization of nitrogen sources by gastrointestinal tract bacteria. In: Hentges DJ (ed) Human intestinal microflora in health and disease. Academic Press, London, pp 167–187

Just A, Jørgensen H, Fernandez JA (1981) The digestive capacity of the caecum-colon and the value of the nitrogen absorbed from the hind-gut for protein synthesis in pigs. Br J Nutr 46:209–219

Kaneko K, Nishida K, Yatsuda J, Osa S, Koike G (1986) Effect of fiber on protein, fat and calcium digestibilities and fecal cholesterol excretion. J Nutr Sci 32:317–325

Kelsay JL, Clark WM, Herbst BJ, Prather ES (1981) Nutrient utilization by human subjects concerning fruits and vegetables as sources of fiber. J Agric Food Chem 29:461–465

Kies C, Fox HM (1978) Fiber and protein nutritional status. Cereal Foods World 23:249–252

Kritchevsky D (1988) Dietary fiber. Ann Rev Nutr 8:301–328

Liener IE, Kakade ML (1980) Protease inhibitors. In: Liener GE (ed) Toxic constituents of plant foods. Academic Press, New York, pp 7–71

Low AG (1979) Studies on digestion and absorption in the intestines of growing pigs. 6. Measurements of the flow of amino acids. Br J Nutr 41:147–156

Low AG, Zebrowksa T (1989) Digestion in pigs. In: Bock H-D, Eggum BO, Low AG, Simon O, Zebrowska T (eds) Protein metabolism in farm animals. Oxford University Press, Oxford, pp 53–121

Low AG, Sambrook IE, Yoshimoto JT (1978) Studies on the true digestibility of nitrogen (N) and amino acids in growing pigs. EAAP 29th Annual Meeting, Stockholm

MacFarlane GT, Allison C (1986) Utilisation of protein by human gut bacteria. FEMS Microbiol Ecol 38:19–24

MacFarlane GT, Cummings JH, Allison C (1986) Protein degradation by human intestinal bacteria. J Gen Microbiol 132:1647–1656

MacFarlane GT, Allison C, Gibson SAW, Cummings JH (1988) Contribution of the microflora to proteolysis in the human large intestine. J Appl Bacteriol 64:37–46

Mason VC (1984) Metabolism of nitrogenous compounds in the large gut. Proc Nutr Soc 43:45–53

Mason VC, Just A, Bech-Andersen S (1976) Bacterial activity in the hind-gut of pigs. 2. Its influence on the apparent digestibility of nitrogen and amino acids. Z Tierphysiol Tierernährg u Futtermittelkde 36:310–324

Mason VC, Kragelund Z, Eggum BO (1982) Influence of fibre and Nebacetin on microbial activity and amino acid digestibility in the pig and rat. Z Tierphysiol Tierernährg u Futtermittelkde 48:241–252

Meier H, Poppe S (1977) Zum Einfluss der Rohfaser aut die wahre Verdaulichkeit der Aminosäuren. Vth international symposium on amino acids, Budapest

Meinl M, Kreienbring F (1985) Investigations into the bacterial contribution in pig faeces. Arch f Tierernährg 35:33–44

Miller TL, Weaver GA, Wolin M (1984) Methanogens and anaerobes in a colon segment isolated from the normal fecal stream. Appl Environ Microbiol 48:449–450

Misir R, Sauer WC (1982) Effect of starch infusion at the terminal ileum on nitrogen balance and apparent digestibilities of nitrogen and amino acids in pigs fed meat-and-bone and soyabean meal diets. J Anim Sci 55:599–607

Mistunaga T (1974) Some properties of protease inhibitor in wheat grain. J Nutr Sci Vitaminol 20:153–159

Mitaru BN, Blair R (1984) The influence of dietary fibre sources on growth, feed efficiency and digestibilities of dry matter and protein in rats. J Sci Food Agric 35:625–631

Mongeau R, Sarwar G, Peace RW, Brassard R (1989) Relationship between dietary fiber levels and protein digestibility in selected foods as determined in rats. Plant Foods Hum Nutr 39:45–51

Mosenthin R (1984) Blood urea as a source of nitrogen for bacteria in the intestine of the pig. Proceedings of the VII international symposium on amino acids, Polish Scientific Publishers, Warsaw, pp 396–400

Mosenthin R, Henkel H (1983) Effects of dietary fibre content on nitrogen metabolism in pigs. In: Protein metabolism and nutrition. Les colloques de l'INRA No 16, Paris

Prins RA (1977) Biochemical activities of gut microorganism. In: Clarke RT, Banchop T (eds) Microbial ecology of the gut. Academic Press, New York, pp 73–183

Radha V, Geervani P (1984) Utilisation of protein and calcium in adult women on cereal legume diets containing varying amounts of fibre. Nutr Rep Intr 30:859–864

Radha V, Geervani P (1985) Influence of neutral detergent fibre and protein in Bengal Gram (*Cicer arietinum*) on the utilization of proteins by albino rats. J Sci Food Agric 36:1212–1218

Raczynski G, Eggum BO, Chwalibog A (1982) The effect of dietary composition on transit time in rats. Z Tierphysiol Tiernährg u Futtermittelkde 47:160–167

Rémésy C, Demigné C (1989) Specific effects of fermentable carbohydrates on blood urea flux and ammonia absorption in the rat cecum. J Nutr 119:560–565

Sandberg A-S, Ahderinne R, Andersson H, Hallgren B, Hulten L (1983) The effect of citrus pectin on the absorption of nutrients in the small intestine. Hum Nutr Clin Nutr 37C:171–183

Shah N, Atallah MT, Mahoney RR, Pellett PL (1982) Effect of dietary fiber components on fecal nitrogen excretion and protein utilization in growing rats. J Nutr 112:658–666

Shah N, Mahoney RR, Pellet PL (1986) Effect of guar gum, lignin and pectin on proteolytic enzyme levels in the gastrointestinal tract of the rat: a time-based study. J Nutr 116:786–794

Sheard NF, Schneeman BO (1980) Wheat bran's effect on digestive enzyme activity and bile acid levels in rats. J Food Sci 45:1645–1648

Stephen AM, Cummings JH (1980) Mechanism of action of dietary fibre in the human colon. Nature 284:283–284

Vandergrift WL, Knabe DA, Thanksley TD, Anderson J (1983) Digestibility of nutrients in raw and heated soyaflakes for pigs. J Anim Sci 57:1215–1224

Wisker E, Maltz A, Feldheim W (1988) Metabolizable energy of diets low or high in dietary fiber from cereals when eaten by humans. J Nutr 118:945–952

Zebrowska T (1973) Digestion and absorption of nitrogenous compounds in the large intestine of pigs. Rocznik Nauk Rolniczych 95B(3):85–90

Zebrowska T (1975) The apparent digestibility of nitrogen and individual amino acids in the large intestine of pigs. Rocznik Nauk Rolniczych 97B(1):117–123

Zebrowska T, Buraczewska L, Buraczewski S (1977) The apparent digestibility of amino acids in the small intestine and the whole digestive tract of pigs fed diets containing different sources of protein. Roczniki Nauk Rolniczych 99B(1):87–98

Zebrowska T, Buraczewska L, Horaczynski H (1978) Apparent digestibility of nitrogen and amino acids and utilization of protein given orally or introduced into the large intestine of pigs. Roczniki Nauk Rolniczych 99B:99–105

Zebrowska T, Zebrowska H, Buraczewska L (1980) The relationship between amount and type of carbohydrates entering the large intestine and nitrogen excretion in faeces and urine of pigs. Proceedings 3rd EAAP symposium on protein metabolism and nutrition, pp 222–226 (EAAP publication no. 27)

Zebrowska T, Buraczewska L, Zebrowska H (1984) Influence of crude fibre on apparent digestibility of nitrogen and amino acids in growing pigs. Proceedings of VI international symposium on amino acids. Polish Scientific Publishers, Warsaw, pp 142–146

Chapter 9

The Influence of Dietary Fibre on Lipid Digestion and Absorption

I.T. Johnson

Introduction

Even before dietary fibre had become a major focus for research, there was evidence to show that diets rich in plant cell walls were associated with elevated faecal energy losses in man, and that part of this increase was due to lipids (Widdowson, 1955; Southgate and Durnin, 1970; Baird et al., 1977; Kelsay et al., 1978). Such losses seldom amount to more than 2–4 g/day however, and are of little nutritional significance in themselves.

Nevertheless there is substantial evidence to show that plant cell polysaccharides exert a subtle influence over the rate and site of lipid absorption. The purpose of this chapter is to review the mechanisms underlying this effect and its interactions with systemic lipid metabolism.

Digestion and Absorption of Dietary Fat

In the plants and animals from which human foods are derived, lipids are stored predominantly as long chain triglycerides. These take the form of intracellular oil droplets, stabilised by a surface layer of phospholipids. Cellular membranes also provide a significant source of dietary phospholipids. Western adults consume about 150 g of triglycerides, together with 4–8 g of phospholipids per day. In addition approximately 20 g of endogenous lecithin, which enters the small intestine in bile, must be reabsorbed (Carey et al., 1983).

Since long chain triglycerides and lecithin are virtually insoluble in water, the first stage in the digestion of dietary lipids is the formation of a finely dispersed emulsion. The mechanical energy required for effective emulsification is supplied by the shear forces of gastric and duodenal peristalsis. Phospholipids and other food components act as chemical emulsifiers within the gastric lumen. The process continues in the duodenum, where, in the presence of bile salts, the further dispersion of lipid droplets proceeds to a size range suitable for efficient lipolysis.

Both salivary and pancreatic lipases are of importance in human fat digestion although salivary activity is probably of considerably more significance in the neonate than in adults. Salivary amylase has a pH optimum of 4–4.5 and is, therefore, active in the partially buffered gastric contents. In the rat, gastric lipolysis by lingual lipase has been shown to facilitate subsequent pancreatic lipase activity (Plucinski et al., 1979). Gargouri and co-workers (1986) have recently proposed that human gastric lipase activity releases a significant proportion of fatty acids in the stomach, and thereby promotes lipid emulsification, and facilitates the rapid initiation of pancreatic lipase activity in the duodenum. Hydrolysis of triglyceride by pancreatic lipase, together with hydrolysis of phospholipids and cholesterol esters, by phospholipase A2 and cholesterol esterase respectively, is completed in the duodenum. Pancreatic lipase and phospholipase act at the surface of emulsified lipid droplets, and require the presence of bile salts, calcium, and a protein co-factor, colipase.

The products of lipid hydrolysis are dispersed as liposomes and enriched mixed micelles which diffuse towards the mucosal surface of the duodenum and proximal jejunum. Monoglycerides, free fatty acids, cholesterol and phospholipids are taken up by the enterocytes. Bile salts remain in the jejunal lumen, but are eventually reabsorbed by a carrier-mediated mechanism in the distal ileum, and recirculated to bile via the liver. Before the products of lipolysis can be absorbed, the micelles must traverse a poorly stirred aqueous microclimate, the surface mucous layer overlying the mucosa, and finally the brush-border membrane. This final step appears to occur by passive, unmediated diffusion, although evidence for carrier-mediated diffusion of essential fatty acids at low concentrations has been reported (Chow and Hollander, 1978, 1979).

Several mechanisms operate to reduce the intracellular concentration of free fatty acids and thereby maintain an inwardly directed concentration gradient. Fatty acids with chain lengths of less than 12 carbon units are absorbed predominantly in the unesterified form and pass directly to the liver via the venous portal route (Vallot et al., 1985). A significant proportion of long chain unsaturated fatty acids are taken up by a high-affinity, cytoplasmic binding protein. For fatty acids with chain lengths between 14 and 24 carbon units, the next step is energy dependent re-esterification with 2-monoacylglycerols to form triacylglycerols. Absorbed phospholipids are re-esterified to form phosphatidylcholine. Newly formed oil droplets pass to the rough endoplasmic reticulum, where phospholipids and apolipoproteins are synthesised and incorporated. Functionally complete chylomicrons are formed in the Golgi apparatus by the addition of carbohydrate moieties to the apolipoproteins. These stable particles are extruded by reverse pinocytosis into the extracellular spaces, and eventually enter the mucosal lymphatic vessels.

Although absorption of triacylglycerides is both rapid and virtually complete in healthy human subjects, the complexity of the process makes it vulnerable to rate-controlling interactions at various stages of digestion and transport. Differences in the rate of fat absorption do appear to have important metabolic consequences in man, and may even influence the rate of hepatic oxidation of lipids (Jones et al., 1985). Cholesterol absorption is a much slower and less complete process, and a substantial fraction (20%–50%) of dietary and endogenous cholesterol is lost to the large bowel under normal circumstances (Wilson et al., 1968). The extent of dietary cholesterol absorption is therefore more susceptible to the inhibitory effects of luminal factors such as dietary fibre.

Inhibition of Lipolytic Activity

Inhibition of pancreatic lipase activity by dietary fibre could, in theory, be an effective rate-limiting mechanism for fat absorption, although in normal individuals there is a considerable excess of enzymatic activity. Several groups have provided evidence for an inhibitory effect of dietary fibre in vitro. Schneeman (1978) investigated the activity of purified pancreatic digestive enzymes in the presence of several fibre-rich complex carbohydrates, and observed a general tendency toward inhibition of enzyme activity. Solka floc and xylan were particularly effective inhibitors, in that a 2.5% suspension led to a reduction in lipolytic activity of more than 70%. In contrast, lipase activity was slightly higher in the presence of pectin, although this enhancement was not statistically significant. In a later study, Dunaif and Schneeman (1981) studied the effect of solka floc, wheat bran, oat bran, pectin, xylan and alfalfa on enzyme activity in isolated pancreatic juice collected from human volunteers. Again, solka floc and xylan were found to be particularly effective inhibitors of lipase activity.

Isaksson and co-workers have also reported inhibitory effects of dietary fibre on lipase activity, both in isolated pancreatic juice and in buffered saline (Isaksson et al., 1979, 1982). Contrary to the observations of Schneeman's group however, Isaksson et al. observed a substantial inhibitory effect in the presence of pectins having both high and low degrees of methylic esterification. Guar gum, another polysaccharide with a high viscosity in aqueous solution, was also shown to be inhibitory. Several mechanisms were proposed to account for the inhibitory effects, including sequestration of the enzyme by adsorption, and a reduction in the pH of the duodenal contents. The proposed mechanisms were thought to vary in importance, depending upon the particular source of fibre in question. Part of the strong inhibitory effect of pectin and guar gum was attributed to their high viscosity, and it was shown that another viscous polymer, polyethylene glycol, would also reduce lipase activity in vitro (Isaksson et al., 1982). Koseki et al. (1989) have recently reported that whereas pectin destabilises fat emulsions and inhibits lipase activity in vitro, gum arabic, which is almost entirely non-viscous, has the reverse effects.

The significance of adsorption as a mechanism for the inhibitory effects of non-starch polysaccharides on lipase activity has been investigated in detail by Lairon et al. (1985). Porcine pancreatic lipase and colipase were purified, and their activity in vitro was assayed in the presence of human bile. Under similar conditions, the binding of bile salts, phospholipids, cholesterol and pancreatic lipase to wheat bran, cellulose, xylan, pectin and the ion-exchange resin cholestyramine were determined. The adsorption of lipase by all the fibre fractions was low compared to cholestyramine, and none except wheat bran had a significant effect on lipase activity in the 0%–5% concentration range. However, although wheat bran reduced lipase activity by up to 94% when present at a concentration of 1%, this effect was independent of its limited capacity to adsorb lipase. Moreover, the inhibitory effect was associated primarily with the aqueous phase, and the authors concluded that a soluble protein constituent of bran was probably responsible.

Several attempts have been made to assess the effect of fibre on fat digestion in vivo, but again there is little consistency. Schneeman and Gallaher (1980) fed rats a fibre-free semi-synthetic diet, or the same diet containing 20% cellulose in the form of solka floc, for 10 days. At the end of the feeding period the activities of the major pancreatic digestive enzymes in the small intestinal contents of the fibre-fed rats were significantly lower than those of the controls. The effect was particularly pronounced in the case of pancreatic lipase, for which the activity of the enzyme per unit weight of gut contents was only 10% of that in the control animals. However there was no reduction in the level of lipase activity associated with the mucosa or the pancreatic tissue. In a later experiment Gallaher and Schneeman (1985) studied the distribution of radioactively labelled triglycerides and cholesterol in the small intestinal lumen of rats given a solid test meal containing 20% cellulose. The absorption of triglyceride was delayed, whereas that of cholesterol, which does not require hydrolysis prior to absorption, was unaffected. The authors attributed this effect to a reduction in the rate of triglyceride digestion in the cellulose-fed rats.

In a recent study Borel et al. (1989a) examined the extent of triglyceride hydrolysis in the stomach and small intestine of rats given a liquid test meal by intra-gastric gavage. The test meals were either fibre-free or supplemented with cellulose or xylan at a concentration of 10% of meal solids. They observed no effect of either material on the degree of triglyceride hydrolysis or absorption.

Using similar techniques to those employed to investigate the effect of dietary cellulose, Sheard and Schneeman (1980) studied the influence of wheat bran on digestive enzyme activity in the rat. The wheat bran was incorporated into semi-synthetic feed at a level of 5%. Assuming the total dietary fibre content of wheat bran to have been about 40%, this would have provided the rats with a total fibre intake of only about one-tenth of that administered in the study with purified cellulose. It is perhaps not surprising therefore that intra-luminal lipase activity was not significantly lower in the fibre-fed rats compared to the controls. However, the level of lipase and other digestive enzymes was significantly higher in the pancreatic tissue of the rats fed wheat bran. This may indicate pancreatic adaptation to a high-fibre diet by way of an entero-hepatic feedback mechanism of the type known to exist for trypsin secretion. In a recent study, Dukehart et al. (1989) administered a high-fibre diet to human subjects for four weeks, and measured pancreatic lipase concentration and output, by aspiration of duodenal contents, before and after a test meal. Some evidence for an adaptive increase in lipase activity late in the postprandial period was obtained.

Borel et al. (1989b) used gastric intubation to investigate the effects of wheat bran and wheat germ fractions on lipid digestion and absorption in the rat. Both wheat fractions reduced the gastric hydrolysis of triolein, and modified the mucosal uptake of fatty acids and cholesterol. There was a reduction in labelled triglycerides and cholesterol appearing in the plasma, and loss of lipids to the caecum was increased. The authors concluded that a protein component of both wheat bran and wheat germ could inhibit fat lipolysis. The reduction in the rate of cholesterol absorption which was also observed was attributed to reduced availability of phospholipids, monoglycerides and free fatty acids for incorporation into the mixed micelles which are essential for cholesterol uptake.

The significance of these various studies in relation to the uptake and assimilation of dietary lipid in healthy human subjects is uncertain, but there is some evidence for inhibitory effects in patients with impaired pancreatic function. Isaksson et al. (1984) administered 14-C labelled triolein, together with a preparation of pancreatic enzymes, to patients with complete pancreactectomy. When pectin or wheat bran was included in the meal there was a reduction in $14CO_2$ excretion, suggestive of impaired triglyceride absorption. Dutta and Hlasko (1985) showed that patients with chronic pancreatic insufficiency had increased faecal fat excretion when given a high-fibre diet.

Formation and Composition of Micelles

After a fatty meal the duodenum contains a complex fatty phase consisting of mixed micelles, liquid crystalline vesicles and unilamellar liposomes (Carey et al., 1983). The size and stability of the micelles depends upon the availability of fatty acids and lecithin, and upon the concentration of bile salts in the inter-micellar aqueous phase. Various components of dietary fibre, including lignin, are capable of sequestering bile salts under in vitro conditions, at least in a low pH environment (Eastwood and Hamilton, 1968; Selvendran, 1978). This effect has received considerable attention as a possible mechanism preventing the reabsorption of bile salts (Story, 1986), and it may also interfere with the formation of micelles and thereby reduce the efficiency of fat absorption in the proximal small intestine.

The ability of various components of dietary fibre to bind the constituents of mixed micelles was studied by Vahouny and co-workers, using an in vitro model system (Vahouny et al., 1980). The micelle suspensions contained either taurocholate or taurochenodeoxycholate, together with mono-olein, oleic acid, lecithin and cholesterol. The suspensions were then incubated with wheat bran, cellulose, alfalfa, lignin or guar gum, and also with cholestyramine or DEAE-Sephadex for comparison. Binding was assayed by comparing the proportions of radioactively labelled components present in the centrifuged supernatants before and after exposure to the test materials. As expected, the ion-exchange resins proved to be very effective binders of bile salts, phospholipid and cholesterol. Guar gum bound 28%–38% of each micellar constituent, but the other components of fibre were progressively less effective in the order lignin → alfalfa → wheat bran → cellulose. Falk and Nagyvary (1982) used various other in vitro techniques, including C13 NMR spectroscopy, to show that significant binding between lipid and pectin polymers occurs, principally by way of hydrogen bonding to the methoxycarbonyl groups of the polysaccharide. Under optimal conditions it was estimated that pectin could bind 3.7 times its own weight of micelle constituents.

By measuring the distribution of radioactively labelled bile acids and phospholipids within the small intestinal contents after a test meal, Gallaher and Schneeman (1986) were able to estimate the capacity of ion-exchange resins and various components of fibre to bind lipids in vivo, under physiological conditions. In the presence of cholestyramine, the concentration of bile acids and phospholipids was reduced by about 50% compared with control animals which had received a fibre-free test meal. Guar gum and lignin bound bile acids within the gut contents, whereas cellulose, wheat bran and oat bran did not. However oat bran was observed to bind phospholipids. In a further study, Ebihara and Schneeman (1989) showed that two soluble polysaccharides, guar gum and konjac mannan could bind bile acids in the duodenal lumen, whilst an insoluble material, chitosan, could bind both bile acids and phospholipids.

Although a variety of binding effects of fibre have now been identified, their practical significance in relation to lipid absorption remains doubtful. In the paper of Gallaher and Schneeman (1986) it was shown that only the synthetic drug cholestyramine significantly reduced the solubilisation of lipid in the liquid phase of the gut contents. In the later study of Ebihara and Schneeman (1989), radioactively labelled cholesterol and triglyceride were included in the test meal, and the disappearance of these substrates from the gut lumen was measured. Under these conditions only the two soluble polysaccharides, konjac mannan and guar gum, were found to have significantly delayed the absorption of fat, and both these materials led to an increase in the total volume of fluid in the gut contents. These observations suggest that sequestration of micelle components by dietary fibre does not significantly influence fat absorption. However, non-starch polysaccharides which are both soluble and highly viscous do apparently slow the transport of nutrients by other mechanisms, and there is good reason to suppose that lipids are particularly susceptible to this inhibitory effect.

Effects of Fibre on Intraluminal Lipid Transport

The final step in the intraluminal phase of fat assimilation is the transfer of lipid to the absorptive cells. Fluid layers adjacent to epithelial surfaces tend to be relatively stagnant, even when the bulk fluid phase is efficiently stirred (Diamond, 1966). In the small intestine this effect is exaggerated by the complex morphology of the villi (Wilson and Dietschy, 1974). The composition of this boundary layer is modified by the absorption of solutes and water by the enterocytes. If absorption is rapid, the transfer of solute from the bulk phase lags behind its disappearance from the boundary layer, leading to a reduction in the concentration of transportable solute at the absorptive surface. By varying the rate of luminal mixing, Thomson (1980) demonstrated that the effective thickness of the unstirred water layer was an important rate determinant of fatty acid and cholesterol absorption in vitro. Viscosity, or resistance to flow, is a hydrodynamic property which can also influence mixing in the mucosal fluid environment. There is now substantial evidence to show that soluble components of dietary fibre can influence lipid transport by modifying the characteristics of the intestinal unstirred layer in vivo.

Southgate (1973) first proposed that the presence of a dietary fibre matrix within the partially digested gut contents might reduce the diffusion of nutrients to the gut surface. Some years later Jenkins and co-workers began to explore the role of dietary fibre in the management of diabetes mellitus and showed that soluble non-starch polysaccharides with a high viscosity could reduce the post-prandial blood glucose response to test meals (Jenkins et al., 1978). Various mechanisms were proposed to account for this effect, including a reduction in the rate of gastric emptying (Holt et al., 1979). However, studies with in vitro systems by Johnson and Gee (1980) and by Elsenhans et al. (1980) established that the unstirred water layer associated with the jejunal surface became significantly thicker in the presence of incubation media containing guar gum and other viscous non-starch polysaccharides. Subsequent work with human subjects (Blackburn et al., 1984) and perfused animal intestine (Rainbird et al., 1984; Anderson et al., 1989) has confirmed that the inhibition of carbohydrate absorption by these components of dietary fibre is a true intraluminal effect, brought about by the viscous damping of fluid movement.

The intestinal unstirred water layer is not a simple, stationary film of fluid with a distinct boundary. Nevertheless this concept is a convenient fiction which can be described easily in mathematical terms. The thickness (d) of such an idealised layer can be described by the following equation, in which D is the diffusion coefficient for a particular probe molecule and t(½) is the half-time for the completion of a step-wise change in transmural potential difference induced by a change in the osmotic environment (Wilson and Dietschy, 1974).

$$d = \left[\frac{D . t(\frac{1}{2})}{0.38} \right]^{\frac{1}{2}}$$

This experimental approach has been used by Johnson and Gee (1981, 1982) to study the relationship between unstirred layer resistance and viscosity in small intestinal tissue, using mannitol as the probe molecule. In such experiments it is assumed that the diffusion coefficient (D) for mannitol remains constant in the bathing medium, and that the observed increase in unstirred layer resistance reflects a reduction in convective fluid movement. This assumption appears to be correct for solutes of small molecular weight such as sodium (Edwards et al., 1988). However, for molecules of higher molecular weight, the presence of dispersed polysaccharides in the lumen of perfused intestine has been shown to reduce the diffusion coefficient to a significant extent (Holzheimer and Winne, 1986). This effect may increase in importance for bulky molecular aggregates such as micelles and liquid crystals. Phillips (1986) tested this possibility using a system of unstirred diffusion tubes, and observed a very marked reduction in the rate of micelle diffusion as the concentration of guar increased.

The ability of relatively low concentrations of guar gum to slow the intestinal absorption of mixed micelles containing cholesterol was confirmed by Gee et al. (1983), using isolated segments of small intestine, or perfused loops with an intact mesenteric circulation. During the luminal perfusion experiments a reduction in the rate of water absorption was observed in the presence of guar gum (Gee et al., 1983; Blackburn and Johnson, 1983). It is this phenomenon which probably underlies the increased small intestinal water content consistently observed in animals fed diets enriched with viscous fibre (Trout et al., 1983; Lund et al., 1989). There was also a positive linear relationship between the rates of small intestinal water and cholesterol absorption from the perfused loops. This suggests a coupling between the movement of water and micelles in the vicinity of the mucosa (Gee et al, 1983). In a recent study with both animals and human subjects in vivo, Fuse et al. (1989) investigated the effects of pectin on fatty acid transport. They observed both a significant increase in unstirred water layer resistance, and a reduction in linoleic acid absorption in the presence of pectin.

Sugano et al. (1990) have described studies in which labelled micelles and various sources of dietary fibre were introduced into the stomach of rats and the rates of cholesterol and fatty acid absorption were determined by collecting lymph from an indwelling cannula in the left thoracic duct. Guar gum reduced the rate of absorption of both cholesterol and triglycerides more effectively than cellulose, but less effectively than chitosan. Interestingly, they observed that the inhibitory effect of fibre depended to some extent upon the fatty acid composition of the triglycerides, but the reasons for this were not explored.

There is now a substantial body of data, obtained with a range of techniques, showing delayed absorption of lipids and increased fluid volume in the proximal small intestine after the consumption of viscous fibre supplements. Taken together, these studies suggest that increased bulk viscosity, a reduced diffusion coefficient, and an inhibition of water absorption in the small intestine all act synergistically to reduce the rate of fat absorption in animals fed viscous fibre supplements. It is probable that the same mechanism also functions in the human small intestine under appropriate conditions, and may lead to loss of fat to the large bowel. Some evidence for this is provided by the work of Sandberg et al. (1983), who observed a significant increase in the water and fat content of ileostomy effluent in patients fed 15.5 g of pectin daily. It is unlikely that such large quantities of pectin could be obtained from a conventional diet, but oat β-glucan is a possible source of viscous polysaccharides which might be consumed in sufficient quantities to influence small intestinal function in man (Lund et al., 1989).

The Cellular Phase: Adaptation to Prolonged Fibre Intake

The final stages in lipid uptake and assimilation involve transport through the brush-border membrane, re-esterification of fatty acids to triglycerides and the synthesis and release of chylomicrons into the circulation. These post-luminal processes are not readily susceptible to the direct physico-chemical effects of dietary fibre, but there is some evidence that fibre-rich diets can modify them indirectly through the induction of adaptive changes in the structure and function of the mucosa.

Vahouny and co-workers were the first to investigate the effect of previous dietary fibre intake on the rate of lipid absorption in rats (Vahouny et al., 1978, 1980). The animals were fed for periods of 3 days or 6 weeks on diets containing various sources of insoluble and soluble fibre at levels of up to 15 g/100 g dry weight. At the end of the feeding period a cannula was introduced into the left thoracic duct to allow collection of lymph, and an intra-gastric infusion cannula was used to administer precise quantities of lipids into the proximal alimentary tract. The test dose consisted of a fibre-free micellar suspension containing 3H-cholesterol and 14C-labelled oleate. Under these conditions the observed rates of cholesterol and oleate absorption were lower in all the animals given fibre supplements compared with the control group. There were marked differences in the effects of the various sources of fibre, the most effective apparently being insoluble cellulose. In a similar investigation, Imaizumi et al. (1982) studied the absorption of triolein into mesenteric lymph in rats previously fed diets containing guar gum, and reported reduced absorption of lipid in proximal small intestine, and a compensating increase in the distal region. However, Gee et al. (1983) studied the disappearance of labelled cholesterol from perfused jejunal loops in rats previously fed a diet containing 20 g/kg guar gum, but observed no significant reduction in comparison with control animals.

In a recently published report, the original observations of Vahouny's group have been refined and extended (Vahouny et al., 1988). The experimental design was similar to that of the earlier studies but the acute lipid test meal was introduced directly into the duodenum, rather than into the stomach, to avoid any effects of gastric emptying. Furthermore the fatty acids were given as free oleic acid rather than triolein, to ensure that any observed effects were due to changes in absorption rather than the hydrolysis of triglycerides. Finally, the distribution of the labelled fatty acids and cholesterol amongst the plasma lipoproteins was determined, and the size ranges of chylomicrons were measured. In contrast to the earlier results, pre-feeding of animals with cellulose or alfalfa had no statistically significant effect on the rate of absorption of oleic acid. However diets containing cholestyramine or soluble fibre, such as pectin and guar gum, caused a reduction in lymphatic recovery of oleic acid in the initial period following administration of the test meal. In general there was no effect on 24-hour recovery. All the supplements led to reduced absorption of cholesterol, both in the initial period, and over the 24 hours following the test meal. There were no observed effects on fatty acid distribution, nor on chylomicron size. The authors concluded that the ability of certain dietary fibres to delay or depress nutrient absorption may not be entirely dependent on the physical presence of the fibre.

By what mechanism could the non-digestible residues of plant cell walls influence the rate of nutrient absorption, even when entirely absent from the small intestinal lumen? Surprisingly perhaps, the morphology and functional attributes of the small intestine are very responsive to the intake of dietary fibre. The mucosa is a complex tissue, constantly renewed by proliferation of stem cells in the crypts. Several groups have reported subtle morphological changes in the villous structure of rats fed diets containing various non-starch polysaccharides (Younoszai et al., 1978; Cassidy et al., 1982; Johnson and Gee, 1986). The changes in villous height and basal width which occur in response to soluble polysaccharides are associated with an increase in cell proliferation rate, and a reduction in the expression of mucosal enzyme and carrier activity in the rat (Johnson et al., 1984). Furthermore, Schwartz et al. (1983) have reported that prolonged fibre intake modifies the activity of intracellular enzymes involved in the synthesis of cholesterol and phospholipid in the rat. These adaptive responses to dietary fibre may influence both the uptake of fatty acids and cholesterol, and the rate at which chylomicrons are synthesised and released into the circulation.

The effective thickness of the unstirred water layer depends to some extent upon villous height (Westergaard and Dietschy, 1974). For example, villous height declines progressively along the length of the small intestine, and this accounts for small differences in jejunal and ileal diffusion resistance which have been observed in the rat (Lucas et al., 1983). An increase in villous height of the type observed in rats fed some types of dietary fibre could lead to a concomitant increase in unstirred water layer resistance, but this would tend to be offset by increased surface area. The situation is therefore complex and there is insufficient evidence available to evaluate the effects on lipid transport of purely morphological changes in villous structure. The mucous layer overlying the enterocytes is a further mucosal diffusion barrier. The production of mucus in the small intestine is influenced by dietary fibre intake, perhaps because of greater goblet cell proliferation (Cassidy et al., 1982). It is possible that increased thickness or density of mucus may slow the absorption of fatty acids and cholesterol in a manner analogous to polysaccharide gums (Gee et al., 1983) but again, this remains to be tested. Finally, although the precise molecular interactions by which lipids transfer from micelles into the brush-border are poorly understood, the rate at which this process occurs probably depends upon the fluidity and composition of the plasma membrane itself. Both aspects of brush-border structure are dependent upon dietary fat intake (Brasitus et al., 1985), but it is not known whether the plasma membranes of enterocytes are also sensitive to changes in the rate of crypt-cell proliferation.

Conclusions

There can be little doubt that dietary fibre is able to influence the absorption of dietary lipids under appropriate experimental conditions, but what is the significance of this in relation to human nutrition? The increased faecal excretion of fat seen in healthy subjects eating high-fibre diets is of little nutritional significance, although in patients with reduced pancreatic function, a high-fibre diet may lead to some frank malabsorption of dietary fat. It is probable that the various physico-chemical mechanisms that delay fat absorption in the proximal small intestine will be balanced by increased absorption at more distal sites. The overall effect will be to shift the intraluminal concentration profile for lipids in a distal direction. As a result, the concentration of lipids to which the cells at these sites are exposed will increase, and the proportion of dietary fat absorbed in the proximal intestine will decline. The metabolic effects of this effect have not been properly explored in humans, but several possible consequences can be identified.

Although there are no sharp anatomical boundaries within the small intestine there are important functional differences between proximal and distal sites. Wu et al. (1980) have shown that in the rat, chylomicrons produced from distal regions of the small intestine are larger than those produced in the jejunum, and differ significantly in their phospholipid and apolipoprotein content. If this is true of humans there may be important metabolic effects of delayed fat absorption which require investigation. The intestinal mucosa is itself responsive in various ways to the level of nutrients in the luminal environment. The rate of cell proliferation is partly dependent upon luminal nutrition, and essential fatty acids appear to be particularly important promotors of growth (Maxton et al., 1990). Delayed absorption of lipids may therefore be the key physiological stimulus underlying the trophic response to non-fermentable viscous polysaccharides seen in the rat (Johnson and Gee, 1986). If so, the adaptive reduction in the rate of lipid absorption in response to viscous polysaccharides described by Vahouny et al. (1988) is itself a consequence of the acute effects of these polysaccharides on lipid transport.

Some indirect evidence for an adaptive metabolic response to dietary fibre in humans lies in the so-called "second-meal effect" in which a meal containing viscous fibre eaten at breakfast time delays the absorption of nutrients from a subsequent meal (Jenkins et al., 1980). This may be a manifestation of the "ileal brake" phenomenon, whereby fatty acids infused into the human ileum reduce gastric emptying and delay the oro-caecal transit time (Read et al., 1984). The consumption of viscous fibre in conjunction with a fatty meal may delay nutrient absorption so as to increase the exposure of mucosal receptors to lipids and activate the ileal brake. This in turn could influence both the metabolism of subsequent meals, and the sensations of satiety which they induce (Burley and Blundell, 1990). It is unclear whether conventional foods are capable of exerting such effects. Further research on the behaviour of mixed diets during digestion is needed to explore this issue.

References

Anderson BW, Kneip JM, Levine AS, Levitt MD (1989) Influence of infusate viscosity on intestinal absorption in the rat. An explanation of previous discrepant results. Gastroenterology 97:938–943

Baird IM, Walters RL, Davies PS, Hill MJ, Drasar BS, Southgate DAT (1977) The effects of two dietary fibre supplements on gastrointestinal transit, stool weight and frequency, and bacterial flora and fecal bile acids in normal subjects. Metabolism 26:117–128

Blackburn NA, Johnson IT (1983) The influence of guar gum on the movements of inulin, glucose and fluid in rat intestine during perfusion in vitro. Pflügers Arch 397:144–148

Blackburn NA, Redfern JS, Jarjis H et al. (1984) The mechanism of action of guar gum in improving glucose tolerance in man. Clin Sci 66:329–366

Borel P, Lairon D, Senft M, Garzino P, Lafont H (1989a) Lack of effect of purified cellulose and hemicellulose on the digestion and the intestinal absorption of dietary lipids in the rat. Ann Nutr Metab 33:237–245

Borel P, Lairon D, Senft M, Chautan M, Lafont H (1989b) Wheat bran and wheat germ: effect on digestion and intestinal absorption of dietary lipids in the rat. Am J Clin Nutr 49:1192–1202

Brasitus TA, Davidson NO, Schachter D (1985) Variations in dietary triacylglycerol saturation alter the lipid composition and fluidity of rat intestinal plasma membranes. Biochim Biophys Acta 812:460–472

Burley VJ, Blundell JE (1990) Action of dietary fibre on the satiety cascade. In: Kritchevsky D et al. (ed) Dietary fibre: chemistry, physiology and health effects. Plenum Press, New York, pp 227–246

Carey MC, Small DM, Bliss CM (1983) Lipid digestion and absorption. Ann Rev Physiol 45:651–677

Cassidy MM, Lightfoot FG, Vahouny GV (1982) Morphological aspects of dietary fibre in the intestine. Adv Lipid Res 24:746–752

Chow SL, Hollander D (1978) Arachidonic acid intestinal absorption: mechanism of transport and influence of luminal factors on absorption. Lipids 13:768–776

Chow SL, Hollander D (1979) Linoleic acid absorption in the unanesthetized rat: mechanism of transport and influence of luminal factors on absorption. Lipids 14:378–385

Diamond J (1966) A rapid method for determining voltage-concentration relations across membranes. J Physiol 183:83–100

Dukehart MR, Dutta SK, Vaeth J (1989) Dietary fibre supplementation: effect on exocrine pancreatic secretion in man. Am J Clin Nutr 50:1023–1028

Dunaif G, Schneeman BO (1981) The effect of dietary fibre on human pancreatic enzyme activity in vitro. Am J Clin Nutr 34:1034–1035

Dutta SK, Hlasko J (1985) Dietary fibre in pancreatic disease: effect of high fibre diet on fat malabsorption in pancreatic insufficiency and in vitro study of the interaction of dietary fibre and pancreatic enzymes. Am J Clin Nutr 41:517–525

Eastwood MA, Hamilton D (1968) Studies on the adsorption of bile salts to non-absorbed components of diet. Biochim Biophys Acta 152:165–173

Ebihara K, Schneeman BO (1989) Interaction of bile acids, phospholipids, cholesterol and triglyceride with dietary fibres in the small intestine of rats. J Nutr 119:1100–1106

Edwards CA, Johnson IT, Read NW (1988) Do viscous polysaccharides slow absorption by inhibiting diffusion or convection? Eur J Clin Nutr 42:307–312

Elsenhans B, Sufke V, Blume R, Caspary WF (1980) The influence of carbohydrate gelling agents on rat intestinal transport of monosaccharides and neutral amino acids in vitro. Clin Sci 59:373–380

Falk JD, Nagyvary JJ (1982) Exploratory studies of lipid–pectin interactions. J Nutr 112:182–188

Fuse K, Bamba T, Hosoda S (1989) Effects of pectin on fatty acid and glucose absorption and on thickness of unstirred water layer in rat and human intestine. Digest Dis Sci 34:1109–1116

Gallaher D, Schneeman BO (1985) Effect of dietary cellulose on site of lipid absorption. Am J Physiol 249:G184–G191

Gallaher D, Schneeman BO (1986) Intestinal interaction of bile acids, phospholipids, dietary fibres and cholestyramine. Am J Physiol 250:G420–G426

Gargouri Y, Pieroni G, Riviere C et al. (1986) Importance of human gastric lipase for intestinal lipolysis: an in vitro study. Biochim Biophys Acta 879:419–423

Gee JM, Blackburn NA, Johnson IT (1983) The influence of guar gum on intestinal cholesterol transport in the rat. Br J Nutr 50:215–224

Holt S, Heading R, Carter D, Prescott L, Tothill P (1979) Effect of gel fibre on gastric emptying and absorption of glucose and paracetamol. Lancet i:636–639

Holzheimer G, Winne D (1986) Influence of dietary fibre and intraluminal pressure on absorption and pre-epithelial diffusion resistance (unstirred layer) in rat jejunum in situ. Naun Schmied Arch Pharmacol 334:514–524

Imaizumi K, Tominaga A, Maivatari K, Sugano M (1982) Effect of cellulose and guar gum on the secretion of mesenteric lymph chylomicrons in meal-fed rats. Nutr Rep Int 26:263–269

Isaksson G, Ihse I, Lundquist I (1979) Inhibition of pancreatic enzyme activity by dietary fibres – an in vitro study using human duodenal aspirates. Dan Med Bull 26:19

Isaksson G, Lundquist I, Ihse I (1982) Effect of dietary fibre on pancreatic enzyme activity in vitro. The importance of viscosity, pH, ionic strength, adsorption and time of incubation. Gastroenterology 82:918–924

Isaksson G, Lundquist I, Akesson B, Ihse I (1984) Effects of pectin and wheat bran on intraluminal pancreatic enzyme activity and on fat adsorption as examined with the triolein breath test in patients with pancreatic insufficiency. Scand J Gastroenterol 19:467–472

Jenkins DJA, Wolever TMS, Leeds AR et al. (1978) Dietary fibres, fibre analogues and glucose tolerance: importance of viscosity. Br Med J i:1392–1394

Jenkins DJA, Wolever TMS, Nineham R et al. (1980) Improved glucose tolerance four hours after guar with glucose. Diabetologia 19:21–24

Johnson IT, Gee JM (1980) Inhibitory effect of guar gum on the intestinal absorption of glucose in vitro. Proc Nutr Soc 39:52A

Johnson IT, Gee JM (1981) Effect of gel-forming gums on the intestinal unstirred layer and sugar transport in vitro. Gut 22:398–403

Johnson IT, Gee JM (1982) Influence of viscous incubation media on the resistance to diffusion of the unstirred water layer in vitro. Pflügers Arch 393:139–143

Johnson IT, Gee JM (1986) Gastrointestinal adaptation in response to soluble non-available polysaccharides in the rat. Br J Nutr 55:497–505

Johnson IT, Gee JM, Mahoney RR (1984) Effect of dietary supplements of guar gum and cellulose on intestinal cell proliferation, enzyme levels and sugar transport in the rat. Br J Nutr 52:477–487

Jones PJH, Pencharz PB, Clandinin MT (1985) Whole body oxidation of dietary fatty acids: implications for energy utilization. Am J Clin Nutr 42:769–777

Kelsay JL, Behall KM, Prather ES (1978) Effect of fibre from fruits and vegetables on metabolic responses of human subjects. I. Bowel transit times, number of defecations, fecal weight, urinary excretion of energy and nitrogen and apparent digestibilities of energy, nitrogen and fat. Am J Clin Nutr 31:1135–1149

Koseki M, Tsuji K, Nakagawa Y et al. (1989) Effects of gum arabic and pectin on the emulsification, the lipase reaction and the plasma cholesterol level in rats. Agric Biol Chem 53:3127–3132

Lairon D, Lafont H, Vigne J-L, Nalbone G, Leonardi J, Hauton JC (1985) Effects of dietary fibres on the activity of pancreatic lipase in vitro. Am J Clin Nutr 42:629–638

Lucas ML, Sood L, Gee JM, Johnson IT (1983) Discrepancies in determinations of unstirred layer depth in small intestine. Gut 24:A461

Lund EK, Gee JM, Brown JC, Wood PJ, Johnson IT (1989) Effect of oat gum on the physical properties of the gastrointestinal contents and on the uptake of D-galactose and cholesterol by rat small intestine in vitro. Br J Nutr 62:91–101

Maxton DG, Cynk EU, Thompson RPH (1990) Promotion of growth of the small intestine by dietary essential fatty acids. Eur J Gastroenterol Hepatol 2:131–136

Phillips DR (1986) The effect of guar gum in solution on diffusion of cholesterol mixed micelles. J Sci Food Agric 37:548–552

Plucinski TM, Hamosh M, Hamosh P (1979) Fat digestion in the rat: role of lingual lipase. Am J Physiol 237:541–547

Rainbird AL, Low AG, Zebrowsky T (1984) Effect of guar gum on glucose and water absorption from isolated jejunal loops in conscious growing pigs. Br J Nutr 53:17–24

Read NW, MacFarlane A, Kinsman R et al. (1984) Effect of infusion of nutrient solutions into the ileum on gastrointestinal transit and plasma level of neurotensin and enteroglucagon in man. Gastroenterology 86:274–280

Sandberg A-S, Ahderinne H, Andersson H et al. (1983) The effect of citrus pectin on the absorption of nutrients in the small intestine. Hum Nutr Clin 37C:171–183

Schneeman BO (1978) Effect of plant fibre on lipase, trypsin and chymotrypsin activity. J Food Sci 43:634–635

Schneeman BO, Gallaher D (1980) Changes in small intestinal digestive enzyme activity and bile acids with dietary cellulose in rats. J Nutr 110:584–590

Schwartz SE, Starr C, Bachman S, Holtzapple PG (1983) Dietary fibre decreases cholesterol and phospholipid synthesis in rat intestine. J Lipid Res 24:746–752

Selvendran RR (1978) Bile salt binding sites in vegetable fibre. Chem Ind (Lond) December:428–430

Sheard NF, Schneeman BO (1980) Wheat bran's effect on digestive enzyme activity and bile acid levels in rats. J Food Sci 45:1645–1648

Southgate DAT (1973) Fibre and other unavailable carbohydrates and their effects on the energy value of the diet. Proc Nutr Soc 32:131–136

Southgate DAT, Durnin JVGA (1970) Calorie conversion factors. An experimental reassessment of the factors used in the calculation of the energy value of human diets. Br J Nutr 24:517–535

Story JA (1986) Modification of steroid excretion in response to dietary fibre. In: Vahouny GV, Kritchevsky D (eds) Dietary fibre: basic and clinical aspects. Plenum Press, New York, pp 253–264

Sugano M, Ikeda I, Imaizumi K, Lu Y-F (1990) Dietary fibre and lipid absorption. In: Kritchevsky D et al. (eds) Dietary fibre: chemistry, physiology and health effects. Plenum Press, New York, pp 137–156

Thomson ABR (1980) Influence of site and unstirred layers on the rate of uptake of cholesterol and fatty acids into rat intestine. J Lipid Res 21:1097–1107

Trout DL, Ryan RO, Bickard MC (1983) The amount and distribution of water, dry matter and sugars in the digestive tract of rats fed xanthan gum (41567). Proc Soc Exp Biol Med 172:340–345

Vahouny GV, Roy T, Gallo LL et al. (1978) Dietary fibre and lymphatic absorption of cholesterol in the rat. Am J Clin Nutr 31:S208–S212

Vahouny GV, Tombes R, Cassidy MM, Kritchevsky D, Gallo LL (1980) Dietary fibres: V. Binding of bile salts, phospholipids and cholesterol from mixed micelles by bile acid sequestrants and dietary fibres. Lipids 15:1012–1018

Vahouny GV, Satchithanandam S, Chen I et al. (1988) Dietary fibre and intestinal adaptation: effects on lipid absorption and lymphatic transport in the rat. Am J Clin Nutr 47:201–206

Vallot A, Bernard A, Carlier H (1985) Influence of the diet on the portal and lymph transport of decanoic acid in rats. Comp Biochem Physiol 82A:693–699

Westergaard H, Dietschy JM (1974) Delineation of the dimensions and permeability characteristics of the two major diffusion barriers to passive mucosal uptake in the rabbit intestine. J Clin Invest 54:718–732

Widdowson EM (1955) Assessment of the energy value of human foods. Proc Nutr Soc 14:142–154

Wilson F, Dietschy J (1974) The intestinal unstirred layer: its surface area and effect on active transport. Biochim Biophys Acta 363:112–126

Wilson JD, Lindsey CA, Dietschy JM (1968) Influence of dietary cholesterol on cholesterol metabolism. Ann NY Acad Sci 149:808–821

Wu A-L, Clark SB, Holt PR (1980) Composition of lymph chylomicrons from proximal or distal rat small intestine. Am J Clin Nutr 33:582–589

Younoszai MK, Adedoyin M, Ranshaw J (1978) Dietary components and gastrointestinal growth in rats. J Nutr 108:341–350

Commentary

Mauron: You state in your paper that "the increased faecal excretion of fat seen in healthy subjects eating high-fibre diets is of little nutritional significance".

I think that if somebody eats permanently a high-fibre diet and excretes constantly more fat even in small quantities, this will affect his fat and energy balance in the long run. What is your comment?

Author's reply: I agree that this must be so to a certain extent. However, the literature suggests that such effects are small in comparison with total energy intake.

Edwards: What are the possible effects of delayed and slower lipid absorption on the metabolic response to a lipid load? Where does the lipid end up?

Author's reply: One can speculate that the relatively larger chylomicrons which are produced in the distal small bowel (Wu et al., 1980) may also be metabolised differently by lipoprotein lipase in the peripheral tissues, but I know of no evidence to confirm or refute this.

Sandberg: It is obvious that viscous polysaccharides influence fat absorption. However, different mechanisms may be involved for different kinds of viscous polysaccharides. We studied two kinds of polysaccharides which both increased the viscosity of the meals. Intake of highly methoxylated citrus pectin resulted in a malabsorption of fat and an increased bile acid and cholesterol excretion in human ileostomy subjects. Addition of sodium alginate resulted in a similar degree of fat malabsorption but did not influence bile acid and cholesterol excretion from the human small intestine.

Author's reply: This is an interesting observation, but it is difficult to comment without further information. Perhaps there was a major difference in viscosity under the conditions of shear in the small intestine. Alternatively, there may have been differences in the binding capacity of the two polysaccharides.

Chapter 10

The Influence of Dietary Fibre on Carbohydrate Digestion and Absorption

B. Flourié

Introduction

Acute studies in normal and diabetic subjects with purified fibres have indicated that the blood glucose and endocrine responses to test meals (liquid carbohydrate load or meals) are reduced by addition of fibre, especially viscous fibre, while the effect of particulate fibre such as wheat bran and cellulose appears more variable (Jenkins et al., 1978; Anderson et al., 1979; Levitt et al., 1980; Monnier, 1985; Hamberg et al., 1989a). Longer-term studies with fibre-supplemented diets in diabetic patients have confirmed that viscous fibres improve glycaemic control. However, it is difficult to make the quantity of soluble fibre used in these experiments acceptable; this has stimulated further work with foods rich in fibre. The specific effect of fibre taken as whole foods, as opposed to fibre supplements, in the management of diabetics is not easy to assess because changes in one dietary element can seldom be made without changes in another – studies with fibre in unprocessed foods usually entail fat restriction and higher intake of available carbohydrate in addition to the fibre. Thus, these studies did not indicate the extent to which high fibre or the combination of high fibre and high carbohydrate (particularly low glycaemic index food) in the diet was responsible for improved diabetic control, but they suggested that fibre and carbohydrate could act synergistically; in the context of starchy foods, fibre intake is one of the aspects which may render these foods particularly useful.

In longer-term studies, viscous fibre-supplemented or high-fibre diets may also induce improvement in diabetic control by reducing fasting plasma glucose values and glucose values in response to a glucose load provided without fibre (Munoz et al., 1979; Ray et al., 1983; Osilesi et al., 1985; Hagander et al., 1988). Particulate fibre preparations have been also reported to improve diabetic control, suggesting that mechanisms other than viscous properties may therefore be operating (Brodribb and Humphreys, 1976; Miranda and Horwitz, 1978; Bosello et al., 1980; Nygren et al., 1984).

Acute Effects of Dietary Fibre on Factors Affecting Digestion and Absorption of Carbohydrates

Blood levels of glucose depend on the rate of carbohydrate entry into the small intestine (i.e. gastric emptying), the rate of digestion and intestinal absorption once carbohydrate enters intestine, and the rate of metabolism once glucose is absorbed. The lowering effect of fibre on plasma glucose is not related to a stimulation of insulin secretion, as plasma insulin levels are reduced or unchanged after fibre ingestion. Alternatively, dietary fibre could lower plasma glucose concentrations: (a) by stimulating overall glucose utilisation; (b) by increasing hepatic uptake of ingested glucose thereby reducing the entry of glucose into the systemic circulation – Wahren et al. (1982) have shown in humans, using the hyperglycaemic clamp technique and measuring the net splanchnic glucose uptake, that neither total nor splanchnic utilisation of glucose are enhanced by acute ingestion of guar gum; and (c) by delaying or decreasing glucose absorption from the gut.

In the gastro-intestinal tract, some fibres form a matrix with fibrous characteristics; some fibres, because of their ability to swell within the aqueous medium can trap water and nutrients, especially water-soluble ones such as sugars. The physical characteristics of the small intestinal contents are altered by fibre sources. The bulk or amount of material in the gastro-intestinal tract is greater because fibre is not digestible and hence remains during the transit of digesta through the small intestine. The volume increase is due to the water-holding capacity of certain fibres. The viscosity of the intestinal contents increases due to the presence of fibre sources containing viscous polysaccharides (Bueno et al., 1981; Poksay and Schneeman, 1983; Gallaher and Schneeman, 1986; Rainbird and Low, 1986; Meyer and Doty, 1988). The positive correlation between the degree of viscosity and the lowering effect on plasma glucose supports the premise of the decisive role played by increased viscosity due to some fibres (Jenkins et al., 1978; Ebihara et al., 1981). Comparing guar, pectin, gum tragacanth, methylcellulose and wheat bran, the greatest flattening of the glucose response was seen with guar. This effect was abolished when hydrolysed non-viscous guar was tested (Jenkins et al., 1978).

The changes in the physical characteristics of the intestinal contents may influence gastric emptying, dilute enzymes and absorbable compounds in the gut, protect starch from hydrolysis, slow the diffusion or mobility of enzymes, substrates and nutrients to the absorptive surface. These effects result in the slower appearance of glucose in the plasma following a meal.

Influence of Dietary Fibres on Gastric Emptying

As the rate of gastric emptying modulates the rate of nutrient absorption from the small intestine, the ability of certain fibres to delay gastric emptying has been associated with blunting of the glycaemic response to a glucose load.

Dietary fibre may affect gastric filling, which might in turn slow gastric emptying. Duncan et al. (1983) reported that subjects required more time to chew their food when selecting from a menu with food high in dietary fibre as compared with a low-fibre menu. A meal of wholemeal bread took 45 minutes to eat, whereas white bread took 34 minutes (McCance et al., 1953). Haber et al. (1977) showed that 60 g of available carbohydrate as 482 g apples, 482 g apple puree, and as 444 ml apple juice took 17.2, 5.9 and 1.5 minutes to eat, respectively.

McCance et al. (1953) used barium sulphate as a marker and showed that after white bread the marker remained in the stomach for longer than for wholemeal bread. Whether the bread remained associated with the marker is uncertain. Using a gamma camera, Grimes and Goddard (1977) found that solids from white and wholemeal breads emptied at the same rate but liquids left the stomach faster when given with white bread. When wheat bran was added to a solid/liquid meal, we did not find, however, any difference in the gastric emptying rate of liquids, assessed by intubation techniques (Cortot et al., 1981).

In most studies of the effect of purified viscous fibres on gastric emptying, only the emptying of liquids has been measured. Holt et al. (1979), studying eight healthy volunteers, added 10 g pectin and 16 g guar gum to 400 ml orange juice labelled with [113]In-DTPA and showed that more marker remained in the stomach at 30 minutes after the meal than remained after the control meal. Subsequent studies have confirmed that large doses of viscous fibre carefully mixed in liquid carbohydrate meals prolonged gastric emptying (Blackburn et al., 1984a; Torsdottir et al., 1989). It appears, however, from these studies that viscous fibres affect gastric emptying of liquid in most but not all healthy subjects (Lawaetz et al., 1983; Blackburn et al., 1984a; Jarjis et al., 1984).

The emptying of the solid components of a meal is probably of greater importance in the regulation of carbohydrate digestion-absorption since they contain starch, which is the main source of glucose under normal dietary conditions. In studies investigating the effects of viscous fibre on gastric emptying of a solid/liquid meal, emptying of liquid phase of the meal is reduced (Ray et al., 1983; Flourié et al., 1985; Sandhu et al., 1987) but the effects on solid phase are controversial. Rainbird and Low (1986) have performed prominent work in pigs fitted with gastric cannulas, but their results were inconclusive. Guar gum reduced the rate of gastric emptying of dry matter and glucose (primarily in the form of starch) one hour after feeding, but when expressed on a half-time basis the emptying of dry matter and glucose was not significantly slower than for the control meal. These authors concluded that the solid and liquid phases of a meal emptied from the stomach at the same rate in the presence of guar gum. In contrast, Meyer et al. (1986) have shown that the viscosity of the aqueous medium diminished the selective retention of large particles in the stomach of dogs. This hydrodynamic effect which accelerated the gastric emptying of indigestible solids or large particles of digestible solids (steak and chicken liver) has not been demonstrated for insoluble carbohydrate such as starch. In healthy subjects, pectin supplementation (15 g) caused a significant prolongation of gastric emptying half-time of both liquid and solid meals (egg sandwich meal method) (Sandhu et al. 1987). This result has been recently confirmed in non-diabetic obese subjects (Di Lorenzo et al., 1988). In non-insulin-dependent diabetic patients, Ray et al. (1983) found that both liquids and solids were delayed by guar gum (6 g) and wheat bran (3 g) ingested for two months, whereas a comparable amount (5 g guar gum and 10.5 wheat bran) did not influence the total gastric emptying time of wheatmeal porridge in healthy subjects (Rydning et al., 1985).

The mechanism by which purified viscous fibres slow gastric emptying is not clear. Gastric emptying of a meal is regulated by its volume, viscosity, osmolarity, chemical composition, caloric content, pH and gastro-intestinal hormone release. It could be proposed that changes in the release of gut hormones might cause, rather than result from, the changes in gastric emptying and intestinal absorption. Several gastro-intestinal hormones have been implicated in the regulation of gastric emptying. For instance, insulin is known to augment gastric contractions by virtue of its hypoglycaemic action, whereas glucagon reduces gastric motility (Kelly et al., 1980). It seems unlikely that changes in blood level of insulin or glucagon can explain the delay in gastric emptying caused by pectin, since gastric emptying can be delayed without consistent changes in blood hormones (Sandhu et al., 1987; Villaume et al., 1988). In our study (Flourié et al., 1985), gastrin and motilin releases were reduced after addition of 10 and 15 g pectin to the meal, but the largest differences in their levels were found later than the changes in gastric emptying. Because it is known that viscous fibres do not significantly change the volume, chemical composition, caloric content, osmolarity or pH of gastric contents, it has been suggested that they delay gastric emptying by increasing the viscosity of the meals.

In support of this mechanism are the studies showing than an increase in viscosity caused by fibre like guar gum and pectin, and also potato granules delays gastric emptying (Leeds et al., 1979; Ebihara et al., 1981; Ehrlein and Pröve, 1982). How viscous fibres affect the gastro-duodenal motor activity remains to be elucidated. In dogs, Pröve and Ehrlein (1982) showed that the depth of antral indentation during maximal contraction as measured by fluoroscopy and induction coils was deeper with the low-viscosity meal than with the medium- and high-viscosity meals (potato granules). These authors suggested that meals of higher viscosity would be retropulsed and gastric emptying would be delayed by this mechanism. In this study, no difference in amplitude or frequency of antral contractions with liquid meals of different viscosity was noted. In dogs, Bueno et al. (1981) have observed, however, changes in the pattern of the postprandial activity in the antrum: guar gum significantly increased the frequency of antral contractions, wheat bran and cellulose had no effect. In contrast, Russell and Bass (1985) showed that fibre meals with high viscosity slowed gastric emptying, but did not affect antro-duodenal motility in dogs. Likewise, in men who received a meal containing 15 g pectin, Sandhu et al. (1987) did not observe any consistent effect on gastro-duodenal motility recorded by a manometric method, which could be, however, too insensitive to detect motility changes in the antrum especially after meals. These data suggest that viscous fibres might delay gastric emptying by a mechanism other than a change in gastro-duodenal motility. In normal man, when a solid meal is eaten the fundus fills, whereas a liquid meal flows rapidly into the antrum. Addition of pectin to a liquid meal results in a prolonged passage of the meal through the stomach (Leeds, 1982; Lawaetz et al., 1983). Viscous fibres may cause the stomach to handle the liquid meal in the manner of a solid or a thick liquid meal. Since there is no obvious difference in the antro-duodenal motility between meals of different viscosities, the delay of gastric emptying with increasing viscosity may be due to larger resistance of the viscous chyme to flow or to tonal changes of the fundus.

In the study by Holt et al. (1979), the viscous fibre flattened the plasma paracetamol curve, and there was a continuing delayed absorption long after gastric emptying, evidenced by the gentler decay slope and also the similar 24-hour urinary recovery rates. Furthermore, in subsequent detailed studies no correlation was found between the change in individual blood glucose response and the change in the gastric emptying half-time induced by viscous fibres (Ray et al., 1983; Blackburn et al., 1984a; Jarjis et al., 1984; Flourié et al., 1985; Edwards et al., 1987). These observations strongly suggest that delayed gastric emptying is not the only mechanism whereby viscous fibres decrease postprandial glycaemia.

Influence of Dietary Fibres on Small Intestinal Digestion and Absorption

For digestion and absorption to proceed, enzymes and substrates must be able to interact and the end products of digestion must reach the mucosal surface for final hydrolysis and absorption.

Reduction of Enzyme–Substrate Interaction

Available evidence suggests that the fibres have little, if any, direct acute effect on the secretory function of the exocrine pancreas (Sommer and Kasper, 1980), suggesting that the primary effect of the fibre on carbohydrate digestion is exerted in the intestinal lumen. In the lumen, the enzymes and substrates may be diluted with the addition of non-digestible material or the fibre may interfere with the interaction of enzymes and substrates by other mechanisms.

Evidence from in vitro studies and from duodenal aspirates suggests that most of the fibre derivatives tested can alter the activities of pancreatic amylase (Dunaif and Schneeman, 1981; Isaksson et al., 1982). The inhibitory effects of fibre on pancreatic enzyme activities have been attributed to various factors including pH changes, ion-exchange properties, enzyme inhibitors and adsorption. Rather than a chemical enzyme fibre interaction, the presence of fibre and its particulate and viscous nature probably impedes enzyme–substrate interaction.

In vitro studies using pooled human pancreatic juice and human saliva demonstrated that there were differences in the rates at which starchy foods were digested. In general, the rates of release of the products of starch digestion related well to the glycaemic responses to the same foods tested in normals and diabetics, and a modest relationship was seen between the rate of digestion and the fibre content of the foods tested (Jenkins et al., 1987a). The slow rate of digestion of some starchy foods is not due to their fibre content, but may be related to the presence of fibre in a form that restricts starch gelatinisation or access of the hydrolytic enzymes to the starch. The slow rate of digestion of legumes may be related to the entrapment of starch in fibrous thick-walled cells, which prevent its complete swelling during cooking (Würsch et al., 1986). In addition, resistance of starch to pancreatic hydrolysis may result from the presence of intact cell walls, which survive processing and cooking and insulate starch in such a manner that portions of it cannot be digested or absorbed. In whole rice kernels the external coat, which is rich in fibre, reduces the rate at which the starch in rice can be digested (Snow and O'Dea, 1981). In vitro, coarsely milled wheat flour is digested significantly slower than its finely milled equivalent obtained after mechanical disruption of cell walls (Heaton et al., 1988). Fibres which increase the viscosity could also reduce enzyme–substrate contact. In in vitro studies, mucilaginous and gum fractions of baobab leaves were found to lose enzyme-inhibiting effects when hydrolysed to a non-viscous state (Arnal-Peyrot and Adrian, 1974). The importance of viscosity was also shown in in vitro experiments where amylase activity was reduced by increasing the viscosity of duodenal juice with viscous fibres and PEG, an otherwise inert agent (Isaksson et al., 1982). However, in fibre-rich foods such as beans and lentils, the rate of starch hydrolysis by amylase and amyloglucosidase in vitro was not found to be related to viscosity; it was increased by grinding beans finely before cooking, suggesting that, as for cereals, the cellular structure rather than viscosity is a factor determining the rate of starch hydrolysis (Wong et al., 1985).

Reduction of Diffusion and Intestinal Absorption Rates

There is evidence that viscous fibres can influence accessibility of available carbohydrates to the mucosal surface and slow their absorption.

Using dialysis tubing containing glucose solution to which guar gum and pectin were added, it could be shown that these substances delayed the movement of glucose out of the dialysis bags in proportion to their viscosity. This did not appear to be a chemical binding in that, with time, the concentration on both sides of the dialysis was the same (Jenkins, 1980). Johnson and Gee (1981) studied the effect of different concentrations of guar gum on the uptake of glucose by everted sacs of rat jejunum; there was an inverse relationship between viscosity and glucose uptake. Elsenhans et al. (1980), using everted rat small intestine rings, showed that the uptakes of α-methyl-D-glucoside and D-galactose were inhibited by guar gum, pectin, gum tragacanth, carubin and carrageenan in relation to the viscosity of the solution. The inhibition of uptake was dependent on the presence of the fibre, since it was reversed by washing (Elsenhans et al., 1980). Hydrolysis in mucosal homogenates was also studied with and without guar gum; there were no significant differences of hydrolysis rates, and so no competition for substrate-binding sites on the enzyme (Elsenhans et al., 1981). In contrast, Schwartz and Levine (1980) reported that the glucose absorption was not inhibited by acute supplementation of pectin. In their study, however, the viscosity of the control glucose solution was adjusted to that of the pectin-containing solution by adding gelatin and experiments were performed in anaesthetised laparotomised rats, where, unlike conscious non-laparotomised rats, absorption is independent of perfusate viscosity (Anderson et al., 1989).

The inhibition of uptake by tissues is dependent on the perfusion or shaking rates – increasing shaking increases tissue uptake in the presence of gums as well as in their absence (Elsenhans et al., 1980; Johnson and Gee, 1981; Elsenhans et al., 1984). Johnson and Gee (1981) showed that inhibition was observed in sacs of rat jejunum pre-incubated with guar gum and exposed to glucose in a subsequent guar-free incubation, suggesting that the guar gum may exert its effects when present not in the bulk phase but in a fluid film surrounding the intestinal villi. From this experiment and from the reversibility of the inhibition by either washing the tissue free of polysaccharide or increasing the shaking rates during incubations, it was suggested that the inhibition of intestinal transport of glucose by gelling agents was due to an enlargement of the unstirred water layer (Elsenhans et al., 1980). The results of kinetic experiments showing a distinct effect on the apparent Michaelis constant with no influence on the maximal transport capacity supported this conclusion (Elsenhans et al., 1980).

In healthy volunteers, addition of pectin 6, 10 and 15 g/l to solution containing glucose perfused in jejunal loops under steady-state conditions caused a respective 10%, 14% and 24% reduction in the rate of glucose absorption (Flourié et al., 1984). In this study, the electrical technique was applied to measure the thickness of the unstirred layer. Although pectin gel itself may decrease slightly the diffusion coefficient of molecules used to induce the change in potential difference, pectin was found to increase the thickness of the unstirred layer. Propantheline bromide was administered to reduce the variation in the electrical record caused by jejunal motility; this may have led to over-estimation of the thickness of unstirred layer. These results recently confirmed with pectin (Fuse et al., 1989) were, however, not found with guar gum. In a similar study, Blackburn et al. (1984a), indeed, demonstrated that the reduction of glucose absorption by guar gum was due to an impairment of mixing from the bulk phase rather than an increase in the thickness of the unstirred layer. Thus, in addition to the possibility that viscous fibres may acutely alter the transport characteristics of glucose at the mucosal surface, they may also interfere with mixing of solute, substrates and their hydrolytic products in the intestinal lumen, the sequestration in the luminal bulk phase retarding the presentation to the absorbing surface.

From in vitro studies with dialysis bags containing guar/glucose mixtures under conditions of constant stirring, Blackburn et al. (1984a) have suggested that a viscosity-related reduction in solute movement may occur throughout the lumen, and be responsible for the inhibitory effect of guar on glucose absorption. The motility of the gut induces radial stirring (from the centre of the lumen toward the brush-border) breaking up the laminar flow pattern observed in laparotomised animals (Anderson et al., 1988). Under normal circumstances, it seems likely that solute movements induced by intestinal motility are largely responsible for bringing nutrients from the bulk phase to the epithelial surface, with diffusion playing an important role only in the unstirred region just adjacent to the epithelium. Increasing the viscosity of the intestinal contents may diminish radial stirring (Anderson et al., 1988).

If viscous fibres reduce luminal mixing, this in turn would reduce the intraluminal enzyme–substrate contact and the access of nutrients to the absorptive epithelium; this would increase the thickness of the unstirred layer since this latter is inversely related to the magnitude of the stir rate. This reduction of mixing effects of intestinal contractions might explain the inhibitory effect of viscous fibre on glucose absorption. In addition, this would impair the action of propulsive contractions and slow intestinal transit. One of the consequences of this conclusion is that the effects of viscous fibre on the small intestinal motility (especially movements resulting in mixing of contents) need further investigation in humans, since increased mixing might overcome any effect on movement in the bulk phase and thickness of the unstirred layer.

Viscous polysaccharides impair intestinal absorption of small molecules like glucose. This action relates mainly to the physical effects of the viscosity on movement of nutrients that are already dissolved in the aqueous phase of chyme. In addition, high viscosity may also affect the movement of solid particles of food that are suspended in the aqueous contents of the gastro-intestinal lumen. By Amidon's hydrodynamic hypothesis high viscosity would slow the transit of fluid and speed the relative transit of particles resulting in gastric emptying of large particles of food (Meyer et al., 1986). Because of poor digestibility of large particles, this in turn might have profound effects on digestion and absorption of nutrients in the small intestine. Meyer and Doty (1988) showed in dogs that guar in a dose-related fashion markedly increased the passage to mid-intestine of large, poorly digestible solid foods (pieces of steak and liver). The digestion and absorption of less solid foods, as starch, were not assessed in this study.

Effect on Small Intestinal Transit and Motor Activity

Transit time or contact time can influence small intestinal absorption of carbohydrates (Holgate and Read, 1983; Chapman et al., 1985). Dietary fibres may affect small intestinal transit time in different ways depending on the kind of fibre administered. Early radiologic studies suggested that transit through the small intestine in humans is more rapid with wholemeal bread than with white bread (McCance et al., 1953). More recent studies have assessed the small intestinal transit using the lactulose hydrogen breath test. Since lactulose is water soluble, it may assess the influence of fibre on the liquid portion of the meal. Lactulose is a non-absorbable and osmotically active disaccharide; it may therefore alter intestinal motility and accelerate transit of liquids. The effect of fibre on starch transit through the small intestine is not known. Jenkins et al. (1978) investigated the action of a variety of fibres on the small intestinal transit time of the head of a 400 ml drink containing glucose (50 g), xylose (25 g) and lactulose (15 g). Addition of 14.5 g of either guar gum (+75 minutes), tragacanth (+30 minutes), or pectin (+15 minutes) delayed transit. Methylcellulose had no effect, while a much larger amount of wheat bran (41.5 g) reduced transit time by 45 minutes. In general, the delaying action of fibres on oro-caecal transit time was directly proportional to the viscosity of the solution. The importance of viscosity was also emphasised by the fact that when guar gum was hydrolysed and rendered non-viscous, the oro-caecal transit time, as measured by hydrogen evolution from lactulose, was more rapid. Hamberg et al. (1989a) showed that wheat bran and also sugar beet fibre decreased oro-caecal transit time of lactulose.

Oro-caecal transit time is, however, composed of gastric emptying and small intestinal transit time; it is therefore not possible by means of the breath hydrogen method to come to a conclusion about small intestinal motility. The incorporation of guar gum into a radiolabelled homogenised meal in rats delayed the delivery of the meal marker from the stomach into the small intestine and also from the small intestine into the colon. The effect of the viscous guar on the stomach to caecum transit time did not occur as a simple consequence of delayed gastric emptying (Brown et al., 1988). Furthermore, guar gum resulted in a slower transit in the mid- but not the proximal intestine (Leeds, 1982). Likewise, in humans guar gum could slow small intestinal transit of the head of a drink of lactulose without having any significant action on gastric emptying assessed by gamma camera (Read, 1986), and guar had a slowing action not in the proximal but in the distal intestine where the viscosity would be greater as more fluid has been absorbed (Blackburn et al., 1984b).

Surprisingly, only a few studies have assessed the effects of fibres on small intestinal motility. The presence of extra nutrients in the ileum may trigger the ileal brake which would contribute to the slowing of small bowel transit by viscous fibres (Read, 1986). Fibre ingestion may alter the release of some gastro-intestinal hormones implicated in the regulation of gastro-intestinal transit. For instance, it was reported recently that the intake of beet fibre bread increased somatostatin response (Hagander et al., 1986). Whether some effects of fibres on intestinal transit and motility are related to changes in hormonal responses are unknown. The increased luminal bulk and viscosity might also induce motor changes. As viscosity increased psyllium and pectin elicited increasing jejunal motor activity in dogs (Russell and Bass, 1986). Bueno et al. (1981) used strain gauges to record small intestinal motor activity in dogs after feeding meals containing 30 g either bran, cellulose or guar gum. There were important differences in the effects of the three fibres. In the intestine, the particulate fibres – bran and cellulose – decreased the number of isolated contractions but increased the number of contractions occurring rhythmically in series. In contrast, guar gum enhanced the occurrence of isolated contractions giving a pattern of uniform small amplitude contractions at a high frequency. As a result, the motility index recorded in the duodenum and jejunum was increased only after meal containing guar. This pattern recorded after guar was associated with a slow transit time through the jejunum; its effect on mixing is not known. In man, it has been shown that small intestinal transit is slowed by guar gum-containing meals, despite the fact that guar gum alone induces propagated clusters of contractions (Welch and Worlding, 1986). These results suggest, therefore, that viscous luminal contents may slow the transit of the meal by resisting the propulsive effects of gastro-intestinal contractions.

Slow Absorption or Malabsorption of Carbohydrates?

Addition of 14.5 g guar gum to a 400 ml glucose/xylose/lactulose drink resulted in a reduced urinary xylose excretion in the first two hours, but there was a compensatory increase from two to eight hours, suggesting that although absorption was delayed, there was no overall impairment (Jenkins et al., 1978). As ingested xylose is not totally recovered in urine, this result has not ruled out increased malabsorption of xylose. By means of breath hydrogen method in man, however, guar gum given with glucose was shown not to cause malabsorption of the glucose up to five hours after the test meal (Jenkins et al., 1977a).

Using the indirect method of breath hydrogen estimation, which may be questioned quantitatively, it has been noted increased wheat starch malabsorption when fibres (from wheat bran, sugar beet and pea) are added to white bread (Hamberg et al., 1989b). Conversely, no influence on the amounts of unabsorbed starch (from white bread and rice) was found in ileostomised patients ingesting wheat bran and pectin (Sandberg et al., 1981, 1983). In these experiments in ileostomised patients, it can be noted that fibres may increase ileal losses of other nutrients, such as nitrogen which may promote hydrogen excretion in breath. Thus, currently there is little evidence that supplementation of diets with fibres causes malabsorption of available carbohydrates. In humans, the hydrodynamic effect of viscous fibres, demonstrated in dogs for large solid pieces of steak and liver (Meyer and Doty, 1988), does not appear to be relevant to starch. Due to their physical properties, supplementation of diets with viscous fibre derivatives reduces enzyme–substrate contact, diffusion and absorption of carbohydrate but induces a slower transit time. This prolonged small intestinal transit would be necessary for the complete absorption of available carbohydrates from the intraluminal contents. Viscous fibres do not induce malabsorption of available carbohydrates but affect their site of absorption. As a greater proportion of nutrients is absorbed from the lower half of the small intestine, viscous fibres create what has been named "lente" carbohydrate.

With fibre-rich foods, the effect of fibre on starch absorption may be different. Levitt et al. (1987) have shown that whole wheat and whole oats give rise to greater hydrogen production related to increased starch malabsorption than do the refined flours. In one ileostomate volunteer, Jenkins et al. (1987b) have tested 20 starchy foods. Measurement (or rather calculation) of available carbohydrates (starch, but also oligosaccharides and endogenous carbohydrates) in ileal effluent demonstrated a wide range of recoveries from 2.7% to 18% from starchy foods and losses related well to the fibre content and the glycaemic responses. The foods that resulted in greater losses of available carbohydrates were lentils, and other legumes, the β-glucan-containing cereals, oat bran, barley and pumpernickel bread where the whole grain structure is preserved. However, this overestimated malabsorption of available carbohydrates did not provide a direct explanation for the lower blood glucose responses seen, since major percentage differences in glycaemic response between foods were only reflected in relatively small percentage differences in the amount of carbohydrate malabsorbed. It is likely that fibres present in whole or partly milled grains and legumes cause a small malabsorption of starch because of incomplete physical access for digestive enzymes in the small intestine. In high-fibre, high-carbohydrate diets, however, other factors (starch nature, processing) than fibre content may be involved in starch malabsorption.

Chronic Effects of Dietary Fibre on Factors Affecting Digestion and Absorption of Carbohydrates

The reduction of urinary glucose and insulin dosage produced by addition of a constant amount of fibre to a constant diet in diabetics is reported to be progressive (Jenkins et al., 1979). Furthermore, fibre-supplemented or high-fibre diets appear to induce improvements in glucose metabolism that cannot be related to the rate of glucose absorption, as they reduce fasting plasma glucose values obtained after a 12-hour fast (Ray et al., 1983; Osilesi et al., 1985;

Hagander et al., 1988). This suggests that the effect of fibre on carbohydrate metabolism may be related not only to the acute interaction of fibre and food in the gastro-intestinal tract but also to subsequent alterations in metabolism and/or alimentary structure and function.

Chronic ingestion of fibre may modify carbohydrate and lipid metabolism. Through reducing the rate of digestion of starchy foods postprandially, fibres blunt many gut hormone responses and prolong free fatty acid and ketone body suppression. In addition to fibres, increased starch losses to the colon may enhance production of short chain fatty acids. Fibre intake may enhance tissue sensitivity to insulin, in part through short chain fatty acids. Propionate stimulates the rate of glycolysis in isolated rat hepatocytes and inhibits the rate of glyconeogenesis. Thus, some of the favourable effects of fibre intake on glucose metabolism may be mediated by these metabolic products, and, hence, in part through the possible malabsorption of available carbohydrates induced by fibre (Anderson, 1986).

In addition to changes in carbohydrate metabolism induced by long-term consumption of fibre, there is evidence mainly in animals that adaptive changes in intestinal structure and function may occur and influence digestion and absorption of carbohydrate.

In healthy man, after four weeks of pectin supplementation the gastric emptying of a meal ingested without pectin is delayed, whereas plasma glucose and hormone responses are not affected. This adaptive effect of intestinal pectin ingestion on gastric emptying is reversible within three weeks, its mechanism is unknown and it did not occur after cellulose supplementation (Schwartz et al., 1982). In insulin-dependent diabetics, a similar effect of pectin on gastric emptying was found but glucose tolerance after chronic pectin supplementation to the meal ingested without pectin was enhanced (Schwartz et al., 1984).

Certain fibre preparations exert secretagogue and trophic effects on the pancreas (Poksay and Schneeman, 1983; Isaksson et al., 1982). Wheat bran supplementation for four weeks increased pancreatic juice flow rate and amylase output in dogs (Stock-Damgé et al., 1983). In rats, amylase activities were elevated in the pancreas after two weeks of wheat bran supplementation, and supplementation with viscous fibres for two weeks affected pancreatic secretion and amylase output (Schneeman et al., 1982; Ikegami et al., 1990). These effects appear due to an enlargement of the pancreas (Poksay and Schneeman, 1983; Ikegami et al., 1990). Since the acute effects of fibres may lead to inhibition of pancreatic enzyme activity or decrease in enzyme–substrate interactions, their chronic effects on pancreatic function could be an adaptive response to an increased need for enzymes.

The morphologic development of the small intestine can be dramatically influenced by dietary fibre supplements in rats. In addition, it is also clear that a variety of insoluble and soluble fibres given to adult animals can influence intestinal length and weight, and modify the morphology of mucosa, cell turnover and mucus secretion (Schneeman et al., 1982; Sigleo et al., 1984; Vahouny, 1987). All these changes could be adaptations to handle the greater bulk of material in animals fed fibres as well as to compensate for delay in absorption. In rats, adding guar to the diet resulted in villous hypertrophy selectively in the ileum (Imsidumi et al., 1982; Johnson et al., 1984); this may be triggered by the displacement of undigested and/or unabsorbed food to more distal intestinal sites. Morphological changes caused by fibres would be expected to affect glucose absorption. For instance, the increased production of mucus could contribute to the thickness of the unstirred layer and modify the carbohydrate diffusion barrier at the intestinal surface. Use of a rat mucosal ring technique has produced some evidence for a reduction of maximal transport capacity for glucose in the proximal small gut after feeding of guar gum-containing diets (Leeds, 1982; Johnson et al., 1984). In rats, Schwartz and Levine (1980) have shown that feeding pectin or cellulose for five weeks resulted in impairment of absorption of glucose by the proximal jejunum as measured by a perfusion technique; however, it is possible that some of the impairment of absorption may have been due to residual fibre overlying the mucosa. Carefully washed intestinal tissue from rats fed pectin or cellulose for four weeks has not exhibited diminished transport rates for 3-0-methylglucose (Sigleo et al., 1984). One effect of reduced glucose transport would be to improve glucose tolerance when tested with glucose alone. An improvement of glucose tolerance has been indeed demonstrated in volunteers maintained on a self-selected or controlled diets supplemented with insoluble or soluble fibres, and who have ingested glucose alone after a 12-hour fast (Brodribb and Humphreys, 1976; Munoz et al., 1979). This effect has not been, however, found after six weeks of pectin in three volunteers maintained on a controlled diet (Jenkins et al., 1977b). Furthermore, in intestinal perfusion studies performed in healthy volunteers chronic pectin ingestion (20 g/day/four weeks) did not impair jejunal absorption of glucose (Schwartz et al., 1982). In humans, morphological changes have not been described and their expected influence, if any, on glucose transport has yet to be assessed. Thus, other mechanisms than reduced intestinal glucose absorption must be activated to promote glucose utilisation.

Conclusion

Current evidence suggests that fibres and fibre derivatives can exert acute and chronic effects on the bioavailability of carbohydrates from the gastro-intestinal tract. Acutely, several factors contribute to explain the slow absorption of carbohydrates with viscous fibres: reduced rate of gastric emptying, altered enzyme–substrate interactions and motility in the small intestine, poorer mixing of digesta in the gut lumen, slower diffusion from the gut to the epithelial cells. Viscous fibres do not appear to exert these effects by acting on secretory functions and processes of hydrolysis and transport; they act by modifying the physical characteristics of gastro-intestinal contents. The higher viscosity would spread the absorption across a longer time-span and this would explain the flat glucose tolerance curves seen after viscous fibre ingestion.

Long-term use of high-fibre or fibre supplemented diets may be accompanied by lower postprandial glucose values that result from events occurring within the gastro-intestinal tract and by long-term improvement in glucose metabolism (changes in hepatic glucose metabolism and enhanced tissue sensitivity to insulin) that may be related to the gastro-intestinal events or to other mechanisms. The possibility that fibres induce adaptive changes in the gastro-intestinal tract, and in carbohydrate digestion and absorption requires further studies in humans.

References

Anderson JW (1986) Dietary fibre in nutrition management of diabetes. In: Vahouny GV, Kritchevsky D (eds) Dietary fibre: basic and clinical aspects. Plenum Press, New York, pp 343–360

Anderson JW, Midgley WR, Wedman B (1979) Fibre and diabetes. Diabetes Care 2:369–379

Anderson BW, Levine AS, Levitt DG, Kneip JM, Levitt MD (1988) Physiological measurement of luminal stirring in perfused rat jejunum. Am J Physiol 17:G843–G848

Anderson BW, Kneip JM, Levine AS, Levitt MD (1989) Influence of infusate viscosity on intestinal absorption in the rat. Gastroenterology 97:938–943

Arnal-Peyrot F, Adrian J (1974) Role des gommes et des mucilages sur la digestibilité. Cas de la feuille de baobab (*Adamsonia digitata*). Ann Nutr Alim 28:505–521

Blackburn NA, Redfern JS, Jarjis H et al. (1984a) The mechanism of action of guar gum in improving glucose tolerance in man. Clin Sci 66:329–336

Blackburn NA, Holgate AM, Read NW (1984b) Small intestinal contact area – another mechanism by which gum reduces postprandial hyperglycaemia in man. Br J Nutr 52:197–204

Bosello O, Ostuzzi R, Armellini F, Micciolo RM, Ludovico AS (1980) Glucose tolerance and blood lipids in bran fed patients with impaired glucose tolerance. Diabetes Care 3:46–49

Brodribb AJM, Humphreys DM (1976) Diverticular disease. Part III. Metabolic effect of bran in patients with diverticular disease. Br Med J i:428–430

Brown NJ, Worlding J, Rumsey RDE, Read NW (1988) The effect of guar gum on the distribution of a radiolabelled meal in the gastrointestinal tract of the rat. Br J Nutr 59:223–231

Bueno L, Praddaube F, Fioramonti J, Ruckebush Y (1981) Effect of dietary fibre on gastrointestinal motility and jejunal transit time in dogs. Gastroenterology 80:701–707

Chapman RW, Sillery JK, Graham MM, Saunders DR (1985) Absorption of starch by healthy ileostomates: effects of transit time and of carbohydrate load. Am J Clin Nutr 41:1244–1248

Cortot A, Jobin G, Flourié B, Bernier JJ (1981) Effets du son de blé sur la digestion normale d'un repas. In: Les fibres céréalières dans l'alimentation humaine. Ronac, Paris, pp 23–34.

Di Lorenzo G, Williams CM, Hajnal F, Valenzuela JE (1988) Pectin delays gastric emptying and increases satiety in obese subjects. Gastroenterology 95:1211–1215

Dunaif G, Schneeman BO (1981) The effect of dietary fibre on human pancreatic enzyme activity in vitro. Am J Clin Nutr 34:1034–1035

Duncan KH, Bacon JA, Weinsier RL (1983) The effects of high and low energy density diets on satiety, energy intake and eating time of obese and non-obese subjects. Am J Clin Nutr 37:763–767

Ebihara K, Masuhara R, Kiriyama S, Manabe M (1981) Correlation between viscosity and plasma glucose- and insulin-flattening activities of pectins from vegetables and fruits in rats. Nutr Rep Int 23:985–992

Edwards CA, Blackburn NA, Craigen L et al. (1987) Viscosity of food gums determined in vitro related to their hypoglycemic actions. Am J Clin Nutr 46:72–77

Ehrlein H-J, Pröve J (1982) Effect of viscosity of test meals on gastric emptying in dogs. Q J Exp Physiol 76:419–425

Elsenhans B, Süfke U, Blume R, Caspary WF (1980) The influence of carbohydrate gelling agents on rat intestinal transport of monosaccharides and neutral amino acids in vitro. Clin Sci 59:373–380

Elsenhans B, Süfke U, Blume R, Caspary WF (1981) In vitro inhibition of rat intestinal surface hydrolysis of disaccharides and dipeptides by guaran. Digestion 21:98–103

Elsenhans B, Zenker D, Caspary WF, Blume R (1984) Guaran effect on rat intestinal absorption. Gastroenterology 86:645–653

Flourié B, Vidon N, Florent C, Bernier JJ (1984) Effects of pectin on jejunal glucose absorption and unstirred layer thickness in normal man. Gut 25:936–941

Flourié B, Vidon N, Chayvialle JA, Palma R, Franchisseur C, Bernier JJ (1985) Effect of increased amounts of pectin on a solid–liquid meal digestion in healthy man. Am J Clin Nutr 42:495–503

Fuse K, Bamba T, Hosoda S (1989) Effects of pectin on fatty acid and glucose absorption and on thickness of unstirred water layer in rat and human intestine. Dig Dis Sci 34:1109–1116

Gallaher D, Schneeman BO (1986) Intestinal interaction of bile acids, phospholipids, dietary fibres, and cholestyramine. Am J Physiol 13:G420–G426

Grimes DS, Goddard J (1977) Gastric emptying of wholemeal and white bread. Gut 18:725–729

Haber GB, Heaton KW, Murphy D, Burroughs L (1977) Digestion and disruption of dietary fibre. Effects on satiety, plasma glucose and serum insulin. Lancet ii:679–682

Hagander B, Asp N-G, Efendic S, Nilsson-Ehle P, Lundquist I, Shersten B (1986) Reduced glycemic response to beet-fibre meal in noninsulin-dependent diabetics and its relation to plasma levels of pancreatic and gastrointestinal hormones. Diabetes Res 3:91–96

Hagander B, Asp N-G, Efendic S, Nilsson-Ehle P, Schersten B (1988) Dietary fibre decreases fasting blood glucose levels and plasma LDL concentration in noninsulin-dependent diabetes mellitus patients. Am J Clin Nutr 47:852–858

Hamberg O, Rumessen JJ, Gudman-Hoyer E (1989a) Blood glucose response to pea fibre: comparisons with sugar beet fibre and wheat bran. Am J Clin Nutr 50:324–328

Hamberg O, Rumessen JJ, Gudman-Hoyer E (1989b) Inhibition of starch absorption by dietary fibre. Scand J Gastroenterol 24:103–109

Heaton KW, Marcus SN, Emmett PM, Bolton CH (1988) Particle size of wheat, maize, and oat test meals: effects on plasma glucose and insulin responses and on the rate of starch digestion in vitro. Am J Clin Nutr 47:675–682

Holgate AM, Read NW (1983) Relationship between small bowel transit time and absorption of a solid meal. Influence of metoclopramide, magnesium sulphate, and lactulose. Dig Dis Sci 28:812–819

Holt S, Heading RC, Carter DC, Prescott LF, Tothill P (1979) Effect of gel fibre on gastric emptying and absorption of glucose and paracetamol. Lancet i:636–639

Ikegami S, Tsuchihashi F, Harada H, Tsuchihashi N, Nishide E, Innami S (1990) Effect of viscous indigestible polysaccharides on pancreatic–biliary secretion and digestive organs in rats. J Nutr 120:353–360

Imsidumi K, Tominaga A, Mawatari K, Sugano M (1982) Effect of cellulose and guar gum on the secretion of mesenteric lymph chylomicrons in meal-fed rats. Nutr Rep Int 26:263–269

Isaksson G, Lundquist I, Ihse I (1982) Effect of dietary fibre on pancreatic enzyme activity in vitro. Gastroenterology 82:918–924

Jarjis HA, Blackburn NA, Redfern JS, Read NW (1984) The effect of ispaghule (Fybogel and Metamucil) and guar gum on glucose tolerance in man. Br J Nutr 51:371–378

Jenkins DJA (1980) Dietary fibre and carbohydrate metabolism. In: Spiller GA, McPherson Kay R (eds) Medical aspects of dietary fibre, Plenum Press, New York, pp 175–192

Jenkins DJA, Leeds AR, Gassull MA, Cochet B, Alberti GMM (1977a) Decrease in postprandial insulin and glucose concentrations by guar and pectin. Ann Intern Med 86:20–23

Jenkins DJA, Leeds AR, Houston H, Hinks L, Alberti KGMM, Cummings JH (1977b) Carbohydrate tolerance in man after six weeks of pectin administration. Proc Nutr Soc 36:60 (abstract)

Jenkins DJA, Wolever TMS, Leeds AR et al. (1978) Dietary fibres, fibre analogues and glucose tolerance: importance of viscosity. Br Med J i:1392–1394

Jenkins DJA, Wolever TMS, Nineham R, Bacon S, Smith R, Hockaday TDR (1979) Dietary fibre and diabetic therapy: a progressive effect with time. Adv Exp Med Biol 119:275–279

Jenkins DJA, Jenkins AL, Wolever TMS, Collier GR, Rao AV, Thompson LU (1987a) Starchy foods and fibre: reduced rate of digestion and improved carbohydrate metabolism. Scand J Gastroenterol 22 (Suppl 129):132–141

Jenkins DJA, Cuff D, Wolever TMS et al. (1987b) Digestibility of carbohydrate foods in an ileostomate: relationship to dietary fibre, in vitro digestibility, and glycemic response. Am J Gastroenterol 82:709–717

Johnson IT, Gee JM (1981) Effect of gel-forming gums on the intestinal unstirred layer and sugar transport in vitro. Gut 22:398–403

Johnson IT, Gee JM, Mahoney RR (1984) Effect of dietary supplements of guar gum and cellulose on intestinal cell proliferation, enzyme levels and sugar transport in the rat. Br J Nutr 52:477–487

Kelly KA (1980) Gastric emptying of liquids and solids: roles of proximal and distal stomach. Am J Physiol 239:G71–G76

Lawaetz O, Blackburn AM, Bloom SR, Aritas Y, Ralphs DNL (1983) Effect of pectin on gastric emptying and gut hormone release in the dumping syndrome. Scand J Gastroenterol 18:327–336

Leeds AR (1982) Modification of intestinal absorption of dietary fibre and fibre components. In: Vahouny GV, Kritchevsky D (eds) Dietary fibre in health and disease. Plenum Press, New York, pp 53–71

Leeds AR, Bolster NR, Andrews R, Truswell AS (1979) Meal viscosity, gastric emptying and glucose absorption in the rat. Proc Nutr Soc 38:44 (abstract)

Levitt NS, Vinik AI, Sive AA, Child PT, Jackson WPU (1980) The effect of dietary fibre on glucose and hormone responses to a mixed meal in normal subjects and in diabetic subjects with and without autonomic neuropathy. Diabetes Care 3:515–519

Levitt MD, Hirsh P, Fetzer CA, Sheahan M, Levine AS (1987) H_2 excretion after ingestion of complex carbohydrates. Gastroenterology 92:383–389

McCance RA, Prior KM, Widdowson EM (1953) A radiological study of the rate of passage of brown and white bread through the digestive tract of man. Br J Nutr 7:98–104

Meyer JH, Doty JE (1988). GI transit and absorption of solid food: multiple effects of guar. Am J Clin Nutr 48:267–173

Meyer JH, Gu Y, Elashoff J, Reedy T, Dressman J, Amidon G (1986) Effects of viscosity and fluid outflow on postcibal gastric emptying of solids. Am J Physiol 13:G161–G164

Miranda PM, Horwitz DL (1978) High fibre diets in the treatment of diabetes mellitus. Ann Intern Med 88:482–486

Monnier L (1985) Intérêt des fibres alimentaires en thérapeutique gastroentérologique et nutritionnelle. Ann Med Interne (Paris) 136:677–681

Munoz JM, Sandstead HH, Jacob RA (1979) Effects of dietary fibre on glucose tolerance of normal men. Diabetes 28:496–502

Nygren C, Hallmans G, Lithner F (1984) Effects of high-bran bread on blood glucose control in insulin-dependent diabetic patients. Diabete Metab 10:39–43

Osilesi O, Trout DL, Glover EE et al. (1985) Use of xanthan gum in dietary management of diabetes mellitus. Am J Clin Nutr 42:597–603

Poksay KS, Schneeman BO (1983) Pancreatic and intestinal response to dietary guar gum in rats. J Nutr 113:1544–1549

Pröve J, Ehrlein H-J (1982) Motor function of gastric antrum and pylorus for evacuation of low and high viscosity meals in dogs. Gut 23:150–156

Rainbird AL (1986) Effect of guar gum on gastric emptying of test meals of varying energy content in growing pigs. Br J Nutr 55:99–109

Rainbird AL, Low AG (1986) Effect of guar gum on gastric emptying in growing pigs. Br J Nutr 55:87–98

Ray TK, Mansell KM, Knight LC, Malmud LS, Owen OE, Boden G (1983) Long-term effects of dietary fibre on glucose tolerance and gastric emptying in noninsulin-dependent diabetic patients. Am J Clin Nutr 37:376–381

Read NW (1986) Dietary fibre and bowel transit. In: Vahouny GV, Kritchevsky D (eds) Dietary fibre. Basic and clinical aspects. Plenum Press, New York, pp 81–100

Russell J, Bass P (1985) Canine gastric emptying of fibre meals: influence of meal viscosity and antroduodenal motility. Am J Physiol 249:G662–G667

Russell J, Bass P (1986) Effects of laxative and nonlaxative hydrophillic polymers on canine small intestinal motor activity. Dig Dis Sci 31:281–288

Rydning A, Berstad A, Berstad T, Hertzenberg L (1985) The effect of guar gum and fibre-enriched wheat bran on gastric emptying of a semi-solid meal in healthy subjects. Scand J Gastroenterol 20:330–334

Sandberg A-S, Andersson H, Hallgren B, Hasselbled K, Isaksson B (1981) Experimental model for in vivo determination of dietary fibre and its effect on the absorption of nutrients in the small intestine. Br J Nutr 45:283–294

Sandberg A-S, Ahderinne R, Andersson H, Hallgren B, Hulten L (1983) The effect of citrus pectin on the absorption of nutrients in the small intestine. Hum Nutr Clin Nutr 37C:171–183

Sandhu KS, El Samahi MM, Mena I, Dooley GP, Valenzuela JE (1987) Effect of pectin on gastric emptying and gastroduodenal motility in normal subjects. Gastroenterology 92:486–492

Schneeman BO (1982) Pancreatic and digestive function. In: Vahouny GV, Kritchevsky D (eds) Dietary fibre in health and disease. Plenum Press, New York, pp 73–83

Schneeman BO, Richter BD, Jacobs LR (1982) Response to dietary wheat bran in the exocrine pancreas and intestine of rats. J Nutr 42:283–286

Schwartz SE, Levine GD (1980) Effects of dietary fibre on intestinal glucose absorption and glucose tolerance in rats. Gastroenterology 79:833–836

Schwartz SE, Levine RA, Singh A, Scheidecker JR, Track NS (1982) Sustained pectin ingestion delays gastric emptying. Gastroenterology 83:812–817

Schwartz SE, Levine RA, Singh A, Scheidecker JB (1984) Chronic pectin ingestion enhances glucose tolerance and delays gastric emptying in diabetics. Gastroenterology 86:1240 (abstract)

Sigleo S, Jackson MJ, Vahouny GV (1984) Effects of dietary fibre constituents on intestinal morphology and nutrient transport. Am J Physiol 246:G34–G39

Snow P, O'Dea K (1981) Factors affecting the rate of starch hydrolysis in food. Am J Clin Nutr 34:2721–2727

Sommer H, Kasper H (1980) The effect of dietary fibre on pancreatic excretory function. Hepatogastroenterology 27:477–483

Stock-Damgé C, Bouchet P, Dentinger A, Aprahamian M, Grenier JF (1983) Effect of dietary supplementation on the secretory function of the exocrine pancreas in the dog. Am J Clin Nutr 38:843–848

Torsdottir I, Alpsten M, Andersson H, Einarsson S (1989) Dietary guar gum effects on postprandial blood glucose, insulin and hydroxyproline in humans. J Nutr 119:1925–1931

Vahouny GV (1987) Effects of dietary fibre on digestion and absorption. In: Johnson LR (ed) Physiology of the gastrointestinal tract, 2nd edn. Raven Press, New York, pp 1623–1648

Villaume C, Flourié B, Beck B, Vidon N, Debry G, Bernier JJ (1988) Insuline et glucagon plasmatiques après ingestion d'un repas enrichi par des doses croissantes de pectine chez l'homme sain. Gastroenterol Clin Biol 12:559–564

Wahren J, Juhlin-Dannfelt A, Björkman O, DeFronzo R, Felig P (1982) Influence of fibre ingestion on carbohydrate utilization and absorption. Clin Physiol 2:315–321

Welch IMcL, Worlding J (1986) The effect of ileal infusion of lipid on the motility pattern in humans after ingestion of a viscous, nonnutrient meal. J Physiol 378:12P (abstract)

Wong S, Traianedes K, O'Dea K (1985) Factors affecting the rate of hydrolysis of starch in legumes. Am J Clin Nutr 42:38–43

Würsch P, Del Vedovo S, Koellreutter B (1986) Cell structure and starch nature as key determinants of the digestion rate of starch in legume. Am J Clin Nutr 43:25–29

Commentary

Edwards: Whether increased mixing can overcome the effect of viscosity will depend on the dose of viscous fibre administered and on the viscosity attained. We showed that in a model of intestinal contractions doubling the contraction rate had no effect on the movement of glucose in the presence of guar but increased the movement of glucose without guar (Edwards et al., 1988).

Reference

Edwards CA, Johnson IT, Read NW (1988) Do viscous polysaccharides slow absorption by inhibiting diffusion or convection? Eur J Clin Nutr 42:307–312

Author's reply: The strength and duration of intestinal motor activity (assessed in vivo in man and not in vitro) is certainly important since glucose is absorbed, although on a longer time-span, irrespective of the dose of viscous fibre ingested.

Chapter 11

The Influence of Dietary Fibre on Mineral Absorption and Utilisation

L. Rossander, A.-S. Sandberg and B. Sandström

Introduction

Fibre and some of the associated substances have strong in vitro mineral binding or complexing capacities and hence fibre has been suspected of impairing mineral absorption. The results of mineral absorption studies of fibre-rich diets in humans are, however, not consistent. The specific characteristics of mineral metabolism introduce a number of methodological difficulties that might have contributed to the conflicting results. Furthermore, in several studies either the content of fibre and other interacting substances has not been adequately analysed or the methods used to study absorption and utilisation have not been sensitive enough to reveal any effects.

Methodological Considerations in Studies of Mineral Absorption in Humans

Characteristic of a number of the minerals and trace elements is that only a small fraction of the dietary content is absorbed and the endogenous intestinal excretion of the mineral is relatively large. Intestinal and faecal minerals are consequently a mixture of non-absorbed elements from the diet and non-reabsorbed endogenous excreted elements. Dietary factors could affect both absorption and reabsorption and maybe also the endogenous excretion of the elements. The conventional balance technique, where absorption is measured as the difference between intake and faecal content, cannot identify these separate effects. A low degree of absorption, in combination with a relatively long colonic transit time in humans, with a subsequent mixture of several days' dietary intake and endogenous excretion, impose specific requirements on the experimental design of balance studies. Turnlund et al. (1982) have shown that in a complete faecal collection of one day's zinc intake the samples can contain zinc from the previous 12 to 30 days' meals. According to Schwartz et al. (1986) an adaptation period of at least 4 weeks on a constant intake followed by a study period of 2–3 weeks is required to obtain reliable data in balance studies for most minerals. Few studies fulfil these criteria. Changes in the intestinal transit time can occur and, great care has to be taken in separating faecal collections according to dietary intake periods. Although the balance studies are improved by a long adaptation period, the adaptation in itself presents a problem. For several minerals body homeostasis is regulated by absorption and excretion and an apparent balance can be maintained over a large range of intakes even if absorption is severely depressed by a food component.

Several of the methodological problems with the conventional balance method can be overcome by use of ileostomised subjects (Sandberg et al., 1982; Sandberg et al., 1983). However, the inability to distinguish between effects on dietary minerals and endogenous minerals remains.

The development of isotope techniques to study mineral absorption has contributed a great deal to an increased understanding of the role of dietary composition in mineral absorption and utilisation. Extrinsic labelling of meals or diets with radioactive isotopes followed by measurement of whole-body retention or enrichment in, for example blood, has been shown to give a valid and precise measurement of the absorption of iron, zinc, calcium and manganese for a range of foods (Hallberg and Björn-Rasmussen, 1972; Arvidsson et al., 1978; Heany and Recker, 1985; Davidsson et al., 1989).

In recent years stable isotope techniques for the measurement of mineral absorption have been developed. The major disadvantage of stable isotopes in comparison with radioactive isotopes is that relatively large amounts of the isotope have to be added to the test diet. For most minerals faecal collections are required. However, compared with balance studies, isotope methods have the great advantage that the measurements are not affected by endogenous excretion of the element.

Due to the many methodological difficulties in the balance technique the following review of the effect of fibre on mineral absorption and utilisation is largely based on observations from studies where isotope techniques have been used. Some well-designed balance studies are also reported.

Effects of Fibre and Fibre-Associated Compounds on Mineral Absorption in Humans

Effect of Non-starch Polysaccharides and Lignin

The results from human studies in which pure fibre fractions have been used indicate that fibre *per se* is relatively inert as regards any effect on mineral availability.

Adding α-cellulose to a basal low-fibre diet produced no effect on zinc absorption in young men using a stable isotope technique (Turnlund et al., 1984). Nor was there a change in iron absorption when cellulose was given with muffins baked with wheat flour compared with plain muffins, using the extrinsic radioiron technique (Cook et al., 1983). Addition of high amounts of refined cellulose (16 g/day) significantly decreased calcium balance in women (Slavin and Marlett, 1980).

Pectin added to a low-fibre diet in metabolic balance studies of ileostomised patients had no effect on zinc, calcium and magnesium absorption but had a negative effect on iron absorption (Sandberg et al., 1983). When pectin was put into cakes made of wheat flour (Cook et al., 1983) using the radioisotope technique, no effect was found on iron absorption. In another study, using the same technique, pectin with both a high and low degree of methoxylation in plain white wheat bread had no effect on iron absorption (Rossander, 1987). Nor was there any effect on iron absorption when guar gum or ispaghula were given in the same kind of white bread made from flour of low extraction (55%) (Hallberg L, Rossander-Hulthén L, Brune M, unpublished work). Adding psyllium, as a source of hemicellulose, resulted in negative zinc balances at high levels of hemicellulose (24.2 g/day) (Kies et al., 1979). Psyllium may, however, also contain other potential inhibitors of zinc absorption, such as phytate. The addition of beet pulp (an isolated fibre source of hemicellulose, cellulose and pectin) to a bread or meat-based meal had no effect on zinc absorption (Sandström et al., 1987b) or on iron absorption (Hallberg L, Rossander-Hulthén L, Brune M, unpublished work) using the radionuclide technique.

A reduced iron absorption was found when cocoa was served with full-cream milk and was interpreted as being an effect of lignin (Gillooly et al., 1984). Cocoa, however, contains only negligible amounts of true lignin but contains other potential antagonists of iron absorption such as phytate and iron-binding phenolic compounds sufficiently high to explain fully the inhibition of iron absorption. Wheat bran contains considerable amounts of lignin. Completely dephytinised bran had no effect on iron absorption (Hallberg et al., 1987). Zinc absorption from a low-phytate bran was high (Sandström, 1987; Hall et al., 1989; Kivistö et al., 1989), and a reduction of the phytate content of bread containing bran improved Zn absorption (Nävert et al., 1985). These observations suggest that the effect, if any, on mineral absorption of lignin as well as hemicellulose is negligible.

Effect of Fibre-Associated Compounds

Phytate

Fibre-rich foods also have a high content of phytate (myoinositol-hexa-phosphate). The concern about the presence of phytate in cereals and legumes arises from the ability of phytate to form insoluble complexes with minerals (calcium, magnesium, iron, zinc and others) at physiological pH values, which may lower the bio-availability of these minerals. The chair conformation of phytate in dilute solutions as deduced by spectroscopic methods (Johnson and Tate, 1969) suggests tremendous chelating potential (Fig. 11.1).

In the early 1920s Mellanby observed that diets poor in vitamin D and rich in cereals greatly reduced mineralisation of bones and teeth in dogs (Mellanby 1925). Subsequent studies with rats demonstrated a clear correlation between the phytate contents of different cereals and the severity of their rachitogenic

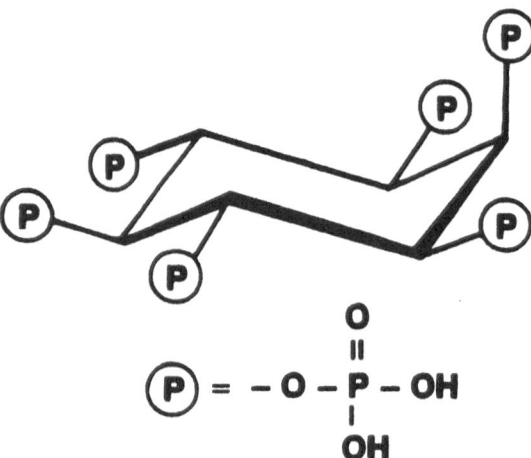

$$P = -O - \overset{\overset{\displaystyle O}{\|}}{\underset{\underset{\displaystyle OH}{|}}{P}} - OH$$

Fig. 11.1. The structure of phytic acid in dilute solution.

effects. An early balance study in humans indicated a negative effect of phytate on absorption of calcium, iron and phosphorus (McCance and Widdowson, 1942).

Single-meal studies using radionuclide techniques as well as stable isotope techniques have confirmed the negative effect of phytate on both iron and zinc absorption in humans. Addition of sodium phytate to a liquid formula to levels found in whole-grain cereal based diets, to white bread to levels found in wholemeal breads as well as to a cow milk infant formula to levels found in soy milk formula resulted in a significant decrease in zinc absorption (Turnlund et al., 1984; Halsted et al., 1972; Nävert et al., 1985; Lönnerdal et al., 1984). Reducing the naturally occurring phytate content in bread by long-term fermentation improved zinc absorption (Nävert et al., 1985) in a dose–effect way which further supports the negative effect of phytate on zinc absorption.

During food processing hydrolysis products of phytate (lower inositol phosphates) can be formed. Added separately to white bread the tetra-inositol phosphate had no effect on zinc absorption while the penta- and hexa-inositol phosphates depressed zinc absorption (Sandström and Sandberg, 1992). However, in processed foods the lower inositol phosphates seem to contribute to the impaired zinc absorption (A-S Sandberg and B Sandström, unpublished observations) in proportion to the number of phosphate groups. It is probable that purified inositol phosphates affect zinc absorption differently than the mixture of inositol phosphates that can be found in processed foods. Fig. 11.2 shows the strong negative correlation between zinc absorption and the sum of inositol tri- to hexa-phosphates in a number of composite meals.

Some conflicting results have been obtained on the effect of dietary phytate on iron absorption. The role of phytate was questioned in an extensive study of humans by Simpson et al. (1981), because of two important observations:

1. A marked reduction of the phytate content of bran by autoenzymatic digestion did not significantly increase the absorption of iron. The reduction in phytate content, however, was not complete in that study. Similar studies done

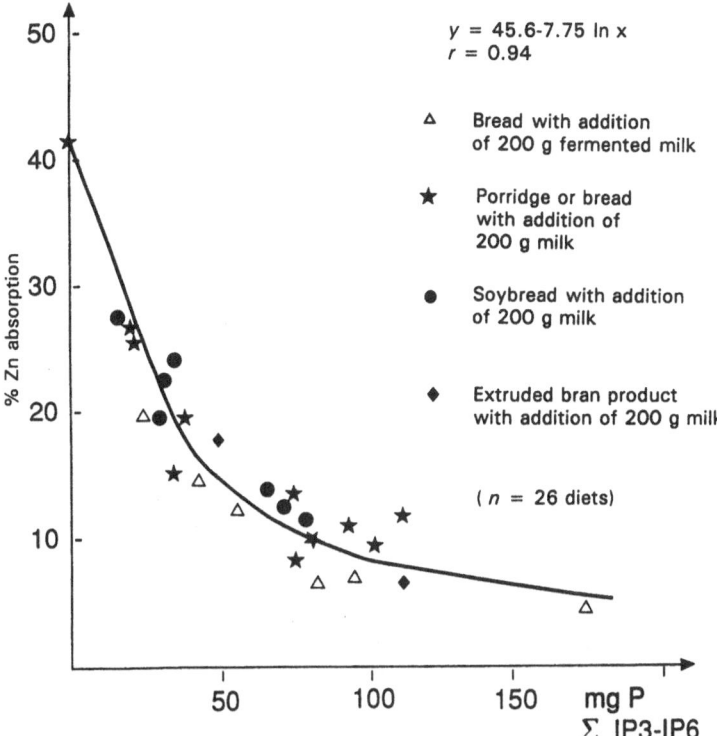

Fig. 11.2. Zinc absorption from composite meals in relation to the level of inositol phosphate-P (sum of IP₃, IP₄, IP₅ and IP₆) (A.-S. Sandberg and B. Sandström, unpublished data). In all cases, the meals included 200 g of milk or fermented milk. The bread meals, with the addition of 200 g fermented milk, contained bran baked in bread with different fermentation times. The fibre content (non-starch polysaccharides) varied from 1–15 g per meal and was not correlated to the zinc absorption. Absorption data from Nävert et al. (1985); Sandström et al. (1987a, 1987c); Kivistö et al (1989).

later strongly indicate that phytates are the main cause of iron absorption inhibition in cereals (Hallberg et al., 1987). Removal of the phytates in bran by endogenous phytase significantly increased the absorption of iron. Moreover, inhibition could be almost completely restored by restituting the phytate content.

2. Iron in monoferric phytate was as absorbable when it was given alone as a simple iron salt. However, less than 5% of the phytates in bran are in the form of monoferric phytate. Adding the other 95% of phytates (in the same amounts as in bran) to white wheat flour inhibited iron absorption to the same extent as the addition of bran (Hallberg et al., 1987). Differences in iron absorption from different batches of rice starch could also be ascribed to differences in the phytate content (Tuntawiroon et al., 1990). The high phytate content of oat meal together with a low phytase activity is also the most probable explanation for the low iron absorption from oats (Rossander-Hulthén et al., 1990). Therefore, there is a strong support for the opinion that phytate and not fibre in cereals is the main iron absorption inhibitory factor. This opinion is supported

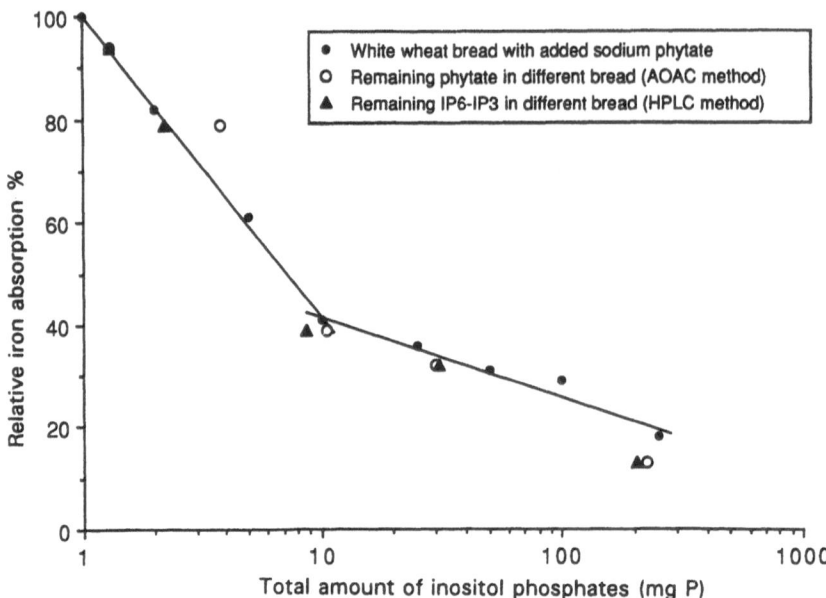

Fig. 11.3. Iron absorption in relation to the content of inositol phosphate (IP$_3$–IP$_6$) in different types of bread (Brune et al., 1992). The relative iron absorption is the ratio between test rolls and control rolls multiplied by 100. The solid lines represent the relationship after adding sodium phytate to the same kind of control rolls (Hallberg et al., 1989). The fibre content of the control rolls was 1 g. It varied from 4 to 18 g for the five different types of bread and was not correlated to the iron absorption.

by the observations that sour dough fermentation of wholemeal rye bread to a very low phytate level gave the same iron absorption as control rolls with a low fibre content and the same low phytate level (Brune et al., 1992) (Fig. 11.3).

When phytate content was held constant during three 24-day balance studies, on white bread, brown bread, wholemeal bread, by sodium phytate addition, no effect on Ca, Zn and Fe retention was seen, suggesting that fibre *per se* does not influence absorption (Andersson et al., 1983).

The inhibition of non-haem iron absorption by phytates is dose-dependent and already with small amounts a strong inhibition is exerted (Hallberg et al., 1989). As is shown in Fig. 11.3, the relationship between iron absorption and phytate seems to be composed of two regression lines with a point of intersection at 10 mg phytate P. The relationship could also be described by a single equation. The reasons for describing the relationship as two regression lines are the very high correlation coefficient ($r = 0.99$) for the high range of phytate P (10–250 mg) and that the point of intersection (10 mg) approximately corresponds to one Fe atom per molecule of inositol hexaphosphate. It is reasonable to assume that the relationship between inhibition of iron absorption and amount of phytate P varies with the iron content of the meals.

Few human data are available on the effects of other minerals. In a balance study of 12 adult men, apparent absorption (intake–faecal excretion) of calcium decreased in a dose-related effect when the diet contained muffins with dephythinised bran with added sodium phytate to increase the molar ratio phytate/calcium from 0.04 to 0.14 and 0.24 (Morris and Ellis, 1985). No effect of phytate has been observed on copper absorption in studies using stable isotopes (Turnlund et al., 1985).

Polyphenols

Phenolic compounds are widely distributed in vegetables, seeds, fruits, cereals, etc. and occur in a wide variety of chemical forms. Recent studies showed that the amount of iron-binding phenolic galloyl (tri-hydroxy-benzene) groups in foods and drinks roughly corresponded to the degree of inhibition of iron absorption (Brune et al., 1989a). Probable phenolic catechol groups in chlorogenic acid (and related substances) also contribute to the effect of phenolic compounds on iron absorption (M. Brune, L. Rossander-Hulthén, L. Hallberg, unpublished observations). Low iron absorption was found from aubergine and spinach (Gillooly et al., 1983), vegetables with a high level of iron-binding polyphenols.

Organic Acids

Many fruits and vegetables are a good source of ascorbic acid and also contain other organic acids.

Ascorbic acid is the main dietary factor that enhances iron absorption (Sayers et al., 1973; Hallberg et al., 1986). Its effect is dose-related and is quite marked in all kinds of diets. A reduction of the natural content of ascorbic acid in a meal reduces the absorption of the non-haem iron content in the whole meal (Hallberg, 1981). Ascorbic acid has a physiological role in iron absorption ensuring conversion of ferric iron in the diet to ferrous iron, which is necessary for absorption (Wollenberg and Rummel, 1987). Ascorbic acid could also have a role in reducing the formation in intestinal lumen of poorly soluble and poorly available ferric complexes with, for example, hydroxyl irons, certain phosphate ions, phytates, and iron polyphenol complexes. Ascorbic acid strongly counteracts the inhibitory effect of phytates and of polyphenols on iron absorption (Hallberg et al., 1989; Tuntawirooh et al., 1990; Siegenberg et al., 1991). No effect of ascorbic acid on zinc absorption has been shown (Solomons et al., 1979; Sandström and Cederblad, 1987).

In some studies *citric acid* has been found to increase non-haem iron absorption (Gillooly et al., 1983). but in others no effect has been found (Hallberg and Rossander, 1984). Addition of citric acid to a phytate-containing soya formula (Lönnerdal et al., 1984) had no effect on zinc absorption. Addition of *malic acid* or *tartaric acid* to a basal rice meal improved the iron absorption (Gillooly et al., 1983). Sauerkraut markedly enhanced iron absorption but this effect cannot be explained by its acidity or its *lactic* or *acetic acid* content (Hallberg and Rossander, 1982a).

Oxalate salts are poorly soluble at intestinal pH and *oxalic acid* is known to decrease calcium absorption in monogastric animals (Allen, 1982). The effect of oxalate on calcium absorption in humans is less clear. Calcium in spinach with a high oxalate content is very poorly absorbed (Heaney et al., 1988) while kale, a low-oxalate vegetable, exhibits excellent calcium absorbability (Heaney and Weaver, 1990). However, studies with calcium oxalate suggest that other factors in spinach contribute to the low calcium absorption (Heaney and Weaver, 1989).

Mineral Absorption from Fibre-Rich Diets

Cereal-Based Diets

Unrefined cereals have a high phytate content and are also rich in minerals. Studies of iron bio-availability have shown poor absorption from most cereals with the exception of highly refined wheat (INACG report, 1982). The fractional iron absorption from cereal-based diets with a high phytate content is low but could to some extent be balanced by a higher iron content (Dobbs and McLean Baird, 1977). The fractional absorption of iron from wholemeal bread was about one-third of that from white bread made from unenriched flour using the radioisotope technique. However, the wholemeal bread contained about four times the content of iron and there was no difference in amounts of iron absorbed. The meal consisted only of bread, but in a meal also containing other iron sources, the phytate would negatively influence the amount of iron absorbed from the whole meal.

In some cereals the content of iron-binding phenolic compounds must also be considered (e.g. red sorghum).

The fractional zinc absorption from cereal-based diets with a high phytate content is low but this is to some extent balanced by a higher zinc content compared with refined diets. However, phytate seems to affect not only small intestinal absorption but also reabsorption of endogenous intestinal losses of zinc. Turnlund et al. (1987) used stable isotopes of zinc to compare diets based on white bread or whole-wheat bread with 7.4 vs. 13.2 mg zinc. More dietary zinc was absorbed from the whole-wheat diet but the endogenous faecal losses were higher and zinc retention did not differ significantly. Similar observations of increased endogenous losses of zinc were also reported after the addition of phytate to a formula diet (Turnlund et al., 1987). The intestinal endogenous losses of iron are slight. On the other hand, small amounts of phytate have a marked inhibitory effect on iron absorption. Van Dokkum et al. (1982) observed in 20-day balance studies an almost constant mineral retention when fibre intake was increased from 9 to 22 g of NDF by addition of 46 g of bran to a low-fibre diet. As the mineral intake also was increased they suggest that the minerals in the bran were not available for absorption. At higher bran intake (35 g NDF/day) iron balance was significantly decreased and balances were negative for Ca, Mg, Fe and Zn but not for Cu. Addition of 26 g of wheat or corn bran in a 30-day balance study of five subjects had no significant negative effect on zinc, iron and copper balances (Sandstedt et al., 1978). When wheat bran (16 g/day) was added to a low-fibre diet in eight ileostomised subjects, apparent absorption of zinc decreased, in relative and absolute amount absorbed, while relative absorption of iron and calcium were unchanged (Sandberg et al., 1982).

Legume-Based Diets

Most legumes have a high phytate content and are also relatively rich in minerals. Iron absorption from soya beans and soya protein products is low (Cook et al., 1981; Morck et al., 1981; Hallberg and Rossander, 1982b) using the extrinsic tag method. Iron absorption, using the same method, from meals based on black beans, lentils, mung beans and split beans was found to be very low, ranging from 0.8% to 1.9% (Lynch et al., 1984).

Studies of meals based on white beans and soya beans indicate that the effect of phytate on zinc absorption is less pronounced in soya beans than in cereals (Sandström and Cederblad, 1980; Sandström et al., 1989) and that legume and animal protein are comparable with the same zinc content. Low zinc absorption from a soya protein-based infant formula has, however, been found (Sandström et al., 1983a). It is possible that this low absorption is to some extent an effect of the processing.

Diets Rich in Vegetables and Fruits

Addition of vegetables like carrots, potatoes and cabbage to a low zinc animal protein meal had no effect on zinc absorption (Sandström et al., 1987b). However, most leafy vegetables as well as tubers and fruits have a low content of zinc and will dilute the zinc density of the diet. The effect on iron absorption of adding vegetables or fruits to a meal depends on the content of phytate, iron-binding polyphenols and especially on the ascorbic acid content. Contrary to the results from isotope studies, balance studies indicate a negative effect on zinc, copper and calcium retention of a diet containing fruits and vegetables (Kelsay et al., 1979a,b). However, in a subsequent balance study, no effect on increasing levels of fruits and vegetables on calcium, magnesium and copper balances were found. Zinc balance decreased, but remained positive as fibre increased (Kelsay et al., 1981).

Interactions Between Dietary Components

Evaluation of the effects of a fibre-rich diet on mineral utilisation is complicated by the many potential interactions between fibres, fibre-associated compounds and nutrients in the diet, and could explain why the effect of an isolated fibre substance in vitro is not always the same as the same fibre component in a mixed diet. The fact that in vitro studies do not include the absorption and utilisation stages also reduces their predictive power.

The protein source and level have been shown to affect both iron and zinc absorption. Meat, fish and poultry have an as yet unidentified positive effect on iron absorption (Layrisse et al., 1973; Björn-Rasmussen and Hallberg, 1979) and an increased level of protein has a positive effect on zinc absorption from a meal containing phytate (Sandström et al., 1980; Sandström et al., 1989). Proteins have many binding sites for minerals as well as for complexing substances and could protect the minerals from binding to unabsorbed substances. On the other hand, if proteins are poorly or slowly digested, absorption of minerals bound to proteins could also be impaired. A reduction in apparent zinc absorption in ileostomised subjects given a soya protein-based diet has been observed concomitant with a reduced protein digestibility (Sandström et al., 1986).

The presence of other minerals is also important for the degree of absorption. Interactions between zinc and iron and manganese and iron are well established (Sandström et al., 1985; Rossander-Hulthén et al., 1991). The level of calcium is of special interest in diets containing phytate. Calcium salts as well as calcium in milk reduce the degradation of phytate in bread (Türk and Sandberg, 1992) and impair the absorption of iron (Hallberg et al., 1991). For zinc, the effect of calcium is more complex and less systematically studied. Animal studies, using high calcium levels have clearly shown a potentiating negative effect of calcium on zinc absorption from a diet containing phytate (Davies and Olpin, 1979). In human subjects, increasing the calcium content of a meal by the addition of milk improved zinc absorption from wholemeal bread (Sandström et al., 1980). Adding milk to a soya protein or white bean-based meal gave a lower fractional zinc absorption although this was counterbalanced by the additional zinc provided by the milk (Sandström et al., 1987c; Sandström et al., 1989). After the addition of calcium to an infant soya formula containing phytate a higher zinc absorption tendency was observed (Lönnerdal et al., 1984).

The Significance of the Phytate Content in the Diet

Ellis et al. (1987) analysed the phytate content in duplicate portions of self-selected diets of North Americans, Asian-Indians and Nepalese. With omnivore North Americans the average intake was approximately 170 mg phytate-phosphorus per day. North American and Asian-Indian vegetarians consumed about twice as much and the average intake for the Nepalese vegetarians was more than 560 mg/day. Cereals formed the major source of phytate for the omnivores in contrast to legumes (soya and lentils) and rice in the vegetarian diets. Intakes close to 560 mg/day have also been reported in East African children (Ferguson et al., 1989) consuming a maize-based diet. An intake of 140-200 mg phytate-phosphorus per day has been calculated for British students and university staff (Wise et al., 1987). If it is assumed that these intakes are divided into four meals, the single meal data presented in Figs. 11.2 and 11.3 indicate that there is a risk of impairment of zinc absorption at an intake of about 150–200 mg phytate-phosphorus/day (50 mg/meal) and for iron at about 30–40 mg/day (10 mg/meal) if no promoting factors are present in the diet.

Thus with the reported phytate intakes the total composition of the diet is crucial for mineral utilisation especially as there does not seem to be any adaptation to a high phytate intake through a more efficient absorption. Iron absorption from bran rolls compared with iron absorption from wheat rolls in a group of strict vegetarians with a high habitual phytate intake did not differ from that of a non-vegetarian control group (Brune et al., 1989b).

Epidemiological observations support the experimentally confirmed negative effect of high phytate diets on mineral availability. Zinc responsive growth impairment has been observed in populations where the staple food is unleavened bread (Halsted et al., 1972).

A poor growth and other indices of a low zinc status is also seen in the West African children eating the above mentioned maize-based diet (Ferguson et al., 1989). Nutritional iron deficiency reaches its greatest prevalence and severity in populations subsisting predominantly on cereal and legume diets (INACG, 1982).

The Influence of Food Processing on Mineral Absorption

Food processing of fibre-rich foods can lead to both positive and negative effects on mineral availability: heat treatment often results in inactivation of the enzyme phytase which hydrolyses phytate, vitamin C can be destroyed during cooking and baking and the structure of polyphenols can be altered. Other food processes, eg soaking, malting and fermentation activate the endogenous phytase and polyphenol-oxidase of plant foods, and during fermentation factors stimulating iron absorption are produced (Sandberg, 1991).

Extrusion Cooking

Heat treatment during extrusion cooking of wheat bran caused inactivation of phytase and was found to decrease apparent absorption of zinc, magnesium and phosphorus in ileostomy subjects (Kivistö et al., 1986) and also zinc absorption measured by isotope technique (Kivistö et al. 1989) when compared with raw bran. This effect was ascribed to the lack of phytate hydrolysis of the extruded bran in the stomach and small intestine of humans (Sandberg et al., 1986; Sandberg et al., 1987). By reducing the phytate content of bran before extrusion cooking, the zinc absorption was increased (Kivistö et al., 1989).

In a balance study using stable isotopes, no effect of extrusion cooking of wheat bran on zinc and iron absorption was found. As some other factors of importance were changed during the study the interpretation of the results are difficult.

Soaking and Malting

Soaking of wheat bran, whole wheat flour and rye flour at optimal conditions for phytase activity resulted in complete phytate hydrolysis (Mellanby, 1950; Sandberg and Svanberg, 1991). Only partial removal of phytate from oats, rice bran and bean was obtained by soaking (Mellanby, 1950; Sandberg and Svanberg, 1991; Tangendjaja et al., 1981; Khokhar and Chauhan, 1986).

Malting is a process during which the whole grain is soaked and then germinated. The amount of phytate in malted grains of wheat, rye and oats intended for the production of flour was only reduced slightly or not at all. However, when the malted cereals were ground and soaked at optimal conditions for wheat phytase there was a complete degradation of phytate (Sandberg, 1991), except for oats which under the conditions studied had a low phytase activity.

Fermentation

Fermentation is an old method for food processing and preservation. Due to the production of lactic acid and other organic acids, the pH is lowered and the phytase activated. Fermentation of maize, soya beans and sorghum reduces the phytate content (Sudarmadju and Markakis, 1977; Lopez et al., 1983; Svanberg and Sandberg, 1988). Scalding or sour dough fermentation of bread containing rye bran and oat flour under optimal pH conditions resulted in almost complete phytate reduction (Larsson and Sandberg, 1991).

Lactic acid-fermented vegetables added to a meal were found to increase the iron absorption (L. Rossander-Hulthén, A.-S. Sandberg, B. Sandström, unpublished observations). The fresh vegetables (carrots, turnips, onions) contained small amounts of phytate, which was hydrolysed during the fermentation. The amount of iron absorbed was increased when the fermented vegetables were added to a white wheat roll (the fractional absorption increased from 13.6 to 23.6) and also when added to phytate-rich meals (wholemeal rye and wheat rolls (the fractional absorption increased from 5.2 to 10.4)). This indicates the formation of iron-promoting factors in lactic acid-fermented vegetables. No differences were found in zinc absorption between a meal containing raw or fermented vegetables.

The Possibility of Predicting Absorption Using In Vitro and Animal Models

In Vitro Studies

The complex nature of mineral absorption from mixed diets has led to attempts to find simpler screening methods to predict the degree of absorption or at least compare absorbability from different foods and diets. It is, however, difficult to design in vitro systems that will accurately predict absorption in humans. Simple binding studies of minerals to fibre may therefore be misleading as transit time, pH, enzyme concentrations and diffusion barriers may all affect the proportion of ingested nutrients absorbed. It is therefore of utmost importance that in vitro systems are validated by in vivo measurements of absorption from the same foods and diets. In vitro systems determining ionisable, soluble or dialysable iron, zinc or calcium in a mixed diet after enzymatic digestion under physiological conditions have been developed (Miller et al., 1981; Narasinga Rao and Prabhavathi, 1978; Sandström and Almgren, 1989; Sandberg et al., 1989; Schwartz and Nevins, 1989).

Plant foods were digested in vitro under simulated physiological conditions and the proportion of iron which diffused across a semi-permeable membrane was used as an index of iron availability (Hazell and Johnson, 1987). The results for iron diffusibility correlated well with literature values for the in vivo absorption of iron from similar foods. A low diffusibility was found for iron in cereals, legumes and nuts and a high diffusibility for fruits and vegetables. The first group contains high levels of phytate and low levels of citrate and ascorbate, whereas the reverse is true for vegetables and fruits.

The effect of sodium phytate on iron solubility was measured under simulated physiological conditions using an in vitro method. This method correlated well ($r = 0.99$) with in vivo measurements of the same foods and diets (Sandberg et al., 1989). Even very small amounts of phytate (inositol hexaphosphate) when added to a white wheat roll with no detectable phytate content was found to have a strong negative effect on iron solubility. This negative effect was, however, obtained only when calcium and magnesium salts were added in physiological amounts with the pepsin solution during the in vitro digestion. Calcium and magnesium are present in the stomach and small intestine during the digestion of food. In vitro studies of soaking, germination, fermentation and addition of phytase indicate that the phytate content of cereals should be reduced to very low levels to prevent a negative effect on iron availability (Svanberg and Sandberg, 1988; Sandberg and Svanberg, 1991). These results are in agreement with human absorption studies (Brune et al., 1992).

Determinations of dialysable zinc at pH 8 after in vitro digestion of phytate-containing meals at simulated physiological conditions (Sandström and Almgren, 1989) was found to correlate reasonably well with in vivo measurements, but the precision was poor.

In vitro studies of polyphenols are few and present major methodological problems because the phenolic compounds are a heterogenous group of compounds in foods and very little is known about which of them are responsible for the inhibiting effect on iron absorption. Thus, the results from these studies are difficult to evaluate. It has, however, been demonstrated that ionisable iron was significantly higher in white ragi (with a low tannin content) compared with brown varieties (with a high tannin content) (Rao and Deosthale, 1988).

Consistent with human absorption studies, in vitro studies suggest an enhancing effect of ascorbic acid on iron availability (Rizk and Clydesdale, 1985; Hazell and Johnson, 1987). Ascorbic acid was added to cereal or soya foods and iron solubility or diffusibility was measured. On the other hand in the same studies in vitro measurements predict that citric acid (Rizk and Clydesdale, 1985; Hazell and Johnson, 1987) should enhance iron availability whereas results from human absorption studies are conflicting (Hallberg and Rossander, 1984; Gillooly et al., 1983). Other organic acids such as lactic acid included in a soya diet were also found to increase iron solubility.

Studies of iron solubility at simulated physiological conditions in meals with a white or wholemeal wheat roll with addition of fresh or fermented vegetables (Svanberg et al., 1990) predicted the enhancing effect on iron absorption found from similar meals with fermented vegetables.

Animal Models

Experimental animals have a number of limitations both as a model for studying mineral absorption in general and also for studying the effects of fibre on mineral absorption. The mineral requirement of a growing animal is much higher than in humans and the metabolism of several elements, for example iron and calcium, differs substantially. The small intestinal and colonic digestion of fibre and fibre-associated compounds could differ in experimental animals compared with humans.

These differences in mineral metabolism exclude the balance technique if animals are to be used to evaluate foods for human consumption. Radioisotope techniques could be used for the screening of the effects of individual dietary components. Liver radiozinc uptake in suckling rats 4 hours after the administration of a labelled infant formula has been found to correlate well with absorption data for human adults using radioisotopes and whole-body retention measurements (Sandström et al., 1983b) with low absorption from a soya formula containing phytate. Adult rats did not show the same differences between diets. The suckling rat model also mimicked the effects of the different inositol phosphates on zinc retention observed in humans (Lönnerdal et al., 1989, Sandström and Sandberg, 1992). In a recent study (Reddy and Cook, 1991) using a dual radioiron method to determine the extent to which iron absorption measurements in the rat can predict non-haem iron bio-availability in humans, factors such as meat, ascorbic acid, bran and soy protein affected iron absorption very little in rats compared with humans. The conclusion was that rats are far less sensitive than humans to dietary influences on non-haem iron absorption and are of limited value in assessing this aspect of human nutrition.

Conclusions

Points of Consensus

Non-starch polysaccharides and lignin in foods do not have any nutritionally significant effect on mineral and trace element absorption, while substances associated with dietary fibre and present in fibre-rich foods are important antagonists and enhancers for the uptake of these nutrients.

A strong negative effect on zinc and iron absorption has consistently been shown for phytate, inositol hexaphosphate, and some of its degradation products. For iron, the absorption depressing effect is pronounced even at low levels of phytate. Some of the phenolic compounds present in vegetable foods impair iron absorption. However, some fibre-rich foods also contain potential enhancers for iron absorption such as ascorbic acid and other organic acids.

The absorption of minerals depends on the total composition of the meal and in a balanced diet containing animal protein, a high intake of fibre-rich foods does not imply a risk of inadequate mineral supply. Strictly vegetarian diets based on unrefined cereals and possibly also some legume-based diets will result in low absorption of zinc and iron. However, the utilisation of zinc and iron and probably other minerals can be improved by food processes such as fermentation or soaking and malting which decrease the phytate content. Fibre-rich foods would then become good sources of iron and zinc as the content of these minerals is high.

A simple measurement of the in vitro binding capacity of minerals is not a good indicator of mineral availability. Other suggested in vitro techniques have to some extent been able to predict mineral utilisation, but need further development.

Due to differences in mineral requirement, metabolism and probably also different digestive capacity of fibre and fibre-associated compounds, the value of animal models for studies of the effect of fibre on mineral absorption and utilisation is questionable.

Implementation of Present Knowledge by the Food Industry and Legislative Bodies

Bio-technological and other food processes should be used to improve the mineral utilisation from phytate-rich foods. The phytate content should be analysed in fibre-rich foods and in isolated and enriched fibre preparations. For industrially prepared fibre-rich foods representing a substantial part of total mineral intake or designed for population groups with a high mineral requirement such as infants, children and adolescents, a high availability of at least iron and zinc should be verified by the manufacturers.

Areas for Future Research

It is still not clear under what dietary conditions, e.g. at what level of calcium and animal protein intake, a diet containing phytate presents a nutritional problem in terms of mineral supply. More knowledge is needed about the utilisation of trace elements from vegetarian-based diets, about the long-term effects on mineral status of increasing the amount of fibre-rich foods in an omnivorous diet as well as the possibility of improving mineral utilisation by changes in food preparation. Research topics of special interest are:

Identification of the iron absorption promoting factor of fermented vegetables

The role of calcium in zinc absorption from diets rich in phytate

The role of fibre-associated substances on calcium absorption and especially from diets low in calcium

Further studies of the degradation products of phytate and their interaction with other food components

The significance of different phenolic compounds for iron absorption; and methods to reduce the content of these compounds in foods

Interactions between polyphenols and phytate
Further studies on mineral absorption from soya products and other legume proteins

The effect of industrial food processing of fibre-rich foods on potential mineral-absorption-depressing substances also needs further study in order to optimise food processes aimed at high mineral availability.

Improvement and validation of in vitro techniques is needed to provide a means of screening foods and predicting mineral utilisation from complete meals.

References

Allen LH (1982) Calcium bioavailability and absorption; a review. Am J Clin Nutr 35:783–808

Andersson H, Nävert B, Bingham SR, Englyst HN, Cummings JH (1983) The effects of breads containing similar amounts of phytate but different amounts of wheat bran on calcium, zinc and iron balance in man. Br J Nutr 50:503–510

Arvidsson B, Cederblad A, Björn-Rasmussen E, Sandström B (1978) A radionuclide technique for studies of zinc absorption in man. Int J Nucl Med Biol 5:104–109

Björn-Rasmussen E, Hallberg L (1979) Effect of animal proteins on the absorption of food iron in man. Nutr Metab 23:192–202

Brune M, Rossander L, Hallberg L (1989a) Iron absorption and phenolic compounds. Importance of different phenolic structures. Eur J Clin Nutr 43:547–558

Brune M, Rossander L, Hallberg L (1989b) Iron absorption: no intestinal adaption to high-phytate intake. Am J Clin Nutr 49:542–545

Brune M, Hallberg L, Rossander-Hulthén L, Sandberg A-S (1992) Iron absorption from bread. Inhibiting effects of cereal fiber, phytate and inositol phosphates with different numbers of phosphate groups. J Nutr (in press)

Cook JD, Morck TA, Lynch SR (1981) The inhibitory effect of soy products on nonheme iron absorption in man. Am J Clin Nutr 34:2622–2629

Cook JD, Noble NL, Morck TA, Lynch SR, Petersburg SJ (1983) Effect of fibre on nonheme iron absorption. Gastroenterology 85:1354–1358

Davidsson L, Cederblad A, Lönnerdal B, Sandström B (1989) Manganese retention in man: a method for estimating manganese absorption in man. Am J Clin Nutr 49:170–179

Davies NT, Olpin SE (1979) Studies on the phytate: zinc molar contents in diets as a determinant of Zn availability to young rats. Br J Nutr 41:591–603

Dobbs RJ, McLean Baird I (1977) Effect of wholemeal and white bread on iron absorption in normal people. Br Med J i:1641–1642

Ellis R, Kelsay JL, Reynolds RD, Morris ER, Moser PB, Frazier CW (1987) Phytate: zinc and phytate X calcium: zinc millimolar ratios in self-selected diets of Americans, Asian Indians, and Nepalese. J Am Diet Assoc 87:1043–1047

Ferguson EL, Gibson RS, Thompson L, Oarpuu S (1989) Dietary calcium, phytate and zinc intakes and the calcium, phytate and zinc molar ratios of the diets of a selected group of East African children. Am J Clin Nutr 50:1450–1456

Gillooly M, Bothwell TH, Torrance JD et al. (1983) The effects of organic acids, phytates and polyphenols on the absorption of iron from vegetables. Br J Nutr 49:331–342

Gillooly M, Bothwell TH, Charlton RW et al. (1984) Factors affecting the absorption of iron from cereals. Br J Nutr 51:37–46

Hall MJ, Downs L, Ene MD, Farah D (1989) Effect of reduced phytate wheat bran on zinc absorption. Eur J Clin Nutr 43:431–440

Hallberg L (1981) Bioavailability of dietary iron in man. Ann Rev Nutr 1:123–147

Hallberg L, Björn-Rasmussen E (1972) Determination of iron absorption from whole diet. A new two-pool model using two radioiron isotopes given as haem and non-haem iron. Scand J Haemotol 9:193–197

Hallberg L, Rossander L (1982a) Absorption of iron from Western-type lunch and dinner meals. Am J Clin Nutr 35:502–509

Hallberg L, Rossander L (1982b) Effect of soy protein on nonheme iron absorption in man. Am J Clin Nutr 36:514–520

Hallberg L, Rossander L (1984) Improvement of iron in developing countries: comparison of adding meat, soy protein, ascorbic acid, citric acid, and ferrous sulphate on iron absorption from a simple Latin American-type of meal. Am J Clin Nutr 39:577–583

Hallberg L, Brune M, Rossander L (1986) Effect of ascorbic acid on iron absorption from different types of meals. Studies with ascorbic acid-rich foods and synthetic ascorbic acid given in different amounts with different meals. Hum Nutr Applied Nutr 40A:97–113

Hallberg L, Rossander L, Skånberg A-B (1987) Phytates and the inhibitory effect of bran on iron absorption in man. Am J Clin Nutr 45:988–996

Hallberg L, Brune M, Rossander L (1989) Iron absorption in man: ascorbic acid and dose-dependent inhibition by phytate. Am J Clin Nutr 49:140–144

Hallberg L, Brune M, Erlandsson M, Sandberg A-S, Rossander-Hulthén L (1991) Calcium: effect of different amounts on nonheme and heme iron absorption in man. Am J Clin Nutr 53:112–119

Halsted JA, Ronaghy HA, Adabi P et al. (1972) Zinc deficiency in man. Am J Med 53:277–284

Hazell T, Johnson IT (1987) In vitro estimation of iron availability from a range of plant foods: influence of phytate, ascorbate and citrate. Br J Nutr 57:223–233

Heaney RP, Recker RR (1985) Estimation of true calcium absorption. Ann Intern Med 103:516–521

Heaney RP, Weaver CM (1989) Oxalate: effect on calcium absorbability. Am J Clin Nutr 50:830–832

Heaney RP, Weaver CM (1990) Calcium absorption from kale. Am J Clin Nutr 51:656–657

Heaney RP, Weaver CM, Recker RR (1988) Calcium absorbability from spinach. Am J Clin Nutr 47:707–709

International Nutritional Anemia Consultative Group (INACG) (1982) Iron absorption from cereals and legumes. A report of the International Nutritional Anemia Consultative Group. New York. The Nutrition Foundation, New York, pp 1–44

Iyer V, Salunkhe DK, Sathe SK, Rockland LB (1980) Quick-cooking beans. II. Phytates, oligosaccharide and anti-enzymes. Qual Plant Foods Hum Nutr 30:45

Johnson LF, Tate ME (1969) Structure of "phytic acids". Can J Chem 47:63–73

Kelsay JL, Behall KM, Prather ES (1979a) Effect of fibre from fruits and vegetables on metabolic responses of human subjects. II. Calcium, magnesium, iron and silicon balances. Am J Clin Nutr 32:1876–1880

Kelsay JL, Jacob RA, Prather ES (1979b) Effect of fibre from fruits and vegetables on metabolic responses of human subjects. III. Zinc, copper, and phosphorus balances. Am J Clin Nutr 32:2307–2311

Kelsay JL, Clark WM, Herbst BJ, Prather ES (1981) Nutrient utilisation by human subjects consuming fruits and vegetables as sources of fibre. J Agric Food Chem 29:461–465

Khokhar S, Chauhan BM (1986) Antinutritional factors in moth bean differences and effects of methods of domestic processing and cooking. J Food Sci 51:591–594

Kies C, Fox HM, Beshgetoor D (1979) Effect of various levels of dietary hemicellulose on zinc nutritional status of men. Cereal Chem 56:133–136

Kivistö B, Andersson H, Cederblad G, Sandberg A-S, Sandström B (1986) Extrusion cooking of a high-fibre cereal product. II. Effects on apparent absorption of zinc, iron, calcium, magnesium and phosphorus in humans. Br J Nutr 55:255–260

Kivistö B, Cederblad A, Davidsson L, Sandberg A-S, Sandström B (1989) Effect of meal composition and phytate content on zinc absorption in humans from an extruded bran product. J Cereal Sci 10:189–197

Larsson M, Sandberg A-S (1991) Phytate reduction in bread containing oat flour, oat bran or rye bran. J Cereal Sci 14:141–149

Layrisse M, Martinez-Torres C, Cook JD, Walker R, Finch CA (1973) Iron fortification of food: its measurement by the extrinsic tag method. Blood 41:333–352

Lönnerdal B, Cederblad A, Davidsson L, Sandström B (1984) The effect of individual components of soy formula and cow's milk formula on zinc bioavailability. Am J Clin Nutr 40:1064–1070

Lönnerdal B, Sandberg A-S, Sandström B, Kunz C (1989) Inhibitory effects of phytic acid and other inositol phosphates on zinc and calcium absorption in suckling rats. J Nutr 119:211–214

Lopez Y, Gordon DT, Fields ML (1983) Release of phosphorus from phytate by natural lactic acid fermentation. J Food Sci 48:953–954

Lynch SR, Beard JL, Dassenko SA, Cook JD (1984) Iron absorption from legumes in humans. Am J Clin Nutr 40:42–47

McCance RA, Widdowson EM (1942) Mineral metabolism of healthy adults on white and brown bread dietaries. J Physiol 101:44–85

Mellanby E (1925) Experimental rickets: the effect of cereals and their interaction with other factors of diet and environment in producing rickets. HMSO, London (Medical Research Council special report series, no. 93)

Mellanby E (1950) Some points in the chemistry and biochemistry of phytic acid and phytase. In: A story of nutritional research. Williams and Wilkins, Baltimore, pp 248–282

Miller DD, Schricker BT, Rasmussen RR, Van Campen D (1981) An in vitro method for estimation of iron availability from meals. Am J Clin Nutr 34:2248–2256

Morck TA, Lynch SR, Skikne BS, Cook JD (1981) Iron availability from infant food supplements. Am J Clin Nutr 34:2630–2634

Morris ER, Ellis R (1985) Bioavailability of dietary calcium. Effect of phytate on adult men consuming nonvegetarian diets. In: Kies C (ed) Nutritional bioavailability of calcium. American Chemical Society, Washington D.C., pp 63–72

Narasinga Rao BS, Prabhavathi T (1978) An in vitro method for predicting the bioavailability of iron from foods. Am J Clin Nutr 31:169–175

Nävert B, Sandström B, Cederblad A (1985) Reduction of the phytate content of bran by leavening in bread and its effect on absorption of zinc in man. Br J Nutr 53:47–53

Rao PU, Deosthale YG (1988) In vitro availability of iron and zinc in white and coloured ragi: role of tannin and phytate. Plant Foods Hum Nutr 38:35–41

Reddy MB, Cook JD (1991) Assessment of dietary determinants of nonheme-iron absorption in humans and rats. Am J Clin Nutr 54:723–728

Rizk SW, Clydesdale FM (1985) Effect of organic acids in the in vitro solubilization of iron from a soy-extended meat patty. J Food Sci 50:577–581

Rossander L (1987) Effect of dietary fibre on iron absorption in man. Scand J Gastroenterol 22 (Suppl 129):68–72

Rossander-Hulthén L, Gleerup A, Hallberg L (1990) Inhibitory effect of oat products on non-haem iron absorption in man. Eur J Clin Nutr 44:783–791

Rossander-Hulthén L, Brune M, Sandström B, Lönnerdal B, Hallberg L (1991) Competitive inhibition of iron absorption by manganese and zinc in humans. Am J Clin Nutr 54:152–156

Sandberg A-S (1991) The effect of food processing on phytate hydrolysis and availability of iron and zinc. In: Friedman (ed.) Nutritional and toxicological consequences of food processing. Plenum Press, New York, pp 499–508

Sandberg A-S, Svanberg U (1991) Effects of phytate hydrolysis by phytase in cereals on in vitro estimation of iron availability. J Food Sci. pp 499–508

Sandberg A-S, Hasselblad C, Hasselblad K, Hulthén L (1982) The effect of wheat bran on the absorption of minerals in the small intestine. Br J Nutr 48:185–191

Sandberg A-S, Ahderinne R, Andersson H, Hallgren B, Hultén L (1983) The effect of citrus pectin on the absorption of nutrients in the small intestine. Human Nutr Clin Nutr 37C:171–183

Sandberg A-S, Andersson H, Kivistö B, Sandström B (1986) Extrusion cooking of a high-fibre cereal product. I. Effects on digestibility and absorption of protein, fat, starch, dietary fibre and phytate in the small intestine. Br J Nutr 55:245–254

Sandberg A-S, Andersson H, Carlsson N-G, Sandström B (1987) Degradation products of bran phytate formed during digestion in the human small intestine. Effect of extrusion cooking on digestibility. J Nutr 117:2061–2065

Sandberg A-S, Carlsson N-G, Svanberg U (1989) Effects of inositol tri-, tetra-, penta- and hexaphosphates on in vitro estimation of iron availability. J Food Sci 54:159–161, 186

Sandsteedt HH, Muñoz JM, Jacob RA et al. (1978) Influence of dietary fibre on trace element balance. Am J Clin Nutr 31:S180–S184

Sandström B (1987) Zinc and dietary fibre. Tricum Symposium. Scand J Gastroenterol 22 (Suppl 129):80–84

Sandström B, Almgren A (1989) Dialyzable zinc after in vitro digestion in comparison with zinc absorption measured in humans. In: Southgate D, Johnson I, Fenwick GR (eds) Nutrient availability: chemical and biological aspects. The Royal Society of Chemistry, Cambridge, pp 238–240

Sandström B, Cederblad A (1980) Zinc absorption from composite meals. II. Influence of the main protein source. Am J Clin Nutr 33:1778–1783

Sandström B, Cederblad A (1987) Effects of ascorbic acid on the absorption of zinc and calcium in man. Int J Vit Nutr Res 57:87–90

Sandström B, Sandberg A-S (1992) Inhibitory effects of isolated inositol phosphates on zinc absorption in humans. Journal of Trace Elements and Electrolytes in Health and Disease (in press)

Sandström B, Arvidsson B, Cederblad A, Björn-Rasmussen E (1980) Zinc absorption from composite meals. I. The significance of wheat extraction rate, zinc, calcium and protein content in meals based on bread. Am J Clin Nutr 33:739–745

Sandström B, Cederblad A, Lönnerdal B (1983a) Zinc absorption from human milk, cow's milk and infant formulas. Am J Dis Child 137:726–729

Sandström B, Keen CL, Lönnerdal B (1983b) An experimental model for studies of zinc availability from milk and infant formulas using extrinsic labeling. Am J Clin Nutr 38:420–428

Sandström B, Davidsson L, Cederblad A, Lönnerdal B (1985) Oral iron, dietary ligands and zinc absorption. J Nutr 115:411–414

Sandström B, Andersson H, Kivistö B, Sandberg A-S (1986) Apparent small intestinal absorption of nitrogen and minerals from soy and meat protein-based diets. A study on human ileostomy subjects. J Nutr 116:2209–2218

Sandström B, Almgren A, Kivistö B, Cederblad A (1987a) Zinc absorption from meals based on rye, barley, oatmeal, triticale and whole-wheat. J Nutr 117:1898–1902

Sandström B, Davidsson L, Kivistö B, Hasselblad C, Cederblad A (1987b) The effects of vegetables and beet fibre on the absorption of zinc from a composite meal. Br J Nutr 58:49–57

Sandström B, Kivistö B, Cederblad A (1987c) Absorption of zinc from soy protein meals in humans. J Nutr 117:321–327

Sandström B, Almgren A, Kivistö B, Cederblad A (1989) Effect of protein level and protein source on zinc absorption in man. J Nutr 119:48–53

Sayers MH, Lynch SR, Jacobs P et al. (1973) The effect of ascorbic acid supplementation on the absorption of iron in maize, wheat and soya. Br J Nutr 24:209–217

Schwartz R, Nevins P (1989) Effects of phytate reduction, fat extraction and level of Ca on Ca and Zn bioavailability. Bio Trace Elem Res 19:93–106

Schwartz R, Apgar BJ, Wien EM (1986) Apparent absorption and retention of Ca, Cu, Mg, Mn and Zn from a diet containing bran. Am J Clin Nutr 43:444–455

Siegenberg D, Baynes RD, Bothwell TH et al. (1991) Ascorbic acid prevents the dose-dependent inhibitory effects of polyphenols and phytates on nonheme-iron absorption. Am J Clin Nutr 53:537–541

Simpson KM, Morris ER, Cook JD (1981) The inhibitory effect of bran on iron absorption in man. Am J Clin Nutr 34:1469–1478

Slavin JL, Marlett JA (1980) Influence of refined cellulose on human bowel function and calcium and magnesium balance. Am J Clin Nutr 33:1932–1939

Solomons NW, Jacob RA, Pineda O, Viteri FE (1979) Studies on the bioavailability of zinc in man. III. Effects of ascorbic acid on the absorption of zinc. Am J Clin Nutr 32:2495–2499

Sudarmadji S, Markakis P (1977) The phytate and phytase of soy bean tempeh. J Sci Food Agric 28:381–383

Svanberg U, Sandberg A-S (1988) Improved iron availability in weaning foods through the use of germination and fermentation. In: Ahlwick D, Moses S, Schmidt OG (eds) Improving young child feeding in Eastern and Southern Africa. Proceedings of a workshop in Nairobi, Kenya, Oct 1987 IDRC, Ottawa, pp 366–373

Svanberg U, Sandberg A-S, Andersson R (1990) Bioavailability of iron in lactic acid fermented foods. In: Zeuthen P et al. (eds) Processing and quality of foods, vol 2. Food biotechnology. Elsevier Applied Science, London, pp 2116–2121

Tangendjaja B, Buckle KA, Wootton M (1981) Dephosphorylation of phytic acid in rice bran. J Food Sci 46:1021–1024

Tuntawiroon M, Sritongkul N, Rossander-Hulthén L et al. (1990) Rice and iron absorption in man. Eur J Clin Nutr 44:489–497

Tuntawiroon M, Sritongkul N, Brune M et el. (1991) Dose-dependent inhibitory effect of phenolic compounds in Food on nonheme-iron absorption in man. Am J Clin Nutr 53:554–557

Turnlund JR, Michel MC, Keyes WR, King JC, Jargen S (1982) Use of enriched stable isotopes to determine zinc and iron absorption in elderly men. Am J Clin Nutr 35:1033–1040

Turnlund JR, King JC, Keyes WR, Gong B, Michel MC (1984) A stable isotope study of zinc absorption in young men: effects of phytate and α-cellulose. Am J Clin Nutr 40:1071–1077

Turnlund JR, King JC, Gong B, Keyes WR, Michel MC (1985) A stable isotope study of copper absorption in young men: effects of phytate and α-cellulose. Am J Clin Nutr 42:18–23

Turnlund JR, Betschart AA, Keyes WR, Acord LL (1987) A stable isotope study of zinc availability in young men from diets with white vs. whole wheat bread or beef vs. soy. Fed Proc 46:879

Türk M, Sandberg AS (1992) Phytate hydrolysis during bread making: effect of addition of phytase from Aspergillus higer. J Cereal Sci (in press)

Van Dokkum W, Wesstra A, Schippers FA (1982) Physiological effects of fibre-rich types of bread.
    I. The effect of dietary fibre from bread on the mineral balance of young men. Br J Nutr
    47:451–460
Wise A, Lockie GM, Liddell J (1987) Dietary intakes of phytate and its meal distribution pattern
    amongst staff and students in a institution of higher education. Br J Nutr 58:337–346
Wollenberg P, Rummel W (1987) Dependence of intestinal iron absorption on the valency state of
    iron. Naunyn Schmiedebergs Arch Pharmacol 336:578–582

Commentary

Southgate: Stable isotopes have important ethical advantages over radio-isotopes and it is not always essential to collect faeces; with the appropriate mass spectrometer precisions high enough to study blood enrichment levels can be reached permitting study of appearance in blood or saliva.

Authors' reply: Even with a mass spectrometer with a high precision, stable isotopes can never be used to label foods and individual meals in the way that is possible with radioisotopes, i.e. extrinsically without changing the native mineral content of the meal. Thus, for stable isotopes one either has to use costly intrinsic labelling procedures which hardly can be applicable for more than a limited number of foods, or one has to accept that stable isotopes measure absorption from an enriched or supplemented meal or diet. Although it is possible theoretically to determine the degree of absorption from isotope ratios in blood, urine or saliva, this approach needs validation. So far it has only been used to some extent for calcium and iron. The advantage with stable isotopes is that they can be used to study turnover rates and net effects of different types of diets and they are also more suitable for multi-element studies.

Regarding the ethical aspects we would like to emphasise that with the sensitive measuring instruments that we have today, the administered activities and thereby the radiation doses can be kept below the natural background radiation level. With access to a sensitive human whole body counter and a skilled radiophysicist who can optimise the measurements, the radiation doses can be lowered even more. Natural background radiation results in a radiation dose of about 4 mSv/year in Sweden (in some places more). Studies using radio-active markers can normally be performed with doses well below 1 mSv, that is at levels which are smaller than variations due to living in houses of different building material. Consequently, this is not a real ethical problem as long as the investigations are performed in a professional manner. From the ethical point of view, it is also important that studies can give clear-cut results.

Chapter 12

Dietary Fibre and Bile Acid Metabolism

F.M. Nagengast

Introduction

Much of the interest in the effects of dietary fibre on bile acid metabolism is derived from the interrelationship of diet and cholesterol metabolism, as well as the role of nutrition in the development of colorectal cancer. Excellent reviews about the effects of fibre components on cholesterol metabolism have been published (Kay and Truswell, 1980; Story, 1980). The association between fibre and gallstones and the intermediate role of bile acids is dealt with in Chap. 14. In this chapter the relation between dietary fibre and bile acid metabolism is focused around the role of bile acids and dietary fibre in the development of colorectal cancer.

Bile Acid Metabolism

Bile acids are the major end products of cholesterol metabolism and synthesised in the liver. The primary bile acids cholic acid (CA) and chenodeoxycholic acid (CDCA) are derived via several intermediate steps from cholesterol and secreted in bile as glycine and taurine conjugates. They serve as cholesterol solubilising agents by the formation of micelles and play an important role in the digestion and adsorption of lipids in the small intestine. More than 95% of the bile acids passing the ileum are readsorbed and return to the liver through the portal vein. An efficient conservation in the so-called entero-hepatic circulation is thus achieved. The proportion of bile acids not adsorbed in the terminal ileum is 2%–5% per cycle and amounts to an average loss of 20% of the bile acid pool with 6–12 entero-hepatic circulations per day. Bile acids that escape adsorption in the ileum, are metabolised in the large bowel by the anaerobic bacterial flora. First, deconjugation takes place and the amino acid molecule on the carboxyl group is removed. Secondly, the primary bile acids CA and CDCA are dehydroxylated and converted into the secondary bile acids deoxycholic acid (DCA) and lithocholic acid (LCA) respectively. Further bacterial degradation in the large bowel and alterations in the liver produce the tertiary bile acids (Fig. 12.1). DCA is partly adsorbed in the colon and enters the entero-hepatic circulation, where it is conjugated in the liver and secreted in bile; LCA is almost

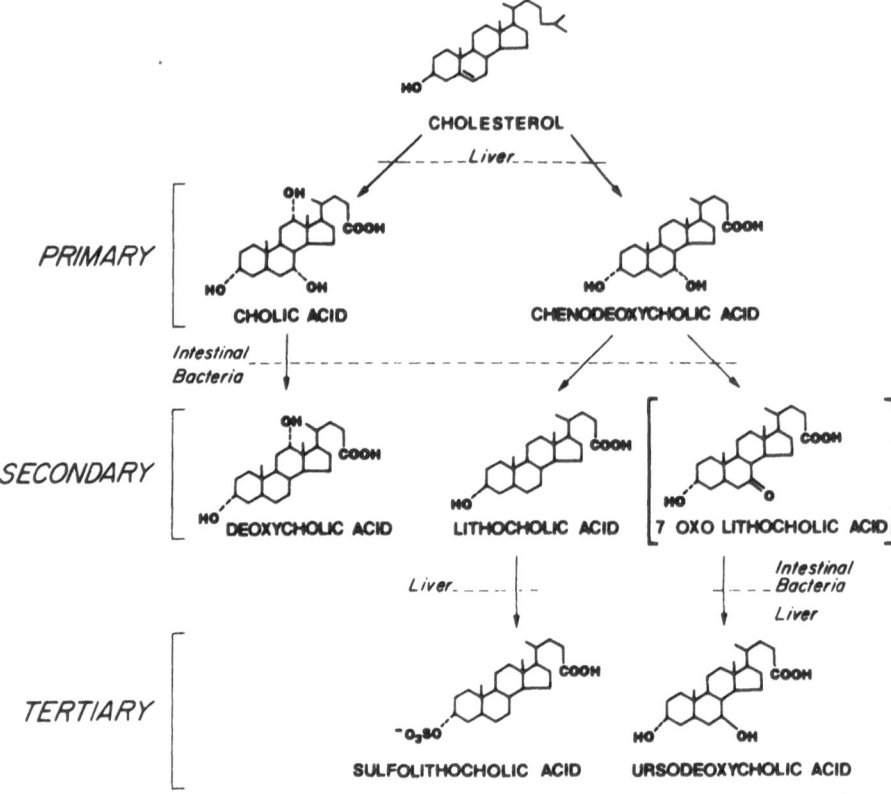

Fig. 12.1. Synthesis and degradation of bile acids in the liver and intestine.

insoluble and very little is reabsorbed. Both secondary bile acids are excreted in the stool and make up to 95% of the total amount of excreted bile acids. In the stool the major part of the bile acids are bound to dietary residue. In the circulating bile acid pool, CA and CDCA each comprise about 30%–40%, DCA about 20%–30% and LCA for less than 5% of the total (Carey, 1982; Nagengast, 1988a).

Colonic Carcinogenesis

Fibre

The incidence of colorectal cancer is high in Western countries and is related to dietary habits (Hill, 1985). Currently it is assumed that dietary factors modulate a genetic susceptibility (Bruce, 1987). In epidemiological observations the consumption of animal fat is positively related to the incidence of colon cancer (vide infra). The intake of fibre is possibly negatively related to this incidence, however, many inconsistencies exist. In a recently published meta-analysis (Trock et al., 1990) of observational epidemiological studies a protective effect of dietary fibre was found in most, but not all studies. One thing that has always to be kept in mind is the reciprocal relation between fat and fibre intake. An interesting substance that recently has drawn more attention but whose role in colonic carcinogenesis is far from clear is "resistant starch". Recently in a case–control study it was found that a high starch diet reduced the relative risk of colonic cancer to 0.82 (Tuyns et al., 1988). There are several possible explanations for the protective effects of fibre and starch. The most consistent are: (1) the stool-bulking effect; (2) the acceleration of gut transit time; (3) the binding of bile acids; and (4) the fermentation of parts of the fibre and probably most of the starch to short chain fatty acids (thereby reducing the formation of secondary bile acids and enhancing the production of butyrate, which has anti-neoplastic properties in vitro).

In most animal experiments a protective effect on colonic carcinogenesis has been shown, however, also in this respect controversies do exist (Castleden, 1977; Fleiszer et al., 1978). Besides the influence of fat and fibre, other dietary constituents like trace elements and vitamins have been suggested as playing a role.

Fat

The hypothesis postulates that a high-fat diet enhances the formation and degradation of bile acids and neutral sterols and that these compounds exert a promoting effect in colonic carcinogenesis (Breuer and Goebell, 1985; Nagengast, 1988a). Indeed, it has been found that dietary fat increases the output and faecal concentration of bile acids (Hill, 1971; Reddy et al., 1975; Cummings et al., 1978) and epidemiological evidence has shown that populations with a high incidence of colorectal cancer and consuming a high fat and animal protein diet, excrete about twice the amount of secondary bile acids (Reddy et al., 1983). The concentration of these bile acids was even more increased. However, other studies in the United States, Great Britain and New Zealand have failed to demonstrate a correlation between a high-fat intake and colorectal cancer incidence (Enstrom, 1975; McMichael et al., 1979). Case–control studies have shown conflicting results in this respect (Wynder and Shigematsu, 1967; Jain et al., 1980).

Dietary Fibre and Bile Acid Metabolism

Dietary fibre is that part of the plant wall matrix which cannot be broken down by human enzymes. The most important resources are wheat, vegetables and fruit. The most important components of fibre are non-cellulose polysaccharides, cellulose and lignin. Different components can exert several physiological effects, which depend on processing, particle size, the source of fibre, and of individual characteristics of the consumer, like transit time and colonic microflora.

In this review, discussion on the effects of fibre on biliary bile acids and bile acid pool sizes will be separated from effects on faecal bile acid excretion. Since animals often have a very different bile acid pattern, only human studies will be reviewed. In many of the published studies the main goal was not the effect of fibre or parts of fibre on bile acid metabolism, but to investigate the role of fibre on cholesterol metabolism. In this respect to increase the excretion of acidic (bile acids) sterols and neutral sterols by consuming dietary fibre was important to lower serum cholesterol levels. Many studies with regard to the effect of dietary fibre on biliary bile acids were initiated, because of the hypothesis that fibre can decrease the cholesterol saturation index (CSI) of bile, which is a major factor in the development of gallbladder bile stones. Since hypothetically deoxycholic acid can increase the CSI, many investigations concentrated on the effect of fibre (or fibre components) on individual biliary bile acids.

Fibre and Biliary Bile Acids

In Table 12.1 a number of studies are shown, in which the effect of different types of dietary fibre on the biliary bile acid pattern is examined. Overall, dietary fibre induces a mild decrease of the deoxycholic acid (DCA) fraction at the expense of chenic acid (CDCA), or in some, of cholic acid (CA). A hypothesis concerning the reciprocal relationship between DCA and CDCA has been put forward (Pomare and Low-Beer, 1975) assuming that DCA inhibits the synthesis of CDCA in the liver. However, some controversy about this hypothesis still exists.

The represented studies show a number of differences regarding the source and type of fibre, the length of the study and the subjects studied. Because of these differences comparison is difficult. Some aspects will be discussed.

Source and Type of Fibre

In most studies 30–60 g of bran per day was used as fibre source. These amounts correspond to about 10–30 g of dietary fibre, depending on the bran quality used. The study with a wheat fibre preparation (Marcus and Heaton, 1986a) concerns the type and amount of fibre comparable to the bran studies. Most studies found a moderate (13%–49%) decline in DCA content and concomitant rise in CDCA content in bile. Some investigators (Tarpila et al., 1978; Marcus and Heaton, 1986a), however, detected that a fall in DCA was accompanied by a rise in the CA percentage in bile, while the CDCA fraction remained constant. The same holds true for the only study that used dietary fibre from several sources like cereals, vegetables and fruit (Thornton et al., 1983). We have recently completed a controlled study with a natural high-fibre diet and came to the same results (Nagengast, 1988b). It is striking that in two studies in which pectin was used, an increase in biliary DCA was found (Miettinen and Tarpila,

Table 12.1. Studies on the effect of dietary fibre on biliary bile acid composition

Reference	Fibre addition			Subjects			Change in bile acid content in bile (%)		
	Source/type	Amount (g/day)	Duration (wk)	Number/sex	Age (yr)	Remarks	CA	CDCA	DCA
Pomare & Heaton (1973)	Wheat bran	33	6–10	5♀		2♀ gallstones	=	+43	−49
Pomare et al. (1976)	Wheat bran	57	4–6	3♀, 3♂	52–56	2♂ gallstones	=	+27	−33
Miettinen & Tarpila (1977)	Pectin	50	2	5	33–60	Normo- and hyperlipidaemia	=	−16[ns]	+7[ns]
McDougall et al. (1978)	Wheat bran	50	4	9		Healthy	=	=	=
Tarpila et al. (1978)	Wheat bran	48–49	26–52	9	51 (35–64)	Diverticulosis	+14	=	−29
Watts et al. (1978)	Wheat bran	30	8	6♀, 5♂	25 (20–42)	5♀ supersaturated bile	+6[nc]	+6[nc]	−24[nc]
Wicks et al. (1978)	Wheat Bran	30	6	12♂	21–24	Healthy	=	+16	−27
Huybregts et al. (1980)	Wheat bran	33	4	7♂	21 ± 2	Healthy	=	=	=
	Wheat bran	31	8	4♂	23 ± 3	Healthy	=	=	=
Thornton & Heaton (1981)	Lactulose	60	6	10♀	46 (42–51)	9♀ supersaturated bile	=	+29	−45
Arffmann et al. (1983)	Oat bran	18	2	6♂	22–26	Healthy	=	+	−
Thornton et al. (1983)	Dietary fibre from corn, vegetables and fruit	14	6	10♀, 3♂	46 (26–64)	Gallstones	+14	=	−13
Hillman et al. (1986)	Pectin	12	4	8	32 ± 8	Healthy	−9	=	+40
	Lignin	12	4	8♀, 2♂	28 ± 8	Healthy	=	=	=
	Cellulose	15	4	9	24 ± 4	Healthy	=	+5	−24
Marcus & Heaton (1986a)	Wheat fibre preparation	10–32	6	16♀, 4♂	49 (38–69)	Constipation 12 supersaturated bile	+9	=	−14
Nagengast et al. (1988a)	Lactulose	0.3 g/kg/day	12	4♂, 5♀	31–54	Healthy	=	+26	−22
				5♂, 5♀	56–81	Healthy	=	+26	−31

CA, cholic acid; CDCA, chenodeoxycholic acid; DCA, deoxycholic acid.
−, decrease; +, increase; =, no change.
ns, not significant; nc, not consistent.

1977; Hillman et al., 1986). An explanation is not clear, but could be caused by one of the physico-chemical properties of pectin. Pectin is a strong gel-former in the small bowel, which could lead to binding of primary bile acids and thus prevent readsorption in the terminal ileum. In the large bowel pectin will be fermented and the liberated bile acids be deconjugated and dehyroxylated to secondary bile acids, like DCA. The reduction of the DCA content in bile by dietary fibre can be explained by several mechanisms, which have recently been reviewed (Heaton, 1987). Theoretically, the most likely explanations are:

1. By adsorption of newly formed DCA in the large bowel to dietary fibre, which has been shown in vitro to occur more strongly for DCA than for the other bile acids (Eastwood and Hamilton, 1968). Also bacteria that feed and multiply on bran are capable of binding bile acids.

2.. By accelerating the transit of colonic contents. This would decrease the absorption of DCA. This effect has also been shown to occur for laxatives. However, no correlation was found between changes in transit time and alterations in DCA pool sizes or percentages (Marcus and Heaton, 1986b).

3. By bacterial fermentation of parts of fibre, which can give rise to the formation of short chain fatty acids and results in a reduction of the intraluminal pH. Such an effect has been found by administering lactulose, a non-absorbable disaccharide, which is completely fermented and can decrease the DCA content in bile as has been shown by several authors (Thornton and Heaton, 1981; Van Berge Henegouwen et al., 1987; Nagengast et al., 1988a). Lowering the pH below 6 would inhibit bacterial 7α-dehydroxylase and thus reduce the formation of the secondary bile acids DCA and LCA. Lowering colonic pH might also limit the adsorption of DCA by precipitation, because it is rather insoluble at low pH.

The effect of fibre on biliary bile acids is slow, since only after 6 weeks a fall in DCA content is seen (Wicks et al., 1978). This favours a metabolic rather than a physical effect.

Subjects

Many factors related to the subjects studied could have influenced the results of the experiments. It is well known that DCA metabolism is age-dependent and in our laboratory it was demonstrated that the dehydroxylation of CA in DCA in the large bowel was age-dependent (Van der Werf et al., 1981). Elderly subjects have a higher DCA and lower CA content in bile than young and middle-aged subjects (Nagengast et al., 1988a). With an initially low DCA percentage in bile (Huybregts et al., 1980) a change after fibre addition is hard to detect. In many of the studies volunteers participated with gallstones or a high cholesterol saturation index. These patients mostly have a higher DCA content, so differences are more likely to occur. In one study (McDougall et al., 1978) only in gallstone patients with a high mean DCA level (31%) a fall after bran was seen, while in the healthy volunteers with a mean DCA level of 19% no effect was observed. One other group (Watts et al., 1978) found a mean decrease of 24% in the biliary DCA content, however this was completely attributable to a significant decrease in three women with a high initial DCA level and high saturation index.

Relation with Other Dietary Factors

In most of the studies concerning the effect of fibre on biliary acids the intake of other food items (like fat) was not controlled for. It is well conceivable that even motivated volunteers who have to consume 30 g bran per day lower their fat intake. This could have had profound consequences on bile acid metabolism.

Dietary Fibre and DCA Kinetics

Surprisingly few studies have looked upon the effect of fibre or its components on the kinetic parameters of bile acid metabolism. The complexity of the formation, adsorption and entero-hepatic circulation of secondary bile acids has been extensively demonstrated (Hoffman et al., 1987; Stellaard and Paumgartner, 1987) and the only way to get a reliable insight into the dynamics of bile acid metabolism is to perform kinetic experiments using radioactive or stable isotopes. However, the availability of these techniques is limited and radioactive isotopes cannot be used any more in experiments with healthy volunteers in most countries.

In studies that have used kinetic experiments different results were shown. Bran can reduce the circulating DCA pool (Pomare and Heaton 1973; Pomare et al., 1976) but a later study with a concentrated bran preparation did not confirm this (Marcus and Heaton, 1986a). In our laboratory also no change in the DCA pool was found; however, a rise in the DCA input was detected in the circulating pool in four volunteers after eight weeks' bran supplementation (Huybregts et al., 1980). It must be remembered that the healthy subjects in the last study were already consuming a high-fibre diet and had small DCA pools to begin with.

In summary, dietary fibre can exert effects on the biliary bile acid composition, which seem largely dependent on the type and source of fibre and the length of administration. Whether in the long term a natural high-fibre diet really can lower the level of circulating secondary bile acids and have a protective effect on gallstone formation and colonic carcinogenesis remains to be seen.

Fibre and Faecal Bile Acids

In Table 12.2 a review of a number of studies is shown concerning the effect of dietary fibre on the concentration and excretion of faecal bile acids. It must be remembered in the interpretation of these studies, that the mechanism whereby secondary bile acids play a promoting role in colonic carcinogenesis is not known at all. The speculative hypothesis is that these bile acids damage the colonic epithelium causing a hyperproliferation in the colonic crypts (Breuer and Goebell, 1985; Stadler et al., 1988). Of course this must be an oversimplification, since it is now well known that many other factors are involved (e.g. genetic, hormonal, growth factors). Assuming the hypothesis is correct, then only soluble bile acids should exert the irritative effect on the colonic mucosa (Rafter et al., 1986, 1987). However, in all studies concerning the effect of fibre

Table 12.2. Studies on the effect of dietary fibre on faecal bile acids

Reference Year	Fibre addition Source/type	Amount (g/day)	Duration (wk)	Subjects Number/sex	Age (yr)	% change in total bile acids in faeces Concentration (mg/g)	Excretion (mg/day)	Remarks
Eastwood et al. (1973)	Wheat bran	16	3	8♂	25–43	−40	= LCA + DCA	
	Cellulose	16	3	4♂	25–43	−42	= LCA + DCA	
Jenkins et al. (1975)	Dietary fibre from wheat	36	3	4♂	21–25	−43[ns]	+40[ns]	
Walters et al. (1975)	Wheat bran	39	12	4♀	.	−38	=	
	Bagasse	10.5	12	9♀	.	=	+50	
Cummings et al. (1976)	Dietary fibre from wheat	28	3	6♂	21–25	−35	+40	
McLean-Baird et al. (1977)	Wheat bran	39	1	2♀, 2♂	65–69	=	=	No significance stated
Kay & Truswell (1977)	Pectin	15	3	5♀, 4♂	21–28	.	+33	
Kay & Truswell (1977)	Oat bran	51	3	5	21–27	−	=	No significance stated
Miettinen & Tarpila (1977)	Pectin	50	2	5♀, 4♂	33–60	.	+57	Normo- and hyperlipidaemia
Raymond et al. (1977)	Dietary fibre from corn, vegetables, fruit	60	4	2♀, 4♂	19–67	.	=	Cholesterol-free diet 3 hyperlipidaemia
		60	4	3♀, 3♂	19–67	.	=	Cholesterol-rich diet 4 hyperlipidaemia
Tarpila et al. (1978)	Wheat bran	48–59	26 52	5♀, 5♂ 5♀, 5♂	51 (35–64) 51 (35–64)	. −58	= −49	Diverticulosis Diverticulosis
Cummings et al. (1979)	Dietary fibre from wheat	31	3	4♂	20–24	−18	+101	
Kretsch et al. (1979)	Dietary fibre from oat	12	15 days	6♂	23–40	=	+111	
	Dietary fibre from corn	93	15 days	6♂	23–40	−49	+111	

Reference	Fibre source	g	Duration	Subjects	Age		Result	Comments
Stasse-Wolthuis et al. (1979)	Dietary fibre from corn, vegetables & fruit (>50% from vegetables & fruit)	33	3	23	20–27	.	+ns°	Low dietary cholesterol
		33	3	23	20–27	.	+ns°	High dietary cholesterol
Huybregts et al. (1980)	Wheat bran	31	8	4♂	23–43	=nc**	=nc°	
Stasse-Wolthuis et al. (1980)	Dietary fibre from vegetables & fruit	25	5	5♀,10♂	18–28	.	=*	
	Citrus pectin	10	5	4♀ / 10♂	18–28	.	=* / +51*	
	Dietary fibre from corn	19	5	6♀ / 10♂	18–28	.	+41* / −23*	
Bell et al. (1981)	Several sorts of bran	26	30 days	4♂	19–54	.	=nc°	Soft or hard wheat bran, corn bran, soya beans, pellicles. No significance stated.
Kirby et al. (1981)	Oat bran	94	10 days	7♂	35–62	Derivatives of CDCA +28, =c	+54	6 Hypercholesterolaemia
Ross & Leklem (1981)	Citrus pectin	15	18 days	8♂	20–27	=	+11ns	

Table 12.2. Continued

Reference Year	Fibre addition Source/type	Amount (g/day)	Duration (wk)	Subjects Number/sex	Age (yr)	% change in total bile acids in faeces Concentration (mg/g)	Excretion (mg/day)	Remarks
Ullrich et al. (1981)	Dietary fibre from corn, vegetables & fruit	37	4 days	8♂	25–32	=	=	
McLean-Ross et al. (1983)	'Gum arabic'	25	3	5♂	30–55	.	=*	
Anderson et al. (1984)	Oat bran	98	3	10♂	34–66	+ns	+65ns	Hypercholesterolaemia not mentioned: concentration/g dry or wet weight
	Dietary fibre from beans	25	3	10♂	39–61	.	−30	
Jacobson et al. (1984)	Wheat bran	50	6	23	45–75	−12	=	No significance stated
Eastwood et al. (1986)	Dietary fibre	9	26	21	50–82	.	=*	
Spiller et al. (1986)	Hard wheat bran	13	13 days	17♀	20 (18–31)	=°	=	
		40	13 days	18♀	20 (18–32)	=°	+65	
		66	13 days	18♀	20 (18–32)	−36°	+60	
Reddy et al. (1987)	Dietary fibre from wheat, oats and rye	11	4	7♀, 8♂	45 ± 4	−50	.	Basal diet: high fat, low fibre. Initially high concentration of faecal bile acids

CA, cholic acid; CDCA, chenodeoxycholic acid; DCA, deoxycholic acid; LCA, lithocholic acid.
–, decrease; +, increase; =, no change; ·, not mentioned.
ns, not significant; nc, not consistent; *, mmol/day; **, mmol/g dry weight; °, mg/g dry weight; , mg/g wet weight.

on faecal bile acids, the total concentration based on dry weight or total excretion is given. The concentration of bile acids in faecal water is normally very low. Only in diarrhoeal conditions does this concentration rise and is then pH dependent (McJunkin et al., 1981).

From Table 12.2 it can be seen that generally consumption of dietary fibre increases the daily output (excretion) and decreases the concentration of faecal bile acids. In almost all studies faecal weight increased, giving the most likely explanation of the result of decreased concentration and increased excretion. As in the biliary bile acid studies differences can be attributed to several factors, some of which will be discussed.

Source and Type of Fibre

Many studies have been carried out with wheat bran or fibre from wheat. In most studies a decreased concentration and similar excretion is found. In one study (Spiller et al., 1986) a dose–response relationship was found. Only at a high dose of wheat bran an effect on faecal bile acids was seen. The importance of the source of fibre is illustrated in one study with oat bran (Kretsch et al., 1979). Oat bran had no effect on the concentration of faecal bile acids, while the excretion increased. An explanation could be the fact that oat bran includes much less cellulose than wheat bran. Cellulose has been shown to decrease the concentration of faecal bile acids (Eastwood et al., 1973). Pectin in rather small quantities (10–15 g) can increase bile acid excretion (Miettinen and Tarpila, 1977). The source of pectin is important in this respect, as was shown in the study where 10 g of pure pectin increased the excretion, but the same doses derived from vegetables and fruit had no effect (Stasse-Wolthuis et al., 1979). It is remarkable that in three studies with doses of 33–60 g fibre from different natural sources (corn, vegetables and fruit) no significant effects could be detected (Raymond et al., 1977; Stasse-Wolthuis et al., 1980; Ullrich et al., 1981). It is conceivable that various components of dietary fibre can have opposite effects, resulting in a net neutral effect.

Duration of the Study

The length of the different investigations varied from four days (Ullrich et al., 1981) to one year (Tarpila et al., 1978), but in most studies the effect of fibre was investigated for 3–6 weeks. In one long-term study after six months no decrease was observed, but after one year a significant decrease in faecal bile acid excretion was observed (Tarpila et al., 1978). From the results in several investigations it is clear that the effect of fibre on colonic function and bile acid metabolism takes several weeks to occur and that by adaptation initial changes can be reversed. No clear understanding exists at this moment whether long-term administration of a natural high-fibre diet can induce changes in bile acid metabolism that would benefit patients at high risk of developing colorectal cancer.

Subjects

What has already been noted in the studies of fibre on biliary bile acids also holds true for the outcome on faecal bile acids. Age, for instance, is such a factor. It has been shown that age-dependent differences exist in the concentration of faecal bile acids (Nagengast et al., 1988b). In the reported studies age varied from 20 to 80 years.

Gender could also influence results. In many studies only men or women were investigated. In one study a sex difference was found, but no valid explanation for this observation was found (Stasse-Wolthuis et al., 1980). The pre-existing health could have had influence. One study (Tarpila et al., 1978) investigated patients with diverticulosis with an initial high faecal bile acid output. Many studies were carried out in hyperlipidaemic patients to study the effect of fibre on serum cholesterol levels since the close interrelationship between cholesterol and bile acid metabolism could have biased the data. A factor that was not accounted for in many studies was the previous nutritional status and consumption pattern of the volunteers. The intake of fibre, fat and cholesterol is especially important, because these nutrients have profound implications on the baseline concentration and excretion of bile acids. Finally, it is important to correct the faecal excretion of bile acids for the individual variation in gut transit time and defecation frequency ("faecal flow"). This is achieved by the administration of non-absorbable markers which are excreted unaltered in the stool. In only a few studies was this fact accounted for.

Individual Bile Acids

In subjects consuming lactulose it has been shown that the dehydroxylation of primary bile acids can be inhibited thereby increasing the output of these compounds and decreasing the level of secondary faecal bile acids (Nagengast et al., 1988a). Fermentation of lactulose in short chain fatty acids and thus a decline in colonic pH is largely responsible for this effect. Despite the fact that parts of dietary fibre can be fermented by colonic bacteria into short chain fatty acids, studies that have looked at individual bile acid output did not find significant changes in favour of primary bile acid excretion. In fact more than 95% of the excreted bile acids on a high-fibre diet consisted of the secondary bile acids DCA and LCA (Nagengast, 1988b). This is probably caused by a slow and incomplete fermentation process.

Conclusions

From the reviewed literature it is clear that dietary fibre has an influence upon bile acid metabolism. Far from clear, however, is if manipulation of bile acids by consuming a high-fibre diet derived from natural sources will decrease the incidence of colorectal cancer. In this respect the lower fat intake that goes along with an increase in fibre consumption could well have much more beneficial effects. One of the problems in determining the exact influence of fibre on bile acid metabolism is the complex interaction between so many components that are derived from the breakdown of fibre and their physico-chemical properties. Dietary intervention studies in patients at high risk for colonic cancer (patients with adenomas, longstanding ulcerative colitis, familial colon cancer syndromes) could give more insight into this problem. It is obvious that we know little about the mechanism whereby bile acids manipulate colonic carcinogenesis. More research is needed to clarify the interaction and possible beneficial effects of dietary fibre and also resistant starch on the metabolism of bile acids.

Acknowledgements. Rianne Leenen and Peter Zock, students in Human Nutrition at the Agricultural University of Wageningen, The Netherlands, are gratefully acknowledged for their contribution in reviewing the literature. Ivo van Munster, internist at the Department of Gastrointestinal and Liver Diseases was helpful in critically reviewing the manuscript.

References

Anderson JW, Story L, Sieling B, Lin Chen W, Petro MS, Story J (1984) Hypocholesterolemic effects of oat-bran or bean intake for hypercholesterolemic men. Am J Clin Nutr 40:1146–1155

Arffmann S, Hojgaard L, Giese B, Krag E (1983) Effect of oat bran on lithogenic index of bile and bile acid metabolism. Digestion 28:197–200

Bell EW, Emken EA, Klevay LM, Sandstead HH (1981) Effects of dietary fiber from wheat, corn and soy hull bran on excretion of fecal bile acids in humans. Am J Clin Nutr 34:1071–1076

Breuer N, Goebell H (1985) Bile acids and colonic cancer. Klin Wochenschr 63:97–105

Bruce WR (1987) Recent hypotheses for the origin of colonic cancer. Cancer Res 47:4237–4242

Carey MC (1982) The enterohepatic circulation. In: Arias I, Popper H, Schachter D, Shafritz DA (eds) The liver: biology and pathobiology. Raven Press, New York, pp 429–465

Castleden WM (1977) Prolonged survival and decrease in intestinal tumours in dimethylhydrazine-treated rats fed a chemically defined diet. Br J Cancer 35:491–495

Cummings JH, Hill MJ, Jenkins DJ, Pearson JR, Wiggins HS (1976) Changes in fecal composition and colonic function due to cereal fiber. Am J Clin Nutr 29:1468–1473

Cummings JH, Wiggins HS, Jenkins DJ, Houston H, Jivraj T, Drasar BS, Hill MJ (1978) Influence of diets high and low in animal fat on bowel habit, gastrointestinal transit time, fecal microflora, bile acid, and fat excretion. J Clin Invest 61:953–963

Cummings JH, Hill MJ, Jivraj T, Houston H, Branch WJ, Jenkins DJ (1979) The effect of meat protein and dietary fiber on colonic function and metabolism. I. Changes in bowel habit, bile acid excretion, and calcium absorption. Am J Clin Nutr 32:2086–2093

Eastwood MA, Hamilton D (1968) Studies on the adsorption of bile salts to non-absorbed components of diet. Biochim Biophys Acta 152:165–173

Eastwood MA, Kirkpatrick JR, Mitchell WD, Bone A, Hamilton T (1973) Effects of dietary supplements of wheat bran and cellulose on faeces and bowel function. Br Med J iv:392–394

Eastwood MA, Elton RA, Smith JH (1986) Long-term effect of wholemeal bread on stool weight, transit time, fecal bile acids, fats, and neutral sterols. Am J Clin Nutr 43:343–349

Enstrom JE (1975) Colorectal cancer and consumption of beef and fat. Br J Cancer 32:432–439

Fleiszer D, Murray D, MacFarlane J, Brown RA (1978) Protective effect of dietary fibre against chemically induced bowel tumours in rats. Lancet ii:552–553

Heaton KW (1987) Effect of dietary fibre on biliary lipids. In: Barbara L et al. (eds) Nutrition in gastrointestinal disease. Raven Press, New York, pp 213–222

Hill MJ (1971) The effect of some factors on the faecal concentration of acid steroids, neutral steroids and urobilins. J Pathol 104:239–245

Hill MJ (1985) Cancer of the large bowel: Human carcinogenesis. Br J Surg 72:37–39

Hillman LC, Peters SG, Fisher CA, Pomare EW (1986) Effects of the fibre components pectin, cellulose, and lignin on bile salt metabolism and biliary lipid composition in man. Gut 27:29–36

Hoffmann AF, Cravetto C, Molino G, Belforte G, Bona B (1987) Simulation of the metabolism and enterohepatic circulation of endogenous deoxycholic acid in humans using a physiologic pharmacokinetic model for bile acid metabolism. Gastroenterology 93:693–709

Huybregts AW, Van Berge-Henegouwen GP, Hectors MP, Van Schaik A, Van der Werf SD (1980) Effects of a standardized wheat bran preparation on biliary lipid composition and bile acid metabolism in young healthy males. Eur J Clin Invest 10:451–458

Jacobson EA, Newmark HL, Bright-See E, McKeown-Eyssen G, Bruce WR (1984) Biochemical changes as a result of increased fiber consumption 30:1049–1059

Jain M, Cook GM, Davis FG, Grace MG, Howe GR, Miller AB (1980) A case–control study of diet and colo-rectal cancer. Int J Cancer 26:757–768

Jenkins DJ, Hill MS, Cummings JH (1975) Effect of wheat fiber on blood lipids, fecal steroid excretion and serum iron. Am J Clin Nutr 28:1408–1411

Kay RM, Truswell AS (1977) Effect of citrus pectin on blood lipids and fecal steroid excretion in man. Am J Clin Nutr 30:171–175

Kay RM, Truswell AS (1980) Dietary fiber: effects on plasma and biliary lipids in man. In: Spiller GA, Kay RM (eds) Medical aspects of dietary fiber. Plenum Press, New York, pp 153–173

Kirby RW, Anderson JW, Sieling et al. (1981) Oat-bran intake selectively lowers serum low-density lipoprotein cholesterol concentrations of hypercholesterolemic men. Am J Clin Nutr 34:824–829

Kretsch MJ, Crawford L, Calloway DH (1979) Some aspects of bile acid and urobilinogen excretion and fecal elimination in men given a rural Guatemalan diet and egg formulas with and without added oatbran. Am J Clin Nutr 32:1492–1496

Marcus SN, Heaton KW (1986a) Effects of a new, concentrated wheat fibre preparation on intestinal transit, deoxycholic acid metabolism and the composition of bile. Gut 27:893–900

Marcus SN, Heaton KW (1986b) Intestinal transit, deoxycholic acid and the cholesterol saturation of bile: three interrelated factors. Gut 27:550–558

McDougall RM, Yakymyshyn L, Walker K, Thurston OG (1978) Effect of wheat bran on serum lipoproteins and biliary lipids. Can J Surg 21:433–435

McJunkin B, Fromm H, Sarva RP, Amin P (1981) Factors in the mechanism of diarrhea in bile acid malabsorption: fecal pH: A key determinant. Gastroenterology 80:1454–1464

McLean-Baird J, Walters RL, Davies PS, Hill MJ, Drasar BS, Southgate DAT (1977) The effects of two dietary fiber supplements on gastrointestinal transit, stool weight and frequency, and bacterial flora, and fecal bile acids in normal subjects. Metabolism 26:117–128

McLean-Ross AH, Eastwood MA, Brydon WG, Anderson JR, Anderson DMW (1983) A study of the effects of dietary gum arabic in human. Am J Clin Nutr 37:368–375

McMichael AJ, Potter JD, Hetzel BS (1979) Time trends in colo-rectal cancer mortality in relation to food and alcohol consumption: United States, United Kingdom, Australia and New Zealand. Int J Epidemiol 8:295–303

Miettinen TA, Tarpila S (1977) Effect of pectin on serum cholesterol, fecal bile acids and biliary lipids in normolipidemic and hyperlipidemic individuals. Clin Chim Acta 79:471–477

Nagengast FM (1988a) Bile acids and colonic carcinogenesis. Scand J Gastroenterol 23:76–81

Nagengast FM (1988b) The effect of a natural high fiber diet on fecal and biliary bile acids, fecal pH and whole gut transit time in man. A controlled study. In: Factors influencing secondary bile acid formation in man. Academic Thesis, Nijmengen, The Netherlands, pp 61–71

Nagengast FM, Hectors MPC, Buys WCAM, van Tongeren JHM (1988a) Inhibition of secondary bile acid formation in the large intestine by lactulose in healthy subjects of two different age groups. Eur J Clin Invest 18:56–61

Nagengast FM, Van der Werf SDJ, Lamers HL, Hectors MPC, Buys WC, Van Tongeren JHM (1988b) Influence of age, intestinal transit time, and dietary composition on faecal bile acid profiles in healthy subjects. Dig Dis Sci 33:673–678

Pomare EW, Heaton KW (1973) Alteration of bile salt metabolism by dietary fibre (bran). Br Med J iv:262–264

Pomare EW, Heaton KW, Low-Beer TS, Espiner HJ (1976) The effect of wheat bran upon bile salt metabolism and upon the lipid composition of bile in gallstone patients. Am J Dig Dis 21:521–526

Pomare R, Low-Beer TS (1975) The selective inhibition of chenodeoxycholate synthesis by chocolate metabolites in man. Clin Sci Mol Med 48:315–321

Rafter JJ, Eng VWS, Furrer R et al. (1986) Effects of calcium and pH on the mucosal damage produced by deoxycholic acid in the rat colon. Gut 27:1320–1329

Rafter JJ, Geltner U, Bruce R (1987) Cellular toxicity of human faecal water: possible role in aetiology of coloncancer. Scand J Gastroenterol (Suppl) 129:245–250

Raymond TL, Connor WE, Lin DS, Warner S, Fry MM, Connor SL (1977) The interaction of dietary fibers and cholesterol upon the plasma lipids and lipoproteins, sterol balance, and bowel function in human subjects. J Clin Invest 60:1429–1437

Reddy BS, Weisburger JH, Wynder EL (1975) Effects of high risk and low risk diets for colon carcinogenesis on fecal microflora and steroids in man. J Nutr 105:878–884

Reddy BS, Ekelund G, Bohe M et al. (1983) Metabolic epidemiology of coloncancer: Dietary pattern and fecal sterol concentrations of three populations. Nutr Cancer 5:34–40

Reddy BS, Sharma C, Simi B et al. (1987) Metabolic epidemiology of coloncancer: Effect of dietary fiber on fecal mutagens and bile acids in healthy subjects. Cancer Res 47:644–648

Ross JK, Leklem JE (1981) The effect of dietary citrus pectin on the excretion of human fecal neutral and acid steroids and the activity of 7α-dehydroxylase and β-glucuronidase. Am J Clin Nutr 34:2068–2077

Spiller GA, Story JA, Wong LG et al. (1986) Effect of increasing levels of hard wheat fiber on fecal weight, minerals and steroids and gastrointestinal transit time in healthy young women. J Nutr 116:778–785

Stadler J, Yeung KS, Furrer R, Marcon N, Himal HS, Bruce WR (1988) Proliferative activity of rectal mucosa and soluble fecal bile acids in patients with normal colons and in patients with colonic polyps or cancer. Cancer Lett 38:315–320

Stasse-Wolthuis M, Hautvast JG, Hermus RJ et al. (1979) The effect of a natural high-fiber diet on serum lipids, fecal lipids, and colonic function. Am J Clin Nutr 32:1881–1888

Stasse-Wolthuis M, Albers HF, van Jeveren JG et al. (1980) Influence of dietary fiber from vegetables and fruits, bran or citrus pectin on serum lipids, fecal lipids, and colonic function. Am J Clin Nutr 33:1745–1756

Stellaard F, Paumgartner G (1987) A new model to assess deoxycholic acid metabolism in health using stable isotope dilution technique. Eur J Clin Invest 17:63–67

Story JA (1980) Dietary fiber and lipid metabolism. In: Spiller GA, Amen RJ (eds) Fiber and human nutrition. Plenum Press, New York, pp 171–184

Tarpila S, Miettinen TA, Metsaranta L (1978) Effects of bran on serum cholesterol, faecal mass, fat, bile acids and neutral sterols, and biliary lipids in patients with diverticular disease of the colon. Gut 19:137–145

Thornton JR, Heaton KW (1981) Do colonic bacteria contribute to cholesterol gall-stone formation? Effects of lactulose on bile. Br Med J 282:1018–1020

Thornton JR, Emmett PM, Heaton KW (1983) Diet and gall stones: Effects of refined and unrefined carbohydrate diets on bile cholesterol saturation and bile acid metabolism. Gut 24:2–6

Trock B, Lanza E, Greenwald P (1990) Dietary fiber, vegetables and coloncancer: Critical review and meta-analyses of the epidemiologic evidence. J Natl Cancer Inst 82:650–661

Tuyns AJ, Kaak R, Haelterman M (1988) Colorectal cancer and the consumption of foods: a case–control study in Belgium. Nutr Cancer 11:189–204

Ullrich IH, Lai HY, Vona L, Reid RL, Albrink MJ (1981) Alterations of fecal steroid composition induced by change in dietary fiber consumption. Am J Clin Nutr 34:2054–2060

Van Berge Henegouwen GP, Van der Werf SDJ, Ruben A (1987) Effect of long-term lactulose ingestion on secondary bile salt metabolism in man: Potential protective effect of lactulose in colonic carcinogenesis. Gut 28:675–680

Van der Werf SDJ, Huybregts AWM, Lamers HLM et al. (1981) Age-dependent differences in human bile acid metabolism and 7α-dehydroxylation. Eur J Clin Invest 11:425–431

Walters RL, Baird IM, Davies PS, Hill MJ, Drasar BS, Southgate DA, Green J, Morgan B (1975) Effects of two types of dietary fibre on faecal steroid and lipid excretion. Br Med J ii:536–538

Watts JM, Jablonski P, Toouli J (1978) The effect of added bran to the diet on the saturation of bile in people without gallstones. Am J Surg 135:321–324

Wicks ACB, Yeates J, Heaton KW (1978) Bran and bile: time course of changes in normal youngg men given a standard dose. Scand J Gastroenterol 13:289–292

Wynder EL, Shigematsu T (1967) Environmental factors of cancer of the colon and rectum. Cancer 20:1520–1561

Chapter 13

Faecal Bulking and Energy Value of Dietary Fibre

E. Wisker and W. Feldheim

Introduction

At first sight there seems to be no correlation between the effect of dietary fibre on faecal bulking and the energy which may be provided to the human metabolism or which may be lost due to the ingestion of dietary fibre. However, an increased consumption of fibre leads to increased stool weights, and thereby also to elevated losses of energy containing organic material. On the other hand, fibre may provide energy, because the short chain fatty acids which result from the fermentation, can be absorbed.

Faecal Bulking Effect of Dietary Fibre

Among the physiological effects of dietary fibre, faecal bulking is one of the best documented. In studies investigating the relation between the intake of dietary constituents and stool weight in free-living people with normal eating habits, it was shown by regression analysis that dietary fibre was the only nutrient which contributed significantly to the enlargement of faecal mass (Eastwood et al., 1984; Davies et al., 1985). This is in agreement with observations by Livesey (1990), who calculated from numerous studies that faecal energy was influenced mainly by the intake of dietary fibre.

Experimentally, an increase in dietary fibre consumption usually results in an increase in stool weight. Cummings (1986) reviewed the influence of various fibres on faecal output and calculated the mean increase ($\pm$ SEM) in faecal weight per gram of fibre consumed in addition to a control diet. Mean increase per gram of fibre was 5.7 $\pm$ 0.5 g (wheat bran), 4.9 $\pm$ 0.9 g (fruits and vegetables), 3.9 $\pm$ 1.5 g (oats), 3.5 $\pm$ 1.5 g (gums and mucilages), 3.4 $\pm$ 0.4 g (corn), 3.0 $\pm$ 0.6 g (cellulose), 2.8 $\pm$ 0.8 g (soya) and 1.3 $\pm$ 0.3 g (pectin), respectively. However, in the studies reviewed by Cummings (1986) intake of fibre was measured by different methods and this may account for some of the differences. Cereal fibres often seem to be more effective than vegetable fibres, when the effects of these fibre sources are compared on the basis of the same analytical method (Cummings et al., 1978; Wisker and Feldheim, 1983; Wisker et al., 1985).

The effect of fibre seems to be dose-dependent. A linear relationship between the intake of fibre and the increase in faecal weight was found when soy fibre (Slavin et al., 1985), and various wheat bran preparations (Spiller et al., 1986; Stephen et al., 1986; Jenkins et al., 1987) were fed. However, the increase in faecal weight per gram of fibre was different. One gram of soy fibre elevated faecal output by 1.5 to 1.8 g (Slavin et al., 1985), one gram of wheat bran fibre increased stool weight by 2.7 g (Jenkins et al., 1987), 4 g (Spiller et al., 1986) and 5 g (Stephen et al., 1986). Some of these differences may again be due to different analytical values. However, these results suggest that different sources of dietary fibre may have different effects on stool output, and that even comparable fibre sources like wheat bran may exert different effects. This may be due to various dietary and non-dietary reasons. It is not possible to draw general conclusions about the relationship between total dietary fibre intake and faecal weight. The physical properties of a fibre source, like the particle size, and the proportion of intact cell wall structures, and also the chemical composition are important. In addition, there are several personal factors which seem to influence stool weight.

Physico-chemical Properties

In the case of faecal bulking, the effects of the particle size in particular have been studied. The particle size of individual fibre sources affects the action of fibre on colonic function. If the same source of fibre is consumed at two different particle sizes, the preparation containing the coarser particles will exert greater effects on stool output. This was seen with wheat bran (Brodribb and Groves, 1978; Heller et al., 1980; Smith et al., 1981; Wrick et al., 1983; Wisker et al., 1986), bran baked into bread (Van Dokkum et al., 1983), but also with breads made from whole meal wheat or rye (Wisker et al., 1986). The greater efficiency of the larger particles may be related to the extent and rate of breakdown of dietary fibre in the colon. Large particles may be degraded more slowly and so are more likely to survive passage through the colon (Cummings, 1986) and may act by themselves and by their water-holding capacity (Stephen and Cummings, 1980). However, grinding had no effect on fermentability in vitro (Van Soest and Robertson, 1976). In vivo, faecal excretion of dietary fibre was not influenced by the particle size of the bran fed with the diet (Van Dokkum et al., 1983). In the case of breads made from whole grain, the intact cell wall structures due to the large particle size may protect parts of the starch from enzymatic breakdown in the small intestine. Non-absorbed starch reaching the colon may act like fermentable fibre in addition to the non-starch polysaccharides.

There are also correlations between the chemical composition and structure of fibre and its influence on stool output. Cummings et al. (1978) found a relation between the bulking capacity of various fibre preparations and their content of pentoses. However, there is no explanation of how pentoses act. Bacon (1979) suggested that the xylose content of a non-starch polysaccharide gives an index of its resistance to fermentation. Pentose-rich fibre sources like wheat bran seem to be less well fermented compared with polysaccharides containing a greater portion of hexoses or uronic acids (Stephen and Cummings, 1980). Probably, the pentose effect is due to the structural characteristics of the cereal cell wall (Selvendran, 1984). Lignification of the outer cell walls of cereal grains may protect these fibre sources from extensive microbial degradation (Selvendran, 1984), although lignification may not be the only explanation for the low fermentability (Cummings, 1981). However, other workers found no immediately discernible correlation between the chemical composition of various fibre sources and their physiological effects (Eastwood et al,. 1986a).

Personality Factors

Wide variations in stool weight were observed between subjects on diets containing similar amounts of dietary fibre (Tucker et al., 1981; Stephen et al., 1986). Eastwood et al. (1984) found that in a population group aged between 18 and 80 on their habitual diet, there was a great variation in faecal wet weight (19 to 278 g/day). In a study with young healthy women of the same age on a controlled diet, Wisker et al. (1990) observed a range of faecal wet weight between 43 and 186 g/day (low fibre control period) and after adding 15 g dietary fibre (carrots) daily to the diet of between 80 and 329 g/day. This suggests that there must be non-dietary factors which influence colonic function. According to the work of Tucker et al. (1981), psychological factors seemed to be as important as dietary ones in accounting for variances in stool production. Transit time has been shown to be related to faecal output (Spiller et al., 1977), and to affect the metabolism of colonic bacteria (Cummings, 1986). Stool weight seems to be related to sex. On similar low-fibre diets, stool production in men was approximately double that of women; this could be explained by differences in transit time (Stephen et al., 1986). Wide variations were also found in the response to a fibre source. Smaller increases were seen in females, in persons with initially low stool weights and in short people (Stephen et al., 1986).

Mechanisms of Action

Several mechanisms seem to be involved in the effect of fibre on faecal bulk. It is well established that dietary fibres are fermented to a varying extent (Cummings, 1981) and thus stimulate bacterial growth. The increased bacterial mass is one of the mechanisms whereby fibre increases stool weight. Those parts of fibre which survive the microbial breakdown alter colonic function by themselves and by holding water (Stephen and Cummings, 1980). However, in vitro water binding of fibre does not correlate with bulking capacities, but fibre sources with water-binding properties that are resistant to fermentation, can exert large effects on stool weight (Eastwood et al., 1983). An increased bulk can shorten the transit rate through the large intestine and lead to an improved efficiency of the bacterial growth (Cummings, 1986). Shorter passage times can also reduce the water absorption from the colon and therefore increase the water content of the stools (Stephen and Cummings, 1980). The gaseous products of fibre fermentation may soften the structure and increase the faecal volume. Which of these mechanisms exerts the greatest effect seems to depend on the source of fibre (Stephen and Cummings, 1980) and on personal factors like the type of gut microflora and the transit time (Cummings, 1984).

Conclusions

Despite the fact that there are analytical methods available which for most foods give comparable values of dietary fibre, and that faecal weight is relatively easy to measure, there is at present no generally accepted concept allowing prediction and explanation of the effects of dietary fibre on stool weight. Of course, dietary fibre is identified as a key factor of faecal bulking, but a lot of details are still unknown. On the basis of the correlation of transit time and faecal wet weight, Spiller et al., (1977) found that there is a critical faecal wet weight beyond which transit times were no longer than two days. According to Spiller (1986), the amount of fibre needed to achieve this stool weight is in the range of 35 to 45 g per day, most of the fibre should be of cereal origin. However, besides the fact that Spiller (1986) did not define how the fibre should be measured, there is not enough scientific background to use these values as a recommended daily fibre intake.

Energy Value of Dietary Fibre

The energy which humans can derive from a food or diet is the metabolisable energy (ME), which is calculated as the gross energy intake minus faecal and urinary energy losses, determined by bomb calorimetry. The digestible energy (DE) which does not consider urinary energy, is estimated as the gross energy intake minus faecal energy. The main sources of energy for the human body are protein, fat and carbohydrate. In early experiments (Rubner, 1885; Atwater and Benedict, 1897) the energy provided by these nutrients was experimentally determined from their heat of combustion and their apparent digestibilities, where the apparent digestibility was calculated as: intake minus faecal excretion of nutrient/intake of nutrient. In the case of protein, corrections for the urinary nitrogen losses were made. On this basis, conversion factors for the nutrients were derived. With these procedures, carbohydrates were calculated by difference, i.e. as the difference between 100 and the sum of the percentage of water, protein, fat and ash. Therefore, this carbohydrate fraction included not only available components like starch and sugars, but also the unavailable carbohydrate. The total fraction was multiplied by a conversion factor, which resulted from the sum of available and unavailable carbohydrate constituents and their apparent digestibility.

As long as fibre intakes were relatively low, i.e. in the range of 5 to 20 g per day, an evaluation of the contribution of dietary fibre to ME and the effect of fibre on the ME delivered by other nutrients was not of great interest. With increasing knowledge of the importance of fibre-rich diets in human nutrition, an increase in fibre intake to a level of about 30 g per day or more is recommended (DGE, 1985). Such fibre levels are already consumed by special groups of individuals (Calkins, 1986; DGE, 1988), and also by people in developing countries (Lubbe, 1971). Diets high in dietary fibre are sometimes considered as an aid to lose body weight (Eyton, 1982). Therefore, in recent years there has been a growing interest in whether and to what extent dietary fibre can contribute to human energy supply and how the energy provided by fibre-rich diets should best be calculated.

Estimation of the Digestible and Metabolisable Energy of Dietary Fibres

In contrast to protein, fat and available carbohydrates, dietary fibre is not hydrolysed by human alimentary enzymes, but is transferred almost completely to the colon (Englyst and Cummings, 1985), where the fibre polysaccharides may be fermented by the colonic bacteria (Cummings, 1984). As reviewed by Cummings (1984), the rate of fermentation is dependent on the chemical composition of fibre components, the water solubility, the lignification of the cell walls, but also on personal factors like the composition and the capacity of the colon microflora and the transit time. On average, about 70% of the dietary fibre in mixed diets consumed by humans will be fermented (Livesey, 1990), however, these values may vary depending on the source of fibre (Southgate and Durnin, 1970; Wisker et al., 1988). The main products of fermentation, the short chain fatty acids, can be absorbed (McNeil et al., 1978) and thus contribute to human energy supply. Theoretically, up to 70% to 75% of the heat of combustion of the polysaccharides may become available for human metabolism (McNeil, 1984). Calculated from the disappearance of dietary fibre from the gut, Cummings (1981) suggested an energy value of about 3 kcal per gram of fermented fibre.

However, the fermentation of fibre cannot be regarded as an isolated event. An elevated intake of fibre is usually associated with an increase in faecal bulk and faecal organic material, and thereby also in faecal energy (Southgate and Durnin, 1970; Wisker et al., 1988). Besides an elevated excretion of fibre, the increase in faecal energy may be due to a conversion of fibre into bacterial matter which is mostly protein and fat, to a decreased availability of dietary nutrients due to fibre and/or to elevated losses of endogenous material (Southgate, 1973; Widdowson, 1978). The additional energy losses are variable, and in some cases may be as large or even larger than the gross energy content of dietary fibre (Southgate and Durnin, 1970; Wisker et al., 1988). Therefore, the apparent digestible energy value of dietary fibre, calculated from its heat of combustion and its apparent digestibility, cannot correctly predict how much energy is actually obtained. The energy value of fibre is more precisely expressed as partial digestible energy value (Kleiber, 1975), which takes into account the additional losses of energy-containing material due to fibre.

Therefore, partial digestible energy values are lower than apparent digestible energy values.

The partial digestible and the partial metabolisable energy values of dietary fibre can be calculated using equations, as suggested by Livesey (1989). These equations are based either on differences in the energy digestibilities in the test and control diets (procedure A) or on differences in the energy lost to faeces (and urine) relative to food dry matter and fibre intake only, which minimises the effects of experimental errors (procedure B).

Procedure A:

$$DEV_s = \Delta H_{c,s}(1 - Z)$$

where $Z = \dfrac{D_{cd} - D_{td}}{E_s/E_{td}} + C$

and $C = (1 - D_{cd})$

Procedure B:

$$DEV_s = \Delta H_{c,s} - \left[\frac{(E_{tf}/M_{td}) - (E_{cf}/M_{cd})}{M_s/M_{td}}\right]$$

$$MEV_s = \Delta H_{c,s} - \left[\frac{((E_{tf} + E_{tu})/M_{td}) - ((E_{cf} + E_{cu})/M_{cd}))}{M_s/M_{td}}\right]$$

DEV_s and MEV_s are the digestible and metabolisable energy values of dietary fibre (kJ/g; kcal/g). D_{cd} and D_{td} are the apparent digestibilities of dietary gross energies for the control diet and test diet respectively (dimensionless). E_{tf}, E_{cf}, E_{tu}, E_{cu}, E_{td}, and E_s are the gross energies in the test faeces, control faeces, test urine, control urine, test diet and dietary fibre, respectively (kJ (kcal) per balance period). $\Delta H_{c,s}$, is the heat of combustion (ΔH_c) of dietary fibre (kJ (kcal)/g) M_{td}, M_{cd} and M_s are the dry masses of the basal portion of the test diet, basal portion of the control diet and dietary fibre, respectively (g).

In a strict sense, these calculation procedures are valid when the test substance, i.e. dietary fibre, is added as supplement to a constant basal diet. When fibre substitutes for another energy source, corrections should be made. However, when the replaced energy source is highly available, corrections are very small and can be omitted for practical purposes (Livesey, 1989). In most of the studies concerning the DE and ME of fibre-rich diets and the energy supplied by fibre, natural foods have been used as fibre sources. This makes the relations more complicated for the following reason: when low fibre foods are substituted by high fibre foods, in most cases there are also changes in other nutrients besides fibre. However, differences in the level of non-fibre nutrients affect faecal energy excretion much less than fibre does (Widdowson, 1955; Livesey, 1990) and therefore have only a small influence on the calculated partial digestible energy value of fibre. Moreover, in studying foods as fibre sources, the heat of combustion of fibre must be calculated, because fibre cannot be isolated in pure form without non-fibre components such as protein.

Several studies have been performed concerning the influence of dietary fibre from various sources on the digestible and metabolisable energy of the diet. Fibre sources that were studied were combinations of different fruits and vegetables, mixed diets containing fruits, vegetables and cereals, different cereal-based diets, and wheat bran. From the data of these experiments, Livesey (1990) calculated the partial digestible energy values of the fibre sources studied. Table 13.1 summarises the results of most of these studies. Values for partial digestible energy were taken from Livesey (1990) unless otherwise indicated. Metabolisable energy values of fibre were not shown in the work of Livesey (1990) and were also not calculated in this paper, because data were not available from all investigations. In a study concerning the ME of diets rich in fruit and vegetable fibres (Wisker and Feldheim, 1990), partial digestible and metabolisable energy values of fibre differed only slightly. An elevated intake of fibre is often associated with an increase in faecal nitrogen excretion (Southgate and Durnin, 1970; Kelsay et al., 1978; Wisker et al., 1988) which might probably be compensated for by a decrease in urinary nitrogen losses (Southgate and Durnin, 1970; Wisker et al., 1987a). However, from the data available, fibre has no significant effect on urinary energy excretion (Southgate and Durnin, 1970; Kelsay et al., 1978; Wisker et al., 1988).

Table 13.1 shows that there is a large range in partial digestible energy values of fibre. Some of these variations may depend on the method of fibre analysis. With the NDF method, only insoluble parts of fibre are measured (Goering and Van Soest, 1970). In the case of fibre from fruits and vegetables, but also from oat bran, measured intakes of fibre would have been higher had total dietary fibre been determined. As a consequence, higher partial digestible energy values would have been calculated (Livesey, 1990). On the other hand, when the dietary fibre values include non-degraded starch, partial digestible energy values of fibre may be too high, because starch, also in vitro resistant starch, is shown to be easily fermented in vivo (Björck et al., 1987), and to yield partial digestible energy values of about 3 kcal/g (Livesey et al., 1990). Besides these possible variations due to methodological reasons, it seems that the partial digestible energy values for cereal fibres were lower than those calculated for fruit and vegetable fibres. These lower values may correlate with the observation that in many cases cereal fibres are more potent enhancers of faecal bulk than fibres from fruits and vegetables (Cummings et al., 1978; Wisker and Feldheim, 1983) and therefore lead to higher faecal energy losses (Wisker et al., 1988; Wisker and Feldheim, 1990). This may be due to a lower apparent digestibility of cereal fibres compared with fruit and vegetable fibres, to non-absorbed starch included into coarse particles of cereal grains (Wisker et al., 1988) or to a decreased transit time and thus to an increased excretion of energy-containing bacterial material (Livesey, 1990).

Partial digestible energy values seem also to be related to the intake of fibre. Negative values are found more commonly when the contribution of fibre to gross energy intake is low, i.e. at low fibre levels. Low fibre intakes seem to be very effective at causing faecal losses of protein and fat, whereas increasing fibre levels seem to be progressively less effective (Livesey, 1990). The contribution of cereal fibre to ME needs further study.

Table 13.1. Intake of dietary fibre from various sources, digestibility of dietary gross energy, and partial digestible energy value of dietary fibre in humans

Source of dietary fibre	Intake of dietary fibre (g/day)		Digestibility of gross energy (%)		Partial digestible energy value of dietary fibre		Literature
	Control diet	High-fibre diet	Control diet	High-fibre diet	kJ/g	kcal/g	
Fruits/ vegetables	3.6 (NDF)[c]	20.0 (NDF)	96.3	91.6	−19	−4.5[a]	Kelsay et al., 1978
	1.9 (NDF)	10.1 (NDF)	96.1	94.7	−5	−1.1[b]	Kelsay et al., 1981
	1.9 (NDF)	19.4 (NDF)	96.1	93.0	−5	−1.2[b]	
	1.9 (NDF)	25.6 (NDF)	96.1	91.2	−8	−2.0[b]	
	6.2	31.9	96.5	92.5	−2	−0.5[a]	Southgate and Durnin, 1970
	16.4	37.4	92.0	88.5	−4	−1.0[b]	Miles et al., 1988
	18.8	52.0	94.7	89.7	+4	+0.9[b]	Wisker and Feldheim, 1990
		64.7			+11	+2.6[a]	Göranzon and Forsum, 1987
Mixed diets	9.7	21.5	96.6	94.3	−14	−3.3[a]	Southgate and Durnin, 1970
	6.2	16.2	96.5	94.9	0	0[a]	
	7.4	20.9	96.8	94.9	+1	+0.2[a]	
	9.6	28.3	96.0	94.1	+4	+1.0[a]	
	28.1	85.6	95.0	90.7	+9	+2.2[a]	Göranzon et al., 1983
Cereals							
Rice	14.8 (NDF)	30.1 (NDF)	94.4	89.3	−21	−5.0[b]	Miyoshi et al., 1986
Mainly barley		48		82	−17	−4.1[a]	Judd, 1982
Mainly wheat		27		90	−13	−3.1[a]	
Whole grain, mainly rye	19.7	48.3	93.2	86.9	−5	−1.2[a]	Wisker et al., 1988
Various		55.7			+1	+0.3[a]	Göranzon and Forsum, 1987
Fibre concentrates							
Oat bran	3.8 (NDF)	11.7 (NDF)	96.8	94.2	−17	−4.1[a]	Calloway and Kretsch, 1978
Oat bran	3.8 (NDF)	12.0 (NDF)	96.8	94.0	−15	−3.6[a]	
Wheat bran	21.2	39.2	95.7	93.1	+4	+0.9[a]	Stevens et al., 1987

[a], values taken from Livesey (1990); [b], , values calculated from original literature; [c] NDF, neutral detergent fibre.

Calculation of the Metabolisable Energy of Fibre-Rich Diets

The ME of a diet can be measured by balance experiments. However, as these studies are not easy to perform in humans for various reasons, procedures were developed for the calculation of the ME of a diet from its chemical composition or its gross energy content. Most of the calculation systems used at present have their origin in the work carried out at the turn of the century by Rubner (1885) and Atwater (Atwater and Benedict, 1897). On the basis of the heat of combustion of the nutrients and their apparent digestibilities, two groups of conversion factors were derived (Atwater's general factors and the specific conversion factors as listed by Merrill and Watt (1955)). In these procedures, dietary fibre is included in the value for total carbohydrates and is therefore multiplied with the conversion factors used for total carbohydrates. In two modifications of the general Atwater factors, that are used in Great Britain (Paul and Southgate, 1978) and in Germany (Amtl. Sammlung von Untersuchungsmethoden, 1988), available carbohydrates are either determined analytically (Great Britain), or are calculated by difference, where the difference is obtained as total carbohydrate minus total dietary fibre (Germany). Concerning these modifications, dietary fibre is regarded as a non-energy providing constituent. On the basis of partial digestible energy values of fibre from various sources, Livesey (1990) proposed to apply a conversion factor of 8.4 kJ (2 kcal) per gram of fibre. This procedure has been called the modified British method.

Furthermore, equations were developed for the calculation of the ME, that are based on the gross energy content of diets. These formulas contain correction factors for the energy and nitrogen losses (Miller and Payne, 1959; Southgate, 1975; Miller and Judd, 1984), and in two cases also for the dietary fibre content of the diet (Southgate, 1975; Miller and Judd, 1984). The various calculation procedures are summarised below:

(1) Specific conversion factors of Merrill and Watt (1955): different conversion factors for the nutrients from different foods
(2) General factors of Atwater: 17 kJ (4 kcal), 37 kJ (9 kcal), 17 kJ (4 kcal) per gram of protein, fat and total carbohydrate by difference respectively
(3) British calculation procedure (Paul and Southgate, 1978): 17 kJ (4 kcal), 37 kJ (9 kcal), 15.7 kJ (3.75 kcal) per gram of protein, fat and available carbohydrate, expressed in monosaccharide equivalents, respectively
(3a) Modified British procedure as proposed by Livesey (1990): as British procedure, but in addition 8.4 kJ (2 kcal) per gram of dietary fibre
(4) German calculation procedure (Amtl. Sammlung von Untersuchungs-methoden, 1988): 17 kJ (4 kcal), 37 kJ (9 kcal), 17 kJ (4 kcal) per gram of protein, fat and available carbohydrate by difference, respectively
(5) Miller and Payne equation (1959): ME (kcal) = 0.95 GE (kcal) − 7.5 N
(6) Miller and Judd equation (1984): ME (kcal) = (0.95 − F') GE (kcal) − 7.5 N
(7) Southgate equation (1975): ME (kcal) = 0.98 GE (kcal) − 6.6 N − DF

In these formulae, GE is the gross energy content of the diet (kcal per day), N and DF correspond to the daily intake of nitrogen and dietary fibre (g), and F' is the dietary fibre (g) per gram of diet dry weight.

Table 13.2. Accuracy of different calculation procedures to predict measured metabolisable energy (ME) of fibre containing diets in humans

Fibre source	Fibre intake (g/day)	ME measured (kcal/day)	% deviation from measured ME							Literature
			ME (M & W)	ME (Atw.)	ME (Brit.)	ME (Germ.)	ME (M & P)	ME (M & J)	ME (Southgate)	
Fruits/vegetables	16.4	2783	+5.2	+ 4.0			−0.8	−4.4	+0.1	Miles et al., 1988
	37.4	2709	+6.8	+ 8.0			+3.1	−4.2	+1.2	Wisker and Feldheim, 1990
	18.8	1831	−0.3	+ 2.5		−1.3	+0.7	−4.4	+0.5	
	52.0	1802	−0.1	+ 9.4		−2.2	+6.6	−7.0	−0.8	Göranzon and Forsum, 1987
	64.7	2280	−2.2	+ 2.6	− 7.9		−0.2		−7.6	Göranzon and Forsum, 1987
Mixed diets	9.7	3210					−1.9		+0.6[a]	Southgate and Durnin, 1970
	21.5	3290					+0.4		+1.5[a]	Southgate and Durnin, 1970
	6.2	2170					−2.1		+0.6[a]	Southgate and Durnin, 1970
	16.2	2260					0		+1.0[a]	Southgate and Durnin, 1970
	7.4	2920					−3.0		−0.4[a]	Southgate and Durnin, 1970
	20.9	2850					−1.1		−0.3[a]	
	9.6	2080					−0.7		+1.4[a]	Southgate and Durnin, 1970
	28.3	2300					+1.1		0 [a]	
	28.1	1971	+2.8	+ 1.2	− 6.1		+0.7		−1.2	Göranzon et al., 1983
	85.6	2166	−3.9	+ 4.3	−13.5		+4.9		−6.8	
Cereal	19.7	1861	+4.5	+ 5.3		+2.1	+2.5		+2.3	Wisker et al., 1987b
	48.3	1932	+6.3	+11.5		+3.2	+9.6		+3.9	
	55.7	2420	+0.4	+ 7.0		−5.4	+4.6		−0.5	Göranzon and Forsum, 1987

[a] The Southgate formula (Southgate, 1975) was derived from the results of this study.

Several studies report calculated values for ME, from others ME could be calculated from the intakes of gross energy, nitrogen, and dietary fibre by the equations of Miller and Payne (1959) and of Southgate (1975). Table 13.2 shows ME of these diets as measured by balance experiments and the accuracy of the different calculation procedures to predict measured ME.

All factorial methods predict the ME of the diets containing lower amounts of fibre with greater precision than the ME of the diets that contained higher levels of fibre. From the data shown in Table 13.1, but also from the paper of Livesey (1990) it is evident that Atwater's factors overestimate measured ME, the British procedure gives an underestimation, whereas the specific factors of Merrill and Watt seem to predict the ME of diets containing high levels of dietary fibre with greater accuracy than other procedures. This may be due to the fact that the specific factors, in contrast to the general factors, were derived from diets that contained relatively large amounts of fibre-containing foods in addition to a basal diet. However, the specific factors are rather difficult to handle in practice. From the values shown in Table 13.2 it appears that the German procedure also gives a good agreement between measured and estimated ME; however, only values for four diets were available.

With the exception of the formula of Miller and Judd (1984), the empirical systems seem to predict the measured ME more adequately than the factorial methods that are shown in Table 13.2, probably because these procedures use directly measured gross energy, whereas the conversion factors use estimated values for the heat of combustion of protein, fat and carbohydrates. However, at high fibre intakes, the Miller and Payne formula gives an overestimation of ME, perhaps because there is no correction factor for dietary fibre. The Southgate equation gives a good agreement between measured and calculated ME, only at very high fibre intakes is there an underestimation. As also shown in the paper of Livesey (1990) the formula of Miller and Judd (1984) gives an underestimation of measured ME. This formula was derived from diets that contained relatively large amounts of cereals, especially barley, and may therefore be unsuitable for the estimation of the ME of diets containing other fibre sources than cereals.

The specific factors of Merrill and Watt (1955) and the Southgate formula (1975) appear to predict ME of fibre-rich diets with the greatest precision. As only very few studies report values for analytically determined available carbohydrates as monosaccharides, there is at present little experience with the modified British procedure as proposed by Livesey (1990). In addition, further knowledge about the partial digestible energy of cereal fibres and of the ME provided by diets containing mostly cereal fibres would be desirable.

References

Amtliche Sammlung von Untersuchungsmethoden & 35 LMGB (1988) 00.018 Beuth, Berlin-Köln

Atwater WO, Benedict FG (1897) Experiments on the digestion of food by man. Conn Agric Exp Stn Storrs Bull 18:154–167

Bacon JSD (1979) Plant cell wall digestibility and chemical structure. Rep Rowett Res Inst 35:99–108

Björck I, Nyman M, Pedersen B, Siljeström M, Asp N-G, Eggum BO (1987) Formation of enzyme-resistant starch during autoclaving of wheat starch: Studies in vitro and in vivo. J Cereal Sci 6:159–172

Brodribb AJM, Groves C (1978) Effect of bran particle size on stool weight. Gut 19:60–63

Calkins BM (1986) Consumption of fibre in vegetarians and nonvegetarians. In: Spiller GA (ed) CRC handbook of dietary fibre in human nutrition. CRC Press, Boca Raton, pp 407–414

Calloway DH, Kretsch MJ (1978) Protein and energy utilisation in men given a rural Guatemalan diet and egg formulas with and without added oat bran. Am J Clin Nutr 31:1118–1126

Cummings JH (1981) Dietary fibre. Br Med Bull 37:65–70

Cummings JH (1984) Microbial digestion of complex carbohydrates in man. Proc Nutr Soc 43:35–44

Cummings JH (1986) The effect of dietary fibre on faecal weight and composition. In: Spiller GA (ed), Handbook of dietary fiber in human nutrition, CRC Press, Boca Raton, pp 211–280

Cummings JH, Branch W, Jenkins DJA, Southgate DAT, Houston H, James WPT (1978) Colonic response to dietary fibre from carrot, cabbage, apple, bran and guar gum. Lancet i:5–9

Davies GJ, Crowder M, Dickerson JWT (1985) Dietary fibre intake of individuals with different eating patterns. J Hum Nutr Appl 39A:139

Deutsche Gesellschaft für Ernährung (1985) Empfehlungen für die Nährstoffzufuhr. 4. Erweiterte Überarbeitung. Umschau Verlag, Frankfurt

Deutsche Gesellschaft für Ernährung (1988) Ernährungsbericht 1988. Henrich, Frankfurt

Eastwood MA, Robertson JA, Brydon WG, MacDonald D (1983) Measurement of water-holding properties of fibre and their faecal bulking ability in man. Br J Nutr 50:539–547

Eastwood MA, Brydon WG, Baird JD, Elton RA, Helliwell S, Smith JH, Pritchard JL (1984) Faecal weight and composition, serum lipids, and diet among subjects aged 18 to 80 years not seeking health care. Am J Clin Nutr 40:628–634

Eastwood MA, Brydon WG, Anderson DMW (1986a) The effect of the polysaccharide composition and structure of dietary fibres on cecal fermentation and faecal excretion. Am J Clin Nutr 44:51–55

Eastwood MA, Elton RA, Smith JH (1986b) Long-term effect of wholemeal bread on stool weight, transit time, faecal bile acids, fats, and neutral sterols. Am J Clin Nutr 43:343–349

Englyst HN, Cummings JH (1985) Digestion of the polysaccharides in some cereal foods in the human small intestine. Am J Clin Nutr 42:778–787

Eyton A (1982) F-plan diet. Penguin Books, Harmondsworth, UK

Goering HK, Van Soest PJ (1970) Forage fibre analysis. ARS/USDA agriculture handbook 379. US Government Printing Office, Washington, DC

Göranzon H, Forsum E (1987) Metabolizable energy in humans in two diets containing different sources of dietary fibre. Calculation and analysis. J Nutr 117:267–273

Göranzon H, Forsum E, Thilen M (1983) Calculation and determination of metabolizable energy in mixed diets to humans. Am J Clin Nutr 38:954–963

Heller SN, Hackler LR, Rivers JM et al. (1980) Dietary fibre: The effects of particle size of wheat bran on colonic function in young adult men. Am J Clin Nutr 33:1734–1744

Jenkins DJA, Peterson RD, Thorne MJ et al. (1987) Wheat fibre and laxation: dose response and equilibration time. Am J Gastroenterol 82:1259–1263

Judd PA (1982) The effects of high intakes of barley on gastrointestinal function and apparent digestibilities of dry matter, nitrogen and fat in human volunteers. J Plant Foods 4:79–88

Kelsay JL, Behall KM, Prather ES (1978) Effects of fibre from fruits and vegetables on metabolic responses of human subjects. I. Bowel transit time, number of defecations, faecal weight, urinary excretions of energy and nitrogen and apparent digestibilities of energy, nitrogen, and fat. Am J Clin Nutr 31:1149–1153

Kelsay JL, Clark WM, Herbst BJ, Prather ES (1981) Nutrient utilisation by human subjects consuming fruits and vegetables as sources of fibre. J Agric Food Chem 29:461–465

Kleiber M (1975) The fire of life. Kreiger, New York

Livesey G (1989) Procedures for calculating the digestible and metabolizable energy values of food components making a small contribution to dietary intake. J Agric Food Sci 48:475–481

Livesey G (1990) Energy values of unavailable carbohydrates and diets. An inquiry and analysis. Am J Clin Nutr 51:617–637

Livesey G, Davies IR, Brown JC, Faulks RM, Southon S (1990) Energy balance and energy values of amylase (EC 3.2.1.1)-resistant maize and pea (*Pisum sativum*) starches in the rat. Br J Nutr 63:467–480

Lubbe AM (1971) Dietary evaluation. A comparative study of rural and urban venda males. S Afr Med J 45:1289–1297

McNeil N (1984) The contribution of the large intestine to energy supplies in man. Am J Clin Nutr 39:338–342

McNeil NI, Cummings JH, James WPT (1978) Short chain fatty acid absorption by the human large intestine. Gut 19:819–822

Merrill AL, Watt BK (1955) Energy value of foods; basis and derivation. US Department of Agriculture. US Government Printing Office, Washington, DC (Agriculture handbook no. 74)

Miles CW, Kelsay JL, Wong NF (1988) Effect of dietary fibre on metabolizable energy of human diets. J Nutr 118:1075–1081

Miller DS, Judd PA (1984) The metabolizable energy value of foods. J Sci Food Agric 35:111–116

Miller DS, Payne PR (1959) A ballistic bomb calorimeter. Br J Nutr 13:501–508

Miyoshi H, Okuda T, Oi Y, Koishi H (1986) Effects of fibre on faecal weight, apparent digestibility of energy, nitrogen and fat, and degradation of neutral detergent fibre in young men. J Nutr Sci Vitaminol 32:581–589

Paul AA, Southgate DAT (eds) (1978) McCance and Widdowson's The composition of foods, 4th rev edn. HMSO, London

Rubner M (1885) Calorimetrische Untersuchungen I und II. Z Biol 21:250–334, 337–410

Selvendran RR (1984) The plant cell wall as a source of dietary fibre: chemistry and structure. Am J Clin Nutr 39:320–337

Slavin JL, Nelson NL, McNamara EA et al. (1985) Bowel function of healthy men consuming liquid diets with and without dietary fibre. J Parent Entr Nutr 9:317–321

Smith AN, Drummond E, Eastwood MA (1981) The effect of coarse and fine Canadian Red Spring Wheat and French Soft Wheat bran on colonic motility in patients with diverticular disease. Am J Clin Nutr 34:2460–2463

Southgate DAT (1973) Fibre and the other unavailable carbohydrates and their effects on the energy value of the diet. Proc Nutr Soc 32:131–136

Southgate DAT (1975) Fibre and other unavailable carbohydrates and energy effects in the diet. In: White PL, Selvey NB (eds) Proceedings of the Western Hemisphere Nutrition Congress IV. Publishing Science Group Inc, Acton, MA, pp 51–55

Southgate DAT, Durnin JVGA (1970) Calorie conversion factors: an experimental reassessment of the factors used in the calculation of the energy value of human diets. Br J Nutr 24:517–535

Spiller GA (1986) Suggestions for a basis on which to determine a desirable intake of dietary fiber. In: Spiller GA (ed) Handbook of dietary fibre in human nutrition. CRC Press, Boca Raton, pp 281–283

Spiller GA, Chernoff MC, Shipley EA, Beigler MA, Briggs GM (1977) Can faecal weight be used to establish a recommended intake of dietary fibre (plantix)? Am J Clin Nutr 30:659–661

Spiller GA, Story JA, Wong LG et al. (1986) Effect of increasing levels of hard wheat fibre on faecal weight, minerals and steroids and gastrointestinal transit time in healthy young women. J Nutr 116:778–785

Stephen AM, Cummings JH (1980) Mechanism of action of dietary fibre in the human colon. Nature 284:283–284

Stephen AM, Wiggins HS, Englyst HN, Cole TJ, Wayman BJ, Cummings JH (1986) Effect of age, sex and level of intake of dietary fibre from wheat on large-bowel function in 30 healthy subjects. Br J Nutr 56:349–361

Stevens J, Levitsky DA, Van Soest PJ, Roberts JB, Kalkwarf HJ, Roe AD (1987) Effect of psyllium gum and wheat bran on spontaneous energy intake. Am J Clin Nutr 46:812–817

Tucker DM, Sandstead HH, Logan GM et al. (1981) Dietary fibre and personality factors as determinants of stool output. Gastroenterology 81:879–883

Van Dokkum W, Pikaar NA, Thissen JTNM (1983) Physiological effects of fibre-rich types of bread. II. Dietary fibre from bread: Digestibility by the intestinal microflora and water holding capacity in the colon of human subjects. Br J Nutr 50:61–74

Van Soest PJ, Robertson JB (1976) Chemical and physical properties of dietary fibre. In: Hawkins WW (ed) Dietary fibre. Proc. Miles Symposium Nutrition Society of Canada, Dalhousie University, Halifax, NS, pp 13–25

Widdowson EM (1955) Assessment of energy value of human foods. Proc Nutr Soc 14:142–154

Widdowson EM (1978) Note on the calculation of the energy value of foods and diets. In: Paul AA, Southgate DAT (eds) McCance and Widdowson's The composition of foods, 4th rev. edn. HMSO, London, pp 322–329

Wisker E, Feldheim W (1983) Einfluß von Ballaststoffen aus Obst, Gemüse oder Brot auf die Darmfunktion von jungen Frauen. Akt Ernähr 5:200–205

Wisker E, Feldheim W (1990) Metabolizable energy of diets low or high in dietary fibre from fruits and vegetables when consumed by humans. J Nutr 120:1331–1337

Wisker E, Feldheim W, Pomeranz Y, Meuser F (1985) Dietary fibre in cereals. In: Pomeranz Y (ed) Advances in cereal science and technology. American Association of Cereal Chemists, pp 169–226

Wisker E, Krumm U, Feldheim W (1986) Einfluß der Partikelgröße von Getreideprodukten auf das Stuhlgewicht von jungen Frauen. Akt Ernähr 11:208–211

Wisker E, Hudtwalker G, Feldheim W (1987a) Untersuchungen zum Kalzium- und Phosphorstoffwechsel beim Menschen. 4. Mitteilung: Einfluß einer veränderten Zufuhr von Phosphat und Ballaststoffen mit der Kost auf die Bilanzen von Phosphor, Kalzium und Magnesium. Akt Ernähr 12:149–153

Wisker E, Maltz A, Feldheim W (1987b) Metabolisierbare Energie von Kostformen mit unterschiedlichem Gehalt an Getreideballaststoffen – Vergleich von gemessenen und berechneten Werten. Getreide Mehl Brot 41:340–344

Wisker E, Maltz A, Feldheim W (1988) Metabolizable energy of diets low or high in dietary fibre from cereals when eaten by humans. J Nutr 118:945–952

Wisker E, Feldheim W, Schweizer TF (1990) Metabolic effects of raw and processed carrots in humans. In: Southgate DAT, Waldron K, Johnson IT, Fenwick GR (eds) Dietary fibre: chemical and biological aspects. Royal Society of Chemistry, Cambridge, pp 318–320

Wrick KL, Robertson JB, Van Soest PJ et al. (1983) The influence of dietary fibre source on human intestinal transit and stool output. J Nutr 113:1464–1479

Commentary

Mauron: Is it fair to say that we do not yet have enough hard data to fix a valuable figure for the average metabolisable energy content of dietary fibre for labelling purposes?

Southgate: One of the difficulties is that the actual value for a particular polysaccharide will depend on the extent to which it is fermented in the large bowel. Thus, cellulose which is only poorly fermented will have an energy value approaching zero, whereas a material such as pectin which is completely fermented will produce around 3 kcal/g. The extent of fermentation will depend on the individual eating the food and the physical form in which the material is eaten.

For a mixed diet I think that 2 kcal/g for a mixture is about right, but for individual constituents this may over- or underestimate the energy. Clearly agreement is needed on methods to assess the energy value of ingredients so that specific factors are available to food producers who wish to use the material as an ingredient.

Section III
Prevention and Treatment of Disease

Chapter 14

Dietary Fibre in the Prevention and Treatment of Gastro-intestinal Disorders

K.W. Heaton

Introduction

The dietary fibre hypothesis came to prominence around 1970 with the publication of a book (Cleave et al., 1969) and several papers (Burkitt, 1969; 1971a, b; Painter and Burkitt, 1971) which adduced an impressive mass of historical and geographical evidence and some convincing arguments relating the consumption of fibre-depleted diets to a wide variety of diseases including several gastro-intestinal ones. During the 1970s and early 1980s more evidence was gathered, many conferences were held and published. Scholarly multi-author tomes seemed to render the hypothesis academically respectable (Trowell and Burkitt, 1981; Trowell et al., 1985). However, the quality of the evidence was far from conclusive and many scientists remained sceptical. Most of the early workers in the field, including the author, underestimated the difficulties of research into the dietary causes of disease and the complexities of fibre itself. Progress in testing the fibre hypothesis has been slow and public interest has moved on to such matters as gene libraries, immunodeficiency viruses and free radicals. Nevertheless much has been learnt and, in a few diseases, the role of a low intake of fibre or, at least, of polysaccharides is becoming moderately clear.

There never was a single fibre hypothesis – rather a family of hypotheses relating protection from diseases to different properties of fibre and fibre-rich diets. In addressing this question, therefore, it is necessary to consider separately each of the diseases mentioned by the early writers. In this chapter I consider each of the gastro-intestinal diseases which have been linked with a fibre-depleted diet and assess the strength of the evidence for such a link and for suggested mechanisms.

Sliding Hiatus Hernia

The idea that straining at stool could displace the stomach through the oesophageal hiatus of the diaphragm into the chest has been around a long time (Muller, 1948). Straining certainly creates a pressure gradient across the diaphragm (Fedail et al., 1979) and must promote gastro-oesophageal reflux but it has not been shown to displace the stomach. The hypothesis that habitual constipation causes hiatus hernia (Burkitt and James, 1973) is completely untested. There are no data on the prevalence of straining at stool in different communities, let alone in people with hiatus hernia and hernia-free controls. Prolonged straining is a feature of irritable bowel syndrome as well as of constipation. Sliding hiatus hernia might be caused by shortening of the oesophageal longitudinal muscle pulling the stomach upwards rather than by pressure from below (Mullard, 1972). There are no data on dietary intakes of people with and without hiatus hernia let alone prospective studies.

Traditionally, doctors have believed that hiatus hernia tends to occur in association with diverticular disease of the colon and gallbladder stones ("Saint's triad") but scientific validation is lacking. There is reasonable evidence of a link between hiatus hernia and gallstones (Capron et al., 1978) which suggests a common aetiological factor but its nature is unknown.

Symptoms in people with hiatus hernia are caused not by the hernia itself but by the frequently associated gastro-oesophageal reflux, which can also occur in the absence of hernia. Recommended treatment of reflux includes correction of constipation but this is based on "common sense" (i.e. untested assumptions) rather than controlled trials. The key elements of the dietary treatment of oesophageal reflux are generally agreed to be reduction in the size and fat content of meals rather than a high-fibre intake. Much research is needed in this area.

Duodenal Ulcer

There are marked differences in the prevalence of duodenal ulcer around the world but these are not related to habitual diet in any consistent way (Tovey, 1985). There is some evidence of a protective factor in whole-grain foods, especially wheat, in that ulcers are less prone to recur on a diet rich in such foods than on one devoid of them (Malhotra, 1978; Rydning et al., 1982). However, English patients with duodenal ulcer do not have a particularly low intake of dietary fibre (Katschinski et al., 1990), a high-fibre diet makes no difference to the healing rate (Rydning and Berstad, 1985) and recent research blames the relapse of duodenal ulcer on colonisation of the gastric antrum and duodenum with *Helicobacter pylori* (Rauws and Tytgat, 1990). It is conceivable that such colonisation is hindered by a diet rich in wholewheat products but there is little reason to look to dietary fibre. Work in rats suggests that the protective factor in diet is a lipid-soluble substance (Tovey, 1985).

There are more promising areas for dietary fibre research than duodenal ulcer.

Gallstones

In the early years of the "fibre hypothesis" it was postulated that gallstones were caused by fibre-depleted diets. Suggested reasons were: (1) the apparent rarity of gallstones in poor, rural, third-world communities; (2) apparently increasing prevalence of gallstones in the 20th century; (3) the association of gallstones with obesity, diabetes and hyperlipidaemia or coronary heart disease; (4) the universal presence of fibre-depleted carbohydrate in experimental gallstone-causing diets in laboratory animals; (5) the ability of such diets to cause adverse changes in bile salt metabolism; (6) a beneficial effect of wheat bran on the composition of bile (Cleave et al., 1969; Heaton, 1973; Burkitt and Tunstall, 1975; Heaton, 1975).

Since those days, much has been learnt about the epidemiology of gallstones, and of biochemical and motility factors in their pathogenesis, and ideas have had to be modified. The present position is outlined below.

Gallstones have certainly become commoner in Europe in the last century and are prevalent in all "Westernised" communities (Heaton, 1988a). Incidence may now be falling in some European countries. There are no good data from poor, rural countries.

Obesity is a major risk factor in women (MacLure et al., 1989) and abdominal obesity is a risk factor in men (Heaton et al., 1991).

The risk of gallstones is related to the biliary content of deoxycholate – a bacterial metabolite of cholate, absorbed from the colon (Marcus and Heaton, 1988) – and biliary deoxycholate levels can be increased by making normal people constipated and decreased by laxative treatment of constipated people (Marcus and Heaton, 1986). Although this suggests that constipation predisposes to gallstones there are as yet no epidemiological data to support this idea.

Case–control studies have yielded mixed results with respect to dietary fibre. Two studies have found a protective effect of a high-fibre intake (Scragg et al., 1984; Heaton et al., unpublished data), two have found a trend in this direction (Attili et al., 1984, 1987) and one found no effect at all (Pixley and Mann, 1988). The inconsistency of these results could be due to the inherent limitations of case–control diet studies. These studies give no indication that cereal fibre is especially protective although it is mostly wheat fibre which has been shown to have beneficial effects on the cholesterol saturation of bile (Heaton, 1987). Some have found a beneficial effect with a diet based on naturally fibre-rich foods without any "bran effect" on bile deoxycholate (Thornton et al., 1983). Indirect support for a protective effect of a naturally fibre-rich diet comes from the relative scarcity of gallstones in vegetarians (Pixley et al., 1985).

Current gallstone research is preoccupied with mechanisms for the crystallisation of cholesterol monohydrate and calcium salts from bile and with gallbladder motility. So far this research has not thrown much light on the diet–gallstones connection except for two findings. Firstly, bile with high levels of deoxycholate is more prone to nucleate crystals of cholesterol, which again points to a colonic factor in gallstone disease. Secondly, missing breakfast seems to increase the risk of gallstones (Capron et al., 1981), perhaps because bile which stays too long in the gallbladder becomes more saturated with cholesterol (Bloch et al., 1980) or because it has more time to form crystals. If constipation predisposes to gallstones then missing breakfast could contribute to gallstones in two more ways. Firstly, since breakfast is the natural stimulus to opening the bowels in many people, missing breakfast may interfere with bowel regularity. Secondly, breakfast is a major contributor to many people's intake of cereal fibre so missing it could entail a drop in the intake of this most laxative element in the diet.

Crohn's Disease

This chronic inflammatory disease can affect any part of the gut but typically it involves the terminal ileum and/or the colon. Its cause is unknown. Accurate data on its incidence are hard to obtain but it seems to be a disease of Westernised countries, especially northern Europe and North America. There have been many case–control studies of dietary intake in Crohn's disease. These have consistently found a high intake of extracted (fibre-depleted) sugars in patients with this disease. Also, on the three occasions when it has been measured, the intake of fresh fruit and vegetables has been low (Heaton, 1988b).

The meaning of these findings is unclear. Some people think the dietary changes are secondary to the disease, that is, they simply reflect the unconscious efforts of patients with Crohn's disease to reduce their abdominal pain and diarrhoea. This sounds plausible but the evidence does not support it. When patients are asked if they have changed their intake of sugars since their symptoms began, they usually say they have decreased it, not increased it. What happens to fruit and vegetable intake when symptoms begin is unknown but, when Italian patients who had been put on a low-fibre diet were encouraged to eat fruit and vegetables freely, they did not get worse (Levenstein et al., 1985). The problem for gastroenterologists is that they do not understand how a high intake of extracted sugars and a low intake of fruit and vegetables fit into the pathogenetic sequence of Crohn's disease, which makes them reluctant to accept a dietary aetiology. This reluctance is understandable but an open mind is more logical than flat rejection because the first step in the pathogenesis of Crohn's disease is quite unknown. A recent hypothesis about the first step is excessive permeability of the mucosa of the upper gut allowing dietary antigens to enter and set off an immune reaction (Hollander, 1988). Sugars can increase intestinal permeability if they are in hypertonic solution (Maxton et al., 1986). Fruit and vegetables might be protective by providing anti-oxidant vitamins to limit free-radical damage or simply by speeding up transit through the ileum and caecum.

Appendicitis

The association of appendicitis with modern urban civilisation has been known for many years. As long ago as 1920, Rendle Short suggested the disease was caused by lack of fibre in the diet (or cellulose as he called it) (Short 1920). More recently, Burkitt (1971a, 1975) produced much epidemiological evidence to support a connection between appendicitis and Westernisation including many anecdotal reports of a sudden increase in the disease when white bread was introduced to groups of people. However, he did not produce evidence for his proposed mechanism (faecoliths or viscous caecal contents blocking the mouth of the appendix) and, when Barker (1985) re-examined the epidemiological time-trends, he found discrepancies in the evidence. In particular the last 35 years have seen a substantial fall in appendicitis rates at a time when dietary fibre intakes were static or even falling. Moreover, the higher rate of appendicitis in Ireland compared with Britain was associated with higher, not lower, consumption of potatoes and cereals (Morris et al., 1987). Unfortunately, case–control studies have not resolved the issue. Three have found a low intake of dietary fibre in cases but two have not (Larner, 1988). The situation is further confused by the findings of Barker et al. (1986). They compared rates of appendicitis in 59 areas of England and Wales with National Food Survey data for those areas and found a negative correlation with non-potato vegetable consumption, especially green vegetables, but a positive correlation with potato consumption.

It is of course possible that different aetiological factors operate at different ages. Barker (1985) believes that, in children, improved hygiene in early life is the major factor, allowing the lymphoid tissue at the base of the appendix to remain immunologically naive so that, when the immune system is eventually challenged by, say, a virus infection in later childhood, it overreacts and the consequent lymphoid hyperplasia occludes the lumen of the appendix. In older people obstruction might be caused by a faecolith or viscous caecal contents in association with constipation.

Constipation

Constipation is the "stalking horse" of the fibre hypothesis, being the one condition in which everyone agrees there is a role for dietary fibre. However, there is considerable doubt as to the relative importance of dietary fibre and other aspects of modern life which can inhibit defecation such as lack of toilet facilities or competition for them, having to rush to work in the morning, travel, irregular habits, stress and unphysiological posture at defecation. Squatting is the "natural" posture and people strain less when they squat than when they sit on a conventional toilet (Fedail et al., 1979).

Constipation is important not just because it is common and uncomfortable but because it may be a risk factor for other diseases: diverticular disease, colorectal cancer and anal problems (haemorrhoids and anal fissure) and, possibly, breast cancer (Petrakis and King, 1981). It has also been suggested that straining at stool leads to venous dilatation in the lower limbs with the consequences of varicose veins and deep vein thrombosis (Burkitt, 1985).

It has become widely accepted that "a low intake of dietary fibre is the major causative factor in the ordinary type of constipation which is so prevalent in Western communities" (Trowell et al., 1985). However, doubts have begun to be expressed. An expert committee considered that "Constipation should probably be regarded as a disorder of colonic or anorectal motility that may respond to the mild laxative action of complex carbohydrate, rather than simply the result of a 'fibre deficient diet' (British Nutrition Foundation, 1990) and a literature review led one gastroenterologist to conclude that the value of bran as a laxative has been exaggerated (Müller-Lissner, 1988).

Part of the problem is that when people say constipation they can mean different things. The hospital gastroenterologist sees mostly severe cases who have already tried and failed with a high-fibre diet and bulking agents. These may be an atypical "hard core" and, certainly, severe constipation in young women is not a fibre-responsive condition but rather a motility disorder (Turnbull et al., 1986). Even with the "ordinary type of constipation" there are difficulties, not least in definition. There is no agreed definition of constipation. It is common to define it as infrequent defecation or frequent straining at stool but it is arbitrary to state a lower limit of normal for frequency of defecation or an upper limit for straining at stool because epidemiological data are lamentably inadequate for bowel habit and totally absent for straining (and for stool consistency). Some data are available for stool weight and transit time in different populations and it is a reasonable assumption that these bear some relationship to straining and infrequent defecation. However, data do not exist to show whether there is such a relationship in the general population. Nor are there data to show that stool weight and transit time are determinants of the symptoms which lead people to say that they are constipated, like weak, unpredictable or unproductive calls to stool, feelings of incomplete evacuation and abdominal bloating. It has, however, been shown that lumpiness of the stool relates to slowness of transit (O'Donnell et al., 1990) and that the lumpier the stool the more likely it is to be associated with straining and feelings of incomplete evacuation (Heaton et al., 1991). It has also been shown that artificially slowing down transit in normal people provokes bloating and abdominal pain (Marcus and Heaton, 1986).

What is the evidence relating stool weight and intestinal transit time to dietary fibre intake within the population? Between-country comparisons cannot be made as data are not available for the distribution of stool weights, transit times and fibre intakes in representative samples of different populations. Only one within-country study has been published – that of Eastwood et al. (1984) from Edinburgh. This involved a more or less random sample of 62 people aged 18 to 80 from that city. Faecal weight ranged from 19 to 278 g/24 hours and dietary fibre intake (Southgate method, from food tables) ranged from 4.3 to 32.6 g/24 hours. The correlation between the two was significant but so weak (Kendal rank correlation coefficient 0.41) that only 17% of the variance in stool output was explained by dietary fibre. However, this was a field study which limited the accuracy of the measurements and may have underestimated the strength of the relationship. In a more tightly controlled study of 51 motivated volunteers with a wider range of fibre intakes (and generally higher intakes of 10–78 g/day) the correlation between fibre intake and faecal weight was extremely close ($r = 0.96$, $P < 0.001$) (Davies et al., 1986). This study was unique in that the authors measured the consistency of the stools using a penetrometer. There was a very good correlation between fibre intake and stool softness ($r = 0.90$, $P < 0.001$). Since it is generally accepted that the ease with which a stool passes depends on its consistency, this study strongly suggests that ease of defecation is dependent on fibre intake.

Extrapolation from this study to the general population must be cautious because it did not include constipated people, indeed few people with low stool weight (the lowest being 54 g/day and the mean about 182 g/day), and the volunteers were exceptionally enthusiastic fibre-eaters, two-thirds of them being vegetarians. But the study does show what is achievable by sufficiently motivated people.

There is of course a mass of data to show that people can increase their faecal output by increasing their fibre intake (Cummings, 1986). This includes people with constipation though it is possible that they respond less well (Müller-

Lissner, 1988). There is good evidence for a linear dose–response curve with wheat bran, whether it is taken raw (Spiller et al., 1986), baked into bread (Stephen et al., 1986) or boiled and processed into a breakfast cereal (Jenkins et al., 1987), the last kind being the least effective. There is no doubt, therefore, that constipation can be prevented and relieved by dietary means if colorectal physiology is intact.

People vary greatly in their reaction to foods, perhaps most of all to fruit and vegetables. Overall, the laxative effect of fibre from fruit and vegetables is slightly less than that from wheat, the mean increase in stool weight per gram of fibre being 4.9 and 5.7 grams respectively (Cummings, 1986). In practice, the difference is more marked because the concentration of fibre in fruit and vegetables is much lower than in cereals.

Cooking reduces the laxative effect of wheat bran (Wyman et al., 1976) and may well do so with other forms of fibre. With wheat bran, particle size is important too (Cummings, 1986). On the other hand, rice bran which is finely particulate, seems to be as effective as a coarser wheat bran (Tomlin and Read, 1988).

Irritable Bowel Syndrome

Irritable bowel syndrome (IBS) is a variable combination of abdominal pain of intestinal origin, bloatedness and symptoms of disturbed defecation (irregularity in timing and stool form, urgency, feelings of incomplete evacuation, excessive straining, passage of mucus), none of the symptoms being explained by anatomical or biochemical disease (Thompson et al., 1989). To some extent the symptoms of IBS are part of everyday life but in patients they are, in general, more frequent and more severe, and bowel habit is objectively different from that of uncomplaining people (Heaton et al., 1991).

Most people develop some IBS symptoms if their intestinal transit is slowed down (Marcus and Heaton, 1987). To the extent that slow transit can be blamed on deficiency of fibre so perhaps can IBS when it is associated with a constipated bowel habit. However, many patients with IBS have "pseudo-constipation", that is, they use the word constipation to express feelings of incomplete evacuation which make them strain after the stool has passed, or to express unproductive calls to stool associated with abdominal discomfort. Moreover, many IBS patients complain of diarrhoea rather than constipation and the mean daily stool weight of IBS patients is much the same as that of healthy people (Hillman et al., 1982). It is not surprising, therefore, that case–control studies have failed to find a particularly low fibre intake in patients with IBS. All the same a sudden fall in fibre intake can almost certainly precipitate IBS in some people.

There was a vogue for treating IBS with bran or a high-fibre diet during the 1970s and 1980s but several controlled trials have shown no difference between the effects of bran and those of a placebo (British Nutrition Foundation, 1990). The placebo response can be substantial and it is becoming increasingly recognised that psychological factors are predominant in most cases of IBS.

Some patients with IBS are made worse by wheat bran (Cann et al., 1984) and 30%–40% are made worse by all wheat products (Jones et al., 1982). This is unlikely to be a reaction to the fibre in wheat since patients react even more often to dairy products (Nanda et al., 1989).

In summary, lack of fibre in the diet can be a cause of IBS but it is probably a relatively uncommon one and, when a high-fibre diet or bran is used in treatment, its placebo effect is the most important effect, except in some patients whose primary problem is constipation.

Diverticular Disease of the Colon

Colonic diverticular disease has a special place in the annals of fibre, as it was the first disease in which a high-fibre intake was claimed to have a therapeutic role (Painter et al., 1972). Fibre treatment seemed logical because the leading theory for the pathogenesis of diverticulosis was that the colon "ruptured itself" in its struggle to propel abnormally small, hard stools (Painter et al., 1965; Painter and Burkitt, 1971). This theory has been tested in several ways and has survived (albeit with some anomalies). A key finding is that diverticulosis is rare in black Africans but common in black Americans (Burkitt et al., 1985). Accurate prevalence data are not available for sufficient populations to enable comparisons to be made between prevalence of diverticular disease and fibre intakes. However, in England the disease is substantially less common in vegetarians (Gear et al., 1979), and vegetarians eat twice as much dietary fibre as the general population; they also pass substantially bulkier and softer stools (Davies et al., 1985, 1986). In Japan, fibre intake has fallen steadily since World War II, and autopsy surveys suggest that the prevalence of diverticular disease has risen (Ohi et al., 1983). Moreover, case–control studies in Japan show people with diverticular disease to have been in the habit of eating less fibre than matched healthy controls (Ohta et al., 1985; Nagahashi et al., 1985). The same is true of Greece, where Manousos et al. (1985) reported a significant reduction in the relative risk of diverticular disease associated with doubled consumption of four fibre-rich food items (brown bread, spinach, lettuce, cucumber).

These case–control studies seem convincing, but are hard to interpret because the cases of diverticulosis were all symptomatic hospital patients. Since only a minority of people with diverticulosis have symptoms, and fewer still are referred to hospital, the results may be biassed and cannot safely be extrapolated to the generality of cases. There is only one case–control study based on asymptomatic cases detected by population screening and the results were not clear-cut (Gear et al., 1979). Fibre intake was lower in cases only if they were over the age of 60, and the authors had to resort to the suggestion that the younger controls were contaminated by people in a pre-diverticular state.

Experimental studies give qualified support to the fibre hypothesis. When groups of rats were given diets containing different amounts of wheat fibre for the whole of their lives, prevalence of colonic diverticulosis was inversely proportional to fibre intake (Fisher et al., 1985). However, even a high-fibre diet (17%) allowed 9.4% of rats to develop diverticulosis, suggesting that other factors are implicated. A similar conclusion was reached by Eastwood et al. (1978) on the basis that 24-hour stool weight was no lower in patients with diverticular disease than in the general population (but the patients were symptomatic and may not be representative).

If starch contributes significantly to faecal bulk one might expect an inverse relationship between starch intake and risk of diverticulosis. This has not so far been reported, but Thornton et al. (1986) found that patients with diverticular disease were unusually efficient at digesting and absorbing the starch in a potato test meal, which should mean that they allow less starch into the colon. More studies along these lines are needed.

Bran, a high-fibre diet, or bulking agents are still considered to be first-line treatment for symptomatic diverticular disease by most gastroenterologists. This is not entirely logical. Placebo-controlled trials are not unanimous, but this may reflect the selection of cases. Bran was clearly superior to placebo in a trial of surgical patients (Brodribb, 1977), but was no better in a trial of medical patients (Ornstein et al., 1981). The latter trial was criticised for having too low a dose of fibre amongst other things, but the real problem may be that symptomatic diverticular disease is just irritable bowel syndrome in a person who happens to have diverticulosis (Thompson et al., 1982, Otte et al., 1986). As already stated, bran is superior to placebo in IBS only when there is a major element of constipation.

If diverticular disease is caused by lack of dietary fibre one might expect a fall in the incidence of the disease and its complications when a population increases its intake of fibre and symptomatic cases are routinely treated with bran. In Scotland these conditions had been fulfilled for about 10 years when Au et al. (1988) examined the time-trends for hospital admissions for diverticular disease in Scotland, but they found no decrease during those years, also no fall in the colectomy rate. It is possible, however, that more than 10 years are needed for such a change to become apparent or that complications are not averted by increased fibre intake.

Cancer of the Large Bowel

This is the second commonest cause of cancer deaths in Western countries and, internationally, its incidence is strongly related to many indices of Westernisation. The possible role of dietary fibre as a protective factor has been intensively investigated since Burkitt (1971b) put forward his hypothesis, but is still unclear. There is no shortage of mechanisms by which fibre (and undigested starch) might be protective (Table 14.1) but as yet no proof that any of them are operative. The epidemiological data are so inconsistent that some experts dismiss them (British Nutrition Foundation, 1990). For example, one huge Australian case–control study concluded there *was* no protective effect – even a trend towards a promoting effect – (Potter and McMichael, 1986) while shortly afterwards another, even larger, one concluded there *was* a protective effect (Kune et al., 1987).

Recently, Trock et al. (1990) reported an aggregate assessment of the strength of evidence from 37 observational epidemiological studies which were considered methodologically sound, namely, 23 case–control studies, one international correlation study, eight within-country correlation studies, two

Table 14.1. Effects of fibre on the large bowel which
have the potential to reduce cancer risk (after
Cummings, 1985)

Dilution of carcinogens (via water-holding capacity)

Provision of a surface for adsorption of carcinogens

Faster transit time, so less contact time

Consequences of fermentation
  lower pH
  production of butyrate (strongly anti-neoplastic)
  reduced microbial metabolism
  lower NH_3 levels

Altered bile acid metabolism

---

cohort studies and three time-trend studies. Thirteen studies were deemed to
give strong support to the fibre hypothesis (nine case–control studies, two
within-country, one cohort and the one international study) in that inverse
associations between fibre intake or surrogates thereof and colon cancer
incidence/mortality were statistically significant and remained so after adjustment for fats, meat or energy. Eight studies were deemed to give moderate
support to the fibre hypothesis (six case–control studies, one within-country and
one time-trend study) because they showed a significant inverse association
between fibre intake and colon cancer risk but they did not control for
confounding by meats or fats. Fourteen studies were deemed equivocal, neither
supporting nor refuting the fibre hypothesis (six case-control studies, five
within-country studies, one cohort and two time-trend studies). Eight of these 14
studies were at least consistent with the fibre hypothesis. Only two studies were
clearly opposed to the fibre hypothesis, that is, they were methodologically
sound and of adequate power but found no protective effect of fibre. Thus of the
37 studies, 29 (78%) provided some evidence consistent with a protective effect
of a high-fibre intake, whereas only eight studies (22%) provided evidence
consistent with no effect or an enhancing effect.

The same authors (Trock et al., 1990), went on to perform meta-analysis on
the 16 case–control studies which reported enough data to allow logarithms of
the odds ratio to be calculated and combined. When certain assumptions were
made, the odds ratio for cancer in people eating the most fibre versus those
eating the least was 0.57 (95% confidence limits 0.50 to 0.64). Some experts
believe that the evidence for a protective effect from vegetables is stronger than
that from fibre. In this meta-analysis, the odds ratio for cancer in people eating
the most vegetables was indeed lower (0.48, 95% confidence limits 0.41 to 0.57).

Epidemiological studies of diet and disease have many limitations but all tend
to produce false negative rather than false positive results. This means that the
true strength of an association is likely to be stronger not weaker than what has
been observed.

If dietary fibre is protective it may be through its stool-bulking effect or
associated with it. This being so there should be an inverse relationship between
the mean stool weight of a community and its incidence of large bowel cancer.
Cummings and Bingham (unpublished data) have collated all published data on
mean stool output of 23 different communities and have shown that there is
indeed a significant inverse relationship between stool weight and colonic cancer
mortality in these populations ($r = 0.78$).

Apart from dietary fibre, the only important component of the diet which probably contributes to faecal weight is starch. Few studies have looked at starch intake in relation to bowel cancer risk. A very large case–control study did so and found that a high starch intake reduced the relative risk to 0.82 (Tuyns et al., 1988). Undigested starch resembles non-starch polysaccharides (fibre) in being fermented by colonic bacteria to short chain fatty acids, including butyrate which has marked anti-neoplastic properties in vitro. Fermentation of starch produces relatively more butyrate than fermentation of non-starch polysaccharide so it is interesting that the faeces of patients with colorectal cancer produce less butyrate than the faeces of controls (Bingham, 1990).

Most colorectal cancers probably arise from adenomatous polyps. There have been few studies of polysaccharide intake in relation to adenoma formation. In Marseilles and in Oslo case–control studies have reported an inverse relation to polysaccharide intake (Macquart-Moulin et al., 1986; Hoff et al., 1986). Moreover, in a prospective controlled trial a large daily dose of wheat bran has been shown to delay the recurrence of polyps after polypectomy (DeCosse et al., 1989). However, this study was done in a very atypical group of patients – people with familial adenomatous polyposis who had undergone colectomy and ileorectal anastomosis – and the findings need to be confirmed in cases of ordinary non-familial adenoma.

In conclusion, the evidence for a protective effect from a fibre-rich diet is substantial but not conclusive.

Conclusions

Consensus

There is still a surprising lack of consensus even on constipation. The laxative properties of dietary fibre are established beyond dispute but other factors are just as important in determining stool output and intestinal transit. In irritable bowel syndrome there is consensus only that treatment with bran helps the symptoms of constipation (which are sometimes prominent). The most acceptable theory for the development of diverticular disease is still Painter's hypothesis that the colon "ruptures itself struggling to handle small, hard faeces" due, in part, to low fibre intake. With regard to large bowel cancer, the weight of evidence favours low faecal output and low fibre intake as causative factors but not the only ones by any means.

Unsolved Matters

These are many, as indicated in the sections on individual diseases. Perhaps the most fundamental are how dietary fibre works to increase faecal bulk and speed up transit and how fibre and emotional factors interact in determining gut function. A major problem is that a realistic blinded placebo is virtually impossible.

Future Research Directions

Gut function is highly susceptible to psychological influences so future treatment trials must be carefully controlled and cautiously interpreted. There is no single type of research which can answer all the unsolved problems but attention should be concentrated on the most powerful type, namely prospective, long-term controlled trials. The mucosal protective role of fermentation products like butyric acid is a promising area of research which needs to be developed. The place of undigested starch deserves much more investigation. The possibility must be considered that the protective effect against large bowel cancer of fruit and vegetables is due as much to their content of anti-oxidant vitamins and minerals as to their content of fibre.

References

Attili AF, The GREPCO Group (1984) Dietary habits and cholelithiasis. In: Capocaccia L, Ricci G, Angelico F, Angelico M, Attili AF (eds) Epidemiology and prevention of gallstone disease. MTP Press, Lancaster, pp 175–181

Attili AF, The Rome Group for the Epidemiology and Prevention of Cholelithiasis (GREPCO) (1987) Diet and gallstones: results of an epidemiologic study performed in male civil servants. In: Barbara L, Bianchi Porro G, Cheli R, Lipkin M (eds) Nutrition in gastrointestinal disease. Raven Press, New York, pp 225–231

Au J, Smith AN, Eastwood MA (1988) Diverticular disease in Scotland over 15 years. Proc R Coll Physicians Edinburgh 18:271–276

Barker DJP (1985) Acute appendicitis and dietary fibre; an alternative hypothesis. Br Med J 290:1125–1127

Barker DJP, Morris J, Nelson M (1986) Vegetable consumption and acute appendicitis in 59 areas in England and Wales. Br Med J 292:927–930

Bingham SA (1990) Diet and large bowel cancer. J R Soc Med 83:420–422

Bloch HM, Thornton JR, Heaton KW (1980) Effects of fasting on the composition of gallbladder bile. Gut 21:1087–1089

British Nutrition Foundation (1990). Complex carbohydrates in foods. Chapman and Hall, London

Brodribb AJM (1977) Treatment of symptomatic diverticular disease with a high-fibre diet. Lancet i:664–666

Burkitt DP (1969) Related disease – related cause? Lancet ii:1229–1231

Burkitt DP (1971a) The aetiology of appendicitis. Br J Surg 58:695–699

Burkitt DP (1971b) Epidemiology of cancer of the colon and rectum. Cancer 28:3–13

Burkitt DP (1975) Appendicitis. In: Burkitt DP, Trowell HC (eds) Refined carbohydrate foods and disease. Some implications of dietary fibre. Academic Press, London, pp 87–97

Burkitt DP (1985) Varicose veins, haemorrhoids, deep-vein thrombosis and pelvic phleboliths. In: Trowell H, Burkitt D, Heaton K (eds) Dietary fibre, fibre-depleted foods and disease. Academic Press, London, pp 317–329

Burkitt DP, James PA (1973) Low-residue diets and hiatus hernia. Lancet ii:128–130

Burkitt DP, Tunstall M (1975) Gallstones: geographical and chronological features. J Trop Med Hyg 78:140–144

Burkitt DP, Clements JL, Eaton SB (1985) Prevalence of diverticular disease, hiatus hernia, and pelvic phleboliths in black and white Americans. Lancet ii:880–881

Cann PA, Read NW, Holdsworth CD (1984) What is the benefit of coarse wheat bran in patients with the irritable bowel syndrome? Gut 25:168–173

Capron J-P, Payenneville H, Dumont M, Dupas J-L, Lorriaux A (1978) Evidence for an association between cholelithiasis and hiatus hernia. Lancet ii:329–331

Capron J-P, Delamarre J, Herve MA, Dupas J-L, Poulain P, Descombes P (1981) Meal frequency and duration of overnight fast: a role in gallstone formation? Br Med J 283:1435

Cleave TL, Campbell GD, Painter NS (1969) Diabetes, coronary thrombosis and the saccharine disease, 2nd edn. Wright, Bristol

Cummings J (1985) Cancer of the large bowel. In: Trowell H, Burkitt D, Heaton, K (eds) Dietary fibre, fibre-depleted foods and disease. Academic Press, London, pp 161–189

Cummings JH (1986) The effect of dietary fibre on fecal weight and composition. In: Spiller GA (ed) CRC handbook of dietary fibre in human nutrition. CRC Press, Boca Raton, pp 211–280

Davies GJ, Crowder M, Dickerson JWT (1985) Dietary fibre intakes of individuals with different eating patterns. Hum Nutr Appl Nutr 39A:139–148

Davies GJ, Crowder M, Reid B, Dickerson JWT (1986) Bowel function measurements of individuals with different eating patterns. Gut 27:164–169

DeCosse JJ, Miller HH, Lesser ML (1989) Effect of wheat fibre and vitamins C and E on rectal polyps in patients with familial adenomatous polyposis. J Natl Cancer Inst 81:1290–1297

Eastwood MA, Smith AN, Brydon WG, Pritchard J (1978) Colonic function in patients with diverticular disease. Lancet i:1181–1182

Eastwood MA, Brydon WG, Baird JD, Elton RA, Helliwell S, Smith JH, Pritchard JL (1984) Fecal weight and composition, serum lipids, and diet among subjects aged 18-80 years not seeking health care. Am J Clin Nutr 40:628–634

Fedail SS, Harvey RF, Burns-Cox CJ (1979) Abdominal and thoracic pressures during defaecation. Br Med J i:91

Fisher N, Berry CS, Fearn T, Gregory JA, Hardy J (1985) Cereal dietary fibre consumption and diverticular disease: a lifespan study in rats. Am J Clin Nutr 42:788–804

Gear JSS, Ware A, Fursdon P et al. (1979) Symptomless diverticular disease and intake of dietary fibre. Lancet i:511–514

Heaton KW (1973) The epidemiology of gallstones and suggested aetiology. Clin Gastroenterol 2:67–83

Heaton KW (1975) Gallstones and cholecystitis. In: Burkitt DP, Trowell HC (eds) Refined carbohydrate foods and disease. Some implications of dietary fibre. Academic Press, London, pp 173–194

Heaton KW (1987) Effect of dietary fibre on biliary lipids. In: Barbara L, Bianchi Porro G, Cheli R, Lipkin M (eds) Nutrition in gastrointestinal disease. Raven Press, New York, pp 213–222

Heaton KW (1988a) Gallstone prevention: clues from epidemiology. In: Northfield T, Jazrawi R, Zentler-Munro P (eds) Bile acids in health and disease. MTP Press, Lancaster, pp 157–169

Heaton KW (1988b) Dietary sugar and Crohn's disease. Can J Gastroenterol 2:41–44

Heaton KW, Ghosh S, Braddon FEM (1991) How bad are the symptoms and bowel dysfunction of patients with irritable bowel syndrome? A prospective, controlled study with special reference to stool form. Gut 32:73–79

Hillman LC, Stace NH, Fisher A, Pomare EW (1982) Dietary intakes and stool characteristics of patients with the irritable bowel syndrome. Am J Clin Nutr 36:626–629

Hoff G, Moen IE, Trygg K et al. (1986) Epidemiology of polyps in the rectum and sigmoid colon. Evaluation of nutritional factors. Scand J Gastroenterol 21:199–204

Hollander D (1988) Crohn's disease – a permeability disorder of the tight junction? Gut 29:1621–1624

Jenkins DJA, Peterson RD, Thorne MJ, Ferguson PW (1987) Wheat fibre and laxation: dose response and equilibration time. Am J Gastroenterol 82:1259–1263

Jones VA, McLaughlan P, Shorthouse M, Workman E, Hunter JO (1982) Food intolerance: a major factor in the pathogenesis of irritable bowel syndrome. Lancet ii:1115–1117

Katschinski BD, Logan RFA, Edmond M, Langman MJS (1990) Duodenal ulcer and refined carbohydrate intake: a case–control study assessing dietary fibre and refined sugar intake. Gut 31:993–996

Kune S, Kune GA, Watson LF (1987) Case–control study of dietary etiologic factors: the Melbourne Colorectal Cancer Study. Nutr Cancer 9:21–42

Larner AJ (1988) The aetiology of appendicitis. Br J Hosp Med, June:540–542

Levenstein S, Prantera C, Luzi C, D'Ubaldi A (1985) Low residue or normal diet in Crohn's disease: a prospective controlled study in Italian patients. Gut 26:989–993

MacLure KM, Hayes KC, Colditz GA, Stampfer MJ, Speizer FE, Willett WC (1989) Weight, diet and the risk of symptomatic gallstones in middle-aged women. N Engl J Med 321:563–569

Macquart-Moulin G, Riboli E, Cornee J, Charnay B, Berthezene P, Day N (1986) Case–control study on colorectal cancer and diet in Marseilles. Int J Cancer 38:183–191

Malhotra SL (1978) A comparison of unrefined wheat and rice diets in the management of duodenal ulcer. Postgrad Med J 54:6–9

Manousos P, Day NE, Tzonou A et al. (1985) Diet and other factors in the aetiology of diverticulosis: an epidemiological study in Greece. Gut 26:544–549

Marcus SN, Heaton KW (1986) Intestinal transit, deoxycholic acid and the cholesterol saturation of bile – three interrelated factors. Gut 27:550–558

Marcus SN, Heaton KW (1987) Irritable bowel type symptoms in spontaneous and induced constipation. Gut 28:156–159

Marcus SN, Heaton KW (1988) Deoxycholic acid and the pathogenesis of gallstones. Gut 29:522–533

Maxton DG, Bjarnason I, Reynolds AP, Catt SD, Peters TJ, Menzies IS (1986) Lactulose 51Cr-labelled ethylenediaminetetra-acetate, L-rhamnose and polyethylene glycol 500 as probe markers for assessment in vivo of human intestinal permeability. Clin Sci 71:71–80

Morris J, Barker DJP, Nelson M (1987) Diet, infection, and acute appendicitis in Britain and Ireland. J Epidemiol Comm Health 41:44–49

Mullard KS (1972) The surgical treatment of diaphragmatic oesophageal hiatus hernia. Ann R Coll Surg Engl 50:73–91

Muller CJB (1948) Hiatus hernia, diverticula and gallstones. Saint's triad. S Afr Med J 22:376–382

Müller-Lissner SA (1988) Effect of wheat bran on weight of stool and gastrointestinal transit time: a meta-analysis. Br Med J 296:615–617

Nagahashi M, Yamazaki N, Ohi G et al. (1985) Dietary fibre intake and diverticular disease of the colon. A case–control study. Nippon Eiseigaku Zasshi 40:781–788

Nanda R, James R, Smith H, Dudley CRK, Jewell DP (1989) Food intolerance and the irritable bowel syndrome. Gut 30:1099–1104

O'Donnell LJD, Virjee J, Heaton KW (1990) Detection of pseudodiarrhoea by simple clinical assessment of intestinal transit rate. Br Med J 300:439–440

Ohi G, Minowa K, Oyama T et al. (1983) Changes in dietary fibre intake among Japanese in the 20th century: a relationship to the prevalence of diverticular disease. Am J Clin Nutr 38:115–121

Ohta M, Ishiguro S, Iwane S et al. (1985) An epidemiological study on relationship between intake of dietary fibre and colonic diseases. Jpn J Gastroenterol 82:51–57

Ornstein MH, Littlewood ER, Baird IM, Fowler J, North WRS, Cox AG (1981) Are fibre supplements really necessary in diverticular disease of the colon? A controlled clinical trial. Br Med J 282:1353–1356

Otte JJ, Larsen L, Andersen JR (1986) Irritable bowel syndrome and symptomatic diverticular disease: different diseases? Am J Gastroenterol 81:529–531

Painter NS, Burkitt DP (1971) Diverticular disease of the colon: a deficiency disease of Western civilisation. Br Med J ii:450–454

Painter NS, Truelove SC, Ardran GM, Tuckey M (1965) Segmentation and the localisation of intraluminal pressures in the human colon, with special reference to the pathogenesis of colonic diverticula. Gastroenterology 49:169–177

Painter NS, Almeida AZ, Colebourne KW (1972) Unprocessed bran in treatment of diverticular disease of the colon. Br Med J ii:137–140

Petrakis NL, King EB (1981) Cytological abnormalities in nipple aspirates of breast fluid from women with severe constipation. Lancet ii:1203–1205

Pixley F, Mann J (1988) Dietary factors in the aetiology of gall stones: a case–control study. Gut 29:1511–1515

Pixley F, Wilson D, McPherson K, Mann J (1985) Effect of vegetarianism on development of gall stones in women. Br Med J 291:11–12

Potter JD, McMichael AJ (1986) Diet and cancer of the colon and rectum: a case–control study. J Natl Cancer Inst 76:557–569

Rauws EAJ, Tytgat GNJ (1990) Cure of duodenal ulcer associated with eradication of *Helicobacter pylori*. Lancet i:1233–1235

Rydning A, Berstad A (1985) Fibre diet and antacids in the short-term treatment of duodenal ulcer. Scand J Gastroenterol 20:1078–1082

Rydning A, Berstad A, Aadland E, Odegaard B (1982) Prophylactic effect of dietary fibre in duodenal ulcer disease. Lancet ii:736–739

Scragg RKR, McMichael AJ, Baghurst PA (1984) Diet, alcohol, and relative weight in gallstone disease: a case–control study. Br Med J 288:1113–1119

Short AR (1920) The causation of appendicitis. Br J Surg 8:171–188

Spiller GA, Story JA, Wong LG et al. (1986) Effect of increasing levels of hard wheat fibre on fecal weight, minerals and steroids and gastrointestinal transit time in healthy young women. J Nutr 116:778–785

Stephen AM, Wiggin HS, Englyst HN, Cole TJ, Wayman BJ, Cummings JH (1986) The effect of age, sex and level of intake of dietary fibre from wheat on large-bowel function in 30 healthy subjects. Br J Nutr 56:349–361

Thompson WG, Patel DG, Tao H, Nair R (1982) Does uncomplicated diverticular disease cause symptoms? Dig Dis Sci 27:605–608

Thompson WG, Dotevall G, Drossman DA, Heaton KW, Kruis W (1989) Irritable bowel syndrome: guidelines for the diagnosis. Gastroenterol Int 2:92–95

Thornton JR, Emmett PM, Heaton KW (1983) Diet and gallstones: effects of refined and unrefined carbohydrate diets on bile cholesterol saturation and bile acid metabolism. Gut 24:2–6

Thornton JR, Dryden A, Kelleher J, Losowsky MS (1986) Does super efficient starch absorption promote diverticular disease? Br Med J 292:1708–1710

Tomlin J, Read NW (1988) Comparison of the effects on colonic function caused by feeding rice bran and wheat bran. Eur J Clin Nutr 42:857–861

Tovey F (1985) Duodenal ulcer. In: Trowell H, Burkitt D, Heaton K (eds) Dietary fibre, fibre-depleted foods and disease. Academic Press, London, pp 229–240

Trock B, Lanza E, Greenwald P (1990) Dietary fibre, vegetables, and colon cancer: critical review and meta-analysis of the epidemiologic evidence. J Natl Cancer Inst 82:650–661

Trowell HC, Burkitt DP (1981) (eds) Western diseases, their emergence and prevention. Edward Arnold, London

Trowell H, Burkitt D, Heaton K (1985) Dietary fibre, fibre-depleted foods and disease. Academic Press, London, p 421

Turnbull GK, Lennard-Jones JE, Bartram CI (1986) Failure of rectal expulsion as a cause of constipation: why fibre and laxatives sometimes fail. Lancet i:767–769

Tuyns AJ, Kaaks R, Haelterman M (1988) Colorectal cancer and the consumption of foods: a case–control study in Belgium. Nutr Cancer 11:189–204

Wyman JB, Heaton KW, Manning AP, Wicks ACB (1976) The effect on intestinal transit and the feces of raw and cooked bran in different doses. Am J Clin Nutr 29:1474–1479

Commentary

Johnson: No doubt there are more promising areas for research on dietary fibre than duodenal ulcer, but a plausible mechanism can be envisaged. Foods such as oats which are rich in soluble non-starch polysaccharides stimulate cell proliferation throughout the small intestine of the rat and pectin improves healing after colonic anastomosis (Rolandelli et al., 1986). If a similar effect occurs in man it may help to maintain the integrity of the mucosa and perhaps assist in the healing of established duodenal ulcer.

At any rate there is evidence for the opposite effect, in that non-steroidal anti-inflammatory drugs reduce mucosal cell proliferation, and have an adverse effect on the healing of ulcers (Levi et al., 1990). The high-fibre diets which have been used in studies with ulcer patients have not included large quantities of soluble fibre.

References:

Levi S, Goodlad RA, Lee CY et al. (1990) Inhibitory effect of non-steroidal anti-inflammatory drugs on mucosal cell proliferation associated with gastric ulcer healing. Lancet ii:840–843

Rolandelli RH, Koruda MJ, Settle RG, Rombeau JL (1986) The effect of enteral feedings supplemented with pectin on the healing of colonic anastomosis in the rat. Surgery 99:703–707

Chapter 15

Dietary Fibre in the Prevention and Treatment of Obesity

S. Rössner

Introduction

Numerous reviews have discussed the fact that the prevalence of obesity is increasing in the Western world and that obesity is rare in populations with a high intake of dietary fibre. Several arguments link obesity with the ingestion of an excessive proportion of fibre-depleted carbohydrates. However, for practical, clinical purposes probably the most important question relates to whether addition of dietary fibre or a change of food composition towards a more fibre-rich diet can be useful as a treatment modality for obesity. The present review will scrutinise the evidence for such an effect. However, since it is methodologically complicated to set up trials to determine the possible role for dietary fibre in obesity therapy, this presentation will start with a discussion of the fibre trial design problems which are generally encountered in the treatment of obesity.

Fibre Trial Design Problems in Obesity

Dietary fibre can be considered as a natural food component in the diet, and a clinical trial can then be designed to compare a low-fibre versus a high-fibre diet. This is methodologically difficult – there is no such thing as a placebo carrot. This means that it is unavoidable that dietary fibre trials in which high- and low-fibre supplemented diets are compared are open to criticism. The additional problem is a classical dilemma in the design of any dietary trial: one food component can hardly be changed in the diet without effects on other components. Furthermore it can be questioned whether from the clinical point of view true double-blind effects can be achieved at all. Effects such as bowel movement frequency, borborygmia, stool consistency and flatus cannot be masked with any placebo.

Instead of only using diets high and low in fibre, a certain degree of blindness in the study design can be obtained if dietary fibre can be added into special food components, such as specially baked bread (Mikkelsen et al., 1979). In a recent study from our group, a potato fibre preparation and a low-fibre wheat control were incorporated into instant soups that were given before the three main meals and made it possible to add as much as 21 g of dietary fibre per day and still retain a reasonable degree of blindness of the trial (Rössner, 1989).

Another alternative is to administer the fibre supplementation in a pharmacological form, such as granulate, tablets or a drink. The advantages of such an approach have recently been described in a Swedish thesis by Ryttig (1990). It is possible to design fibre tablets containing about 0.3 g fibre and to use identical placebo tablets containing only minimal amounts of fibre. Since the placebo tablet by necessity has to contain some substance apart from fibre, it has generally been filled by material such as lactose. This may result in at least two potential design pitfalls: (1) lactose may have some unwanted side effects on patients unaware of a mild alactasic condition; (2) the carbohydrate contents of such tablets will result in a slightly higher energy value of the placebo tablet compared with the fibre. All conditions alike, a difference in daily intake of, for example, 50 kcal/day due to the difference in energy between placebo and dietary fibre tablets could theoretically increase the likelihood of detection of an effect of the dietary fibre on weight loss. In practice it would be impossible to prove that such small differences in energy can account for changes in weight.

An obvious practical problem with tablets is that they each can accommodate only small amounts of fibre. Thus, in some of the Ryttig studies, as many as 20 tablets a day had to be given to increase the dietary fibre intake by 50%, which clearly can make patients reluctant to continue such a programme on a long-term basis and can be expected to reduce patient compliance (Ryttig, 1990).

Another methodological problem concerns the optimal energy allowance during the trial period. Under the assumption that the main effect of the dietary fibre addition is a reduction in energy intake, one could envisage designs, where subjects were given an *ad libitum* diet with fibre/placebo addition. However, in the placebo group this will probably result in an unchanged body weight, which the participant can easily discover. This will in turn lead to an increased likelihood of changes in the diet, to non-compliance or to drop-out. The other extreme assumption would be that fibre affects basal metabolism. If this be the case, fibre or placebo could be given as the only supplement during a period of starvation, and the weight loss of both groups compared.

Most designs that meet standard quality requirements have chosen an intermediate approach and added dietary fibre to a hypocaloric diet. Such a design would lead to weight loss in each subject who follows the trial instructions, but with a higher loss in subjects receiving such fibres which facilitate weight loss.

Generally, acceptable long-term studies on the effect of dietary fibre on weight loss and weight loss maintenance have been designed as double-blind, randomised studies, where placebo and verum have been compared during a hypocaloric study period and after a run-in period. An interesting alternative approach was used by Andersson et al. (1990), who first treated obese women with a hypocaloric diet until they had reached a lower and steady weight level. At this point, placebo/verum was introduced. The trial then continued until a relapse of more than 2 kg compared with previous levels had occurred, and this time interval was used as an endpoint. In the Andersson study, however, the addition of 28 g/day of a sugar beet fibre preparation, mainly consisting of pectic substances, did not affect the rate of body weight relapse.

In the discussion above it has been argued that dietary fibre tablets offer several methodological advantages since they make it possible to design adequate randomised double-blind placebo-controlled clinical trials. However, if one assumes that dietary fibre works through its physical effect on the texture of food on chewing, gastric emptying and intestinal degradation (Heaton, 1973), incorporation of fibre into food products, as suggested by the Mikkelsen et al. (1979) design, for example, would be more appropriate. Such studies seem to be rare in the literature.

Indicators of Success of Obesity Treatment

Although the ultimate goal of treatment for overweight and obesity is to normalise body weight and keep it at the desired level, this does not happen very often in reality. Therefore, it has become increasingly important to individualise treatment to increase the likelihood of a therapeutic success. A mean weight reduction, described as e.g. 5 ± 4 (SD) kg in a group of participants may not seem impressive, but indicates that for some individuals the treatment clearly was of great value for them (Garrow, 1989). The participants that did not lose weight in such a programme obviously should not have remained there but should have been shifted into other programmes, until they began to lose weight as well. Thus mean weight loss values, obtained from formalised trials, may underestimate the true value of a treatment that is helpful to a subpopulation of the participants (Guy-Grand, 1987; Garrow, 1989).

The indicators of success of a certain treatment programme could be envisaged in the following way (Fig. 15.1).

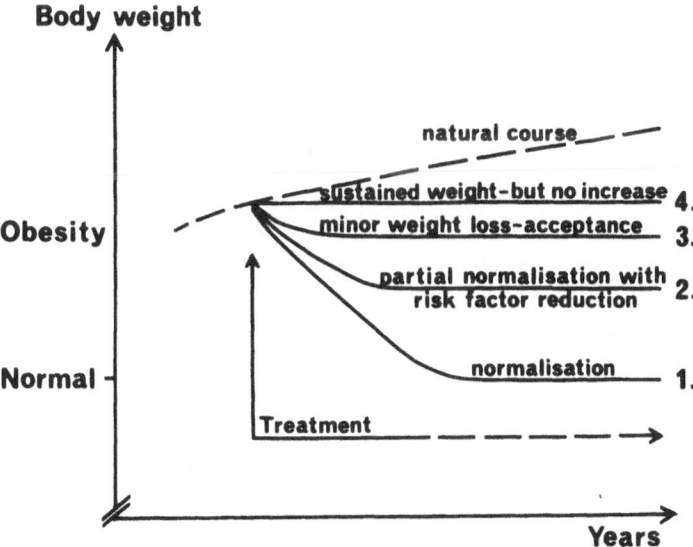

Fig. 15.1. Theoretical outcome of long-term weight-reduction programmes.

1. Sustained weight normalisation will occur (but only occasionally) as the result of treatment for obesity.

2. Maintained weight loss, partly towards a predetermined goal weight, will generally be considered as an acceptable result. Such a weight loss will affect obesity-related risk factors favourably, although body weight is not completely normalised. A weight loss in the range of 5-10 kg will significantly reduce elevated blood pressure in about ⅔ of overweight men (Reisen, 1983). Likewise blood sugar will fall towards normal values, serum triglycerides will drop and HDL-cholesterol will increase (Liu et al, 1985, Rössner and Björvell, 1985). The role of dietary fibre in the treatment of these metabolic abnormalities will be dealt with in other chapters of this publication.

3. Minor weight loss, but increased ability to cope with the obese condition may still be regarded as a very valuable result. In some cases such a seemingly modest weight change may conceal the fact that adipose tissue has been lost and muscular mass gained as a result of increased physical activity, which also will affect carbohydrate and lipid metabolism favourably (Krotkiewski and Björntorp, 1986).

4. Sustained body weight at an obesity level may, unimpressive as it seems, still represent an achievement. Few data are available on the longitudinal development of body weight over a long time, but cross-sectional data as well as longitudinal observations do emphasise that body weight increases considerably with age, in particular in women (Kuskowska-Wolk and Rössner, 1990). A weight-reduction programme that results in only an unchanged body weight for forthcoming decades thus actually represents a certain degree of success.

- Increased saliva production
- Increased chewing
- Reduced energy intake
- Increased gastric filling
- Delayed gastric emptying
- Flattening glucose absorption
- Diminished insulin secretion
- Increased satiation and satiety
- Reduced digestibility
- Reduced energy expenditure
- Increased faecal energy excretion

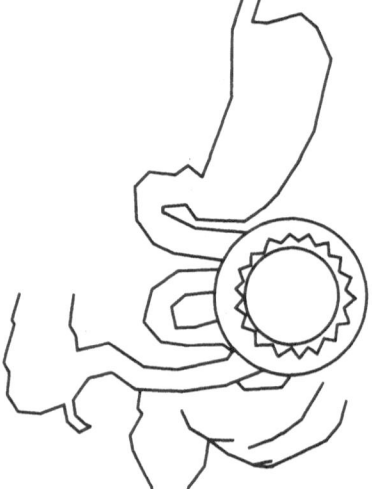

Fig. 15.2. Mode of action of dietary fibre in weight control (Reproduced from Ryttig, 1990.)

5. Finally, programmes that report lowered drop-out rates may also represent one different form of success. Since after 2-3 years there are few studies that have succeeded in keeping more than 20%–30% of the original patients in the programme (Brownell and Kramer, 1989), any programme that can document low drop-out rates will constitute one form of success. Even if weight loss may not have occurred, the fact that obese individuals have stayed with the programme means that such a programme is an important tool to develop further and to add qualities to it. The effect of dietary fibre supplementation, known to be of some help to reduce body weight and maintain that weight loss has been suggested as functioning in this way. The participants in some fibre programmes, such as those of Krotkiewski (1984) and Rössner et al. (1987) preferred to remain on fibre treatment instead of switching over to other potential alternatives, not because of further significant weight loss but because fibre supplementation facilitated adherence to the basic weight-reducing programme.

Dietary Fibre in Obesity

The possible modes of action of dietary fibre in overweight are summarised in Fig. 15.2. Dietary fibre may have several effects throughout the gastro-intestinal tract varying from more simple mechanic interference to complex hormonal interactions. However, the proportional effect of each mode of action in affecting body weight change in the individual is unknown (Ryttig, 1990).

Dietary Fibre and Energy Intake

Table 15.1 (based on data from Ryttig's thesis, 1990) summarises the effects of a fibre pre-load on subsequent food intake. However, the designs of these studies may vary greatly in several respects:

Table 15.1. Effects of dietary fibre intervention on subsequent food intake (modified from Ryttig, 1990)

Reference	Treatment	No. of subjects	Energy intake
Yudkin (1959)	10 g/day	20	Reduced
Duncan et al. (1960)	4.5 g	85	Unchanged
Geliebter (1976)		12	Unchanged
Heaton (1980)	Brown/white bread	13	Reduced
McCance et al. (1953)	Brown/white bread	6	Reduced
Evans and Miller (1975)	10 g/day (soluble and insoluble)	11	Reduced
Porikos and Hagamen (1986)	High/low fibre bread	31	Unchanged
		19	Reduced
Mikkelsen et al. (1979)	Brown/white bread	16	Reduced
Burley et al. (1987b)	High/low fibre	20	Unchanged
Grimes and Gordon (1978)	Brown/white bread	12	Reduced
Bryson et al. (1980)	Brown/white bread	10	Unchanged
Duncan et al. (1983)	7 g/1000 kcal vs	10	Reduced
	1 g/1000 kcal	10	Reduced

Both soluble and insoluble preparations or fibre-enriched food products were used

The studies were both acute and chronic after administration for up to a few weeks

They were carried out in normal weight as well as in obese subjects, who were also of different ages

The overall impression is that several researchers, although certainly not all, have demonstrated that energy intake was reduced after a fibre pre-treatment. A decrease in energy intake has been predominantly observed in overweight subjects, whereas there is more controversy concerning the influence of fibre on energy intake in lean individuals.

Effects of Dietary Fibre on Hunger, Appetite, Satiation and Satiety

Fibre in food products or as supplements may affect the subjective feelings of hunger and satiety during the course of the meal and thus affect energy intake. As indicated by Blundell, many scales measuring these subjective feelings have been constructed without proper validation and the results are open to criticism (Blundell and Burley, 1987). Table 15.2 summarises a number of studies relating fibre intake to hunger, satiety and other subjective feelings related to food intake. An overall impression from this summary is that most investigators demonstrate reduced hunger and related variables with fibre supplementation.

Table 15.2. Effects of dietary fibre on eating behaviour (modified from Ryttig, 1990)

Reference	Treatment	No. of subjects	Eating behaviour
Duncan et al. (1983)	High/low fibre	20	High fibre more satiating
Haber et al. (1977)	Apple preparations	10	Satiation increased with whole fruit
Bolton et al. (1981)	Citrus preparations	10	Satiation increased with whole fruit
Shearer (1976)	Citrus preparations	73 + 60	High-fibre supplement reduced hunger score
Durrant and Royston (1979)	1 g/day	13	No effect
Krotkiewski (1984)	20 g guar gum	21	Soluble, not insoluble fibre, reduced hunger
Hylander and Rössner (1983)	12 g soluble vs. 9 g insoluble fibre	135	Hunger reduced by both fibre types
Burley et al. (1987b)	12 vs. 3 g/day	20	Better fullness with 12 g
Burley et al. (1987a)	30 vs. 3 g/day	16	Suppressed hunger and desire to eat with 30 g

Effects of Dietary Fibre on Weight Loss

Few controlled clinical studies have been carried out showing that supplementation of dietary fibre improves weight loss. In the Krotkiewski study (1984) 9 patients were asked to maintain their dietary habits, while receiving 10 g guar gum twice daily for 8 weeks. The study demonstrated a weight loss of 4.3 kg, from 95.6 to 91.3 kg, but is obviously difficult to evaluate, since no control group was included. In further studies by Krotkiewski and Smith 54 obese patients were given a reduced diet of 1000 kcal/day supplemented with 24 g of fibre as oat bran biscuit for 8 weeks (1985). 42 obese patients receiving the same diet but without fibre served as controls. Weight loss in the fibre group was reported as high as 5.1 ± 1.7 kg/week, compared with 3.8 ± 1.8 kg in the control group. This study was however not blind, as the authors themselves also point out.

Another way to demonstrate effects of dietary fibre on weight loss and diet adherence was further suggested by Krotkiewski and Smith (1985). Withdrawal rates in the fibre-treated group were 24% compared with 36% in controls after 20 weeks, which was reported to be a statistically significant difference.

A few studies with adequate designs have been published that demonstrate that dietary fibre improves weight loss. Tuomilehto et al. (1980) demonstrated that in a 16-week study period 15 g of guar gum daily resulted in a significant weight loss compared with placebo. However, the 32 women under study were normal weight hypercholesterolaemic patients and were instructed to maintain their dietary habits throughout the study. Walsh et al. (1984) treated 20 obese women with 3 g of purified glucomannan or placebo for 8 weeks. The women maintained their diet and exercise habits. Patients on fibre lost a mean of 2.5 kg, whereas in the placebo group surprisingly a weight increase of 0.7 kg was seen during the corresponding time.

The most systematic approach to evaluating the role of dietary fibre supplementation on weight loss and weight maintenance seems to be the data summarised in the Ryttig thesis, originating from our Obesity Unit (1990). In these studies, tablets consisting of combinations of 10%–20% soluble (citrus) and 90%–80% unsoluble (grain) fibres have been used. The studies were double-blind, randomised and placebo-controlled. The results from those studies showing an effect are summarised in Table 15.3. In addition to these, one study in the thesis did not show any such effect (Rössner et al. 1988). Sixty-two females (body mass index = 34.8 kg/m^2) were treated with 6.5 g of a fibre supplement, which however was different from that in the studies in Table 15.3 or a corresponding placebo. A 1600 kcal diet was given for 12 weeks and this design resulted in similar weight losses in both groups. As indicated in Table 15.3, the other seven Ryttig studies demonstrated that fibre supplementation significantly improved weight loss compared with placebo. These studies comprised 45 to 97 patients, who were mildly to moderately obese. The fibre supplementation was up to 7 g/day, the hypocaloric diets up to about 1800 kcal/day, and the treatment period ranging from 8 to 52 weeks. Overall, fibre improved the weight loss obtained by the diet by about 40%. In these studies hunger feelings in fibre groups decreased with time, in contrast to ratings in controls, and the number of withdrawals was significantly lower in fibre-treated patients than in controls.

Table 15.3. Studies in the Ryttig thesis (1990) showing statistically significant effects of dietary fibre on weight reduction

Reference	Energy intake (kJ/day)	Added fibre (g/day)	Number of patients	Duration (weeks)	Initial BMI (kg/m^2)	Mean weight reduction (kg)	
						Fibre	Placebo
Ryttig et al. (1985)	5000	7	89	11	29.0	6.3	4.2
Solum et al. (1987)	5000	6	60	12	26.8	8.5	6.4
Ryttig et al. (1989)	5000/6700/ad lib	7/6/6	97	11/26/52	27.4	3.8	2.8
Ryttig (1990)	5000	6/4	53	24	27.5	8.0	5.8
Rigaud et al. (1990)	7376/7544	7	52	24	29.3	5.3	2.9
Rössner et al. (1987)	5880/4550	5	60	8	36.3	7.0	6.0
Rössner et al. (1987)	6720	7	45	12	35.9	6.2	4.1

Thus, although there are numerous theoretical reasons why dietary fibre might facilitate weight loss in man, as summarised by Krotkiewski and Smith (1985), and such effects have been demonstrated in repeated acute or short-term studies, few studies with a strict and acceptable scientific approach have been able to demonstrate that in clinical reality, these theoretical effects will lead to a further weight reduction or maintenance. In this connection it should be pointed out that recently an expert panel on obesity treatment recommended that studies describing a clinically significant treatment modality should cover a treatment period exceeding one year to qualify for publication (Apfelbaum et al., 1987). Only one of the Ryttig studies barely meets that criterion (Ryttig et al., 1989).

Dietary Fibre in the Prevention of Obesity

In the search for obesity therapy it is always argued and agreed that prevention is important. However, there are not studies of any kind or with any type of intervention modality that have demonstrated whether a certain treatment or intervention will reduce the risk of obesity development. Much historical and anecdotal evidence concerning the beneficial effects of fibre has accumulated, many through the brilliant original observations from Africa; however, none of these studies can be used as strict scientific evidence that a diet rich in fibre will prevent the development of obesity or that a diet which has been supplemented with dietary fibre will protect against overeating. Although it is readily agreed that obesity is the end result of an imbalance between energy intake and expenditure, it still remains uncertain why some individuals develop overweight and obesity and others not. During recent years, more emphasis has been put on the genetic aspects of the condition.

Dietary Fibre, Obesity and Hypertension

This presentation mainly deals with the association between dietary fibre and obesity. It seems, however, important to include a reference here also to the relation between dietary fibre and blood pressure, since this is not covered in any other section of this book and some new data have emerged during the study of dietary fibre in obesity. Surprisingly, the role of dietary fibre in the treatment of hypertension has received little attention, possibly because of the fact that some of the earlier studies showed no effect or that such effects were indistinguishable from the effects of a particular life style in itself that was associated with a high dietary fibre intake (Bursztyn, 1987). The association between obesity and hypertension is well established, but the underlying mechanisms have not been fully clarified. Several factors have been suggested, such as effects via thyroid hormones, insulin, increased sodium with increased energy intake and changes in sympathetic neural activity (Blundell and Burley, 1987). Dietary fibre may influence blood pressure, as will many other dietary factors. Once again, a methodological problem has been to dissociate the effects of dietary changes from those of the fibre. The fact that vegetarians have lower blood pressure than controls can certainly be interpreted in other ways than a reflection of the difference in dietary fibre intake (Margetts, 1987). However, using double-blind randomised placebo-controlled designs, we and others have demonstrated that fibre supplementation significantly reduces diastolic blood pressure in obese normotensive women (Rössner et al., 1988), and that fibre supplementation reduces blood pressure in normal as well as overweight hypertensives (Schlamowitz et al., 1987; Eliasson et al., 1992). Dietary fibre enrichment has also been found to reduce blood pressure in non-insulin-dependent diabetes mellitus (NIDDM) patients (Hagander et al., 1989). Although the blood pressure reduction achieved (about 4–5 mmHg in hypertensives) may seem modest, this type of non-pharmacological therapy can certainly have important health implications if applied in a wider scale (Anonymous, 1980).

Conclusions

Several, although not all, studies with adequate designs have demonstrated that dietary fibre supplementation may reduce food intake. The clinical implication of such studies for obesity remains uncertain.

Several, although not all, studies with adequate design have demonstrated that dietary fibre supplementation may reduce feelings of hunger and appetite and increase feelings of satiation and satiety. The clinical implication of such studies for obesity also remains uncertain.

Several, although not all, studies with adequate design have demonstrated that fibre supplementation may improve weight loss, but only in a few studies over periods up to one year.

It is not clear what amount of fibre, its composition, its administration pattern in relation to time and meals, and basic diet will result in the best clinical effects and in what type of obese patients such effects can be expected.

Based on these inconclusive findings, it is at present difficult to recommend definite actions to be taken by the food industry and legislation bodies as regards the role of dietary fibre in the prevention and treatment of obesity until further scientific evidence has accumulated. The immediate areas of future research have already been indicated above. The importance of long-term studies in the evaluation of clinically significant effects should be stressed.

References

Andersson B, Seidell J, Terning K, Björntorp P (1990) Influence of menopause on dietary treatment of obesity. J Intern Med 227:173–181

Anonymous (1980) Lowering blood pressure without drugs. Lancet ii:459–461

Apfelbaum M, Björntorp B, Garrow J, James P, Jequier E, Stunkard A (1987) Standards for reporting the results of treatment for obesity. Am J Clin Nutr 45:1035–1036

Blundell JE, Burley VJ (1987) Satiation, satiety and the action of fibre on food intake. Int J Obesity 11(suppl):9–25

Bolton RP, Heaton KW, Burroughs LF (1981) The role of dietary fiber in satiety, glucose and insulin: studies with fruit and fruit juice. Am J Clin Nutr 34:211–217

Brownell KD, Kramer FM (1989) Behavioral management of obesity. Med Clin North Am 73:185–201

Bryson R, Dore C, Garrow JS (1980) Wholemeal bread and satiety. J Hum Nutr 34:113–116

Burley VJ, Blundell JE, Leeds AR (1987a) The effect of high- and low-fibre lunches on blood glucose, plasma insulin levels and hunger sensations. Int J Obesity 11(suppl 2):12 (abstract)

Burley VJ, Leeds AR, Blundell JE (1987b) The effects of high- and low-fibre breakfast on hunger, satiety and food intake in a subsequent meal. Int J Obesity 11(suppl 1):87–93

Bursztyn P (1987) Dietary fibre and blood pressure. In: Burztyn P (ed). Nutrition and blood pressure. John Libbey, London, pp 51–61

Duncan LPJ, Rose K, Meiklejohn AP (1960) Phenmetrazine hydrochloride and methylcellulose in the treatment of 'refractory' obesity. Lancet i:1262–1265

Duncan KH, Bacon JA, Weinsier RL (1983) The effects of high and low energy density diets on satiety, energy intake, and eating time of obese and non-obese subjects. Am J Clin Nutr 37:763–767

Durrant ML, Royston P (1979) The effect of preloads of varying energy density and methyl cellulose on hunger, appetite and salivation. Proc Nat Soc 37:87A (abstract)

Eliasson K, Hylander B, Ryttig K, Rössner S (1992) A dietary fibre supplement in the treatment of mild hypertension. Hypertension (in press)

Evans E, Miller DS (1975) Bulking agents in the treatment of obesity. Nutr Metab 18:199–203

Garrow JS (1989) Criteria of success of weight reduction In: Björntorp P, Rössner S (eds) Obesity in Europe 88. John Libbey, London, pp 23–28

Geliebter AA (1976) The effects of equal caloric loads of protein, fat and carbohydrate, and non-caloric loads on food intake in the rat and man. Columbia University. Dissertation Abstracts 3663-B (abstract)

Grimes DS, Gordon C (1978) Satiety value of wholemeal and white bread. Lancet ii:106

Guy-Grand BJP (1987) A new approach to the treatment of obesity. In: Wurtman RJ, Wurtman JJ, (eds) Human obesity. Ann N Y Aca Sci 499:313–317

Haber GB, Heaton KW, Murphy D, Burroughs LF (1977) Depletion and disruption of dietary fibre. Effects on satiety, plasma-glucose, and serum-insulin. Lancet ii:679–682

Hagander B, Asp N-G, Ekman R, Nilsson-Ehle P, Scherstén B (1989) Dietary fibre enrichment, blood pressure, lipoprotein profile and gut hormones in NIDDM patients. Eur J Clin Nutr 43:44–53

Heaton KW, (1973) Effects of increased dietary fibre on intestinal transit. Lancet ii:1278–1280

Heaton KW (1980) Food intake regulation and fiber. In: Spiller GS, Kay RM (eds) Medical aspects of dietary fibre. Plenum Press, New York, pp 223–238

Hylander B, Rössner S (1983) Effects of dietary fibre intake before meals on weight loss and hunger in a weight-reducing club. Acta Med Scand 213:217–220

Krotkiewski M (1984) Effect of guar-gum on body weight, hunger ratings and metabolism in obese subjects. Br J Nutr 52:97–105

Krotkiewski M, Björntorp P (1986) Muscle tissue in obesity with different distribution of adipose tissue: effects of physical training. Int J Obesity 10:331–341

Krotkiewski M, Smith U (1985) Dietary fibre in obesity. In: Leeds AR, Avenell A (eds) Dietary fibre perspectives – reviews and bibliography, 1. John Libbey, London, pp 61–67

Kuskowska-Wolk A, Rössner S (1990) Prevalence of obesity in Sweden: cross-sectional study of a representative adult population. J Intern Med 217:241–246

Liu GC, Coulston AM, Lardinois CK, Hollenbeck CB, Moore JG, Reaven GM (1985) Moderate weight loss and sulfonylurea treatment of non-insulin-dependent diabetes mellitus. Arch Intern Med 145:659–665

Margetts BM (1987) Vegetarian diets and blood pressure. In: Bursztyn P (ed) Nutrition and blood pressure. John Libbey, London, pp 5–15

McCance RA, Orior KM, Widdowson EM (1953) A radiological study of the rate of passage of brown and white bread through the digestive tract of man. Br J Nutr 7:98–104

Mikkelsen O, Makdani DD, Cotton RH, Titcomb ST, Colmey JC, Gatty R (1979) Effects of a high fiber bread diet on weight loss in college-age males. Am J Clin Nutr 32:1703–1709

Porikos K, Hagamen S (1986) Is fibre satiating? Effects of a high fibre preload on subsequent food intake of normal-weight and obese young men. Appetite 7:153–162

Reisen E (1983) Obesity and hypertension; effect of weight reduction In: Robertson JIS (ed) Handbook of hypertension, 1. Elsevier Science Publishers, Amsterdam, New York, Oxford, pp 30–43

Rigaud D, Ryttig KR, Angel LA, Apfelbaum M (1990) Overweight treated with energy restriction and a dietary fibre supplement: a 6-month randomized, double-blind, placebo-controlled trial. Int J Obesity 14:763–770

Rössner S (1989) Effects of potato fiber supplementation on serum lipids, blood sugar, hunger ratings and blood pressure in moderate obesity. 2nd European Congress on Obesity, Oxford (abstract)

Rössner S, Björvell H (1985) Early and late effects of weight loss on lipoprotein metabolism in severe obesity. Atherosclerosis 64:125–130

Rössner, S, van Zweigberg D, Öhlin A, Ryttig KR (1987) Weight reduction with dietary' fibre supplements. Results of two double-blind randomized studies. Acta Med Scand 222:83–88

Rössner S, Andersson IL, Ryttig K (1988) Effects of dietary fibre supplement to a weight reduction program on blood pressure. Acta Med Scand 223:353–357

Ryttig KR (1990) Clinical effects of dietary fibre supplements in overweight and in hypertension. Thesis, Karolinska Institute, Stockholm

Ryttig KR, Larsen S, Haegh L (1985) Treatment of slightly to moderately overweight persons. A double-blind placebo-controlled investigation with diet and fiber tablets (Dumovital). In: Björntorp P, Vahouny GV, Kritchevsky D (eds) Dietary fiber and obesity. Alan R Liss, New York, pp 77–84

Ryttig KR, Tellnes G, Haegh L, Böe E, Fagerthun H (1989) A dietary fibre supplement and weight maintenance after weight reduction. A randomized, double-blind, placebo-controlled study. Int J Obesity 13:165–171

Schlamowitz P, Halberg T, Warnoe O, Wilstrup F, Ryttig K (1987) Treatment of mild to moderate hypertension with dietary fibre. Lancet ii:622–623

Shearer RS (1976) The effects of bulk-producing tablets on hunger intensity in dieting patients. Curr Ther Res 19:433–441

Solum TT, Ryttig KR, Solum E, Larsen S (1987) The influence of a high-fibre diet on body weight, serum lipids and blood pressure in slightly overweight persons. A randomized, double-blind, placebo-controlled investigation with diet and fibre tablets (Dumovital). Int J Obesity 11 (suppl 1): 67–71

Southgate DAT, Bingham S, Robertson J (1978) Dietary fibre in the British diet. Nature 274:51–52

Tuomilehto J, Voutilainen E, Huttonen J, Vinni S, Homan K (1980) Effect of guar gum on body weight and serum lipids in hypercholesterolaemic females. Acta Med Scand 208:45–48

Walsh DE, Yaghoubian V, Behforooz A (1984) Effect of glucomannan on obese patients. A clinical study. Int J Obesity 8:289–293

Yudkin J (1959) The causes and cure of obesity. Lancet ii:1135–1138

Commentary

Heaton: Fibre tablets cannot be used to test the fibre–obesity hypothesis if fibre works through its physical effect on the texture of food, as originally proposed by Heaton (1973). To my knowledge no-one has adequately tested the hypotheses in that paper, namely: (1) that the more food needs to be chewed the less is eaten; (2) that cohesive food, which resists the churning action of the gastric antrum and so remains solid and stays in the stomach longer, is thereby more satiating; (3) that food which has intact cell walls even when it is emptied into the small intestine is more slowly and/or less completely digested and absorbed.

Reference:

Heaton KW (1973) Food fibre as an obstacle to energy intake. Lancet ii:1418–1421

Sandström: Although there are no controlled studies available showing an effect of a diet based on fibre-rich foods on development or treatment of obesity, epidemiological observations strongly suggest a potential role of such a diet in the prevention of obesity. The specific characteristic of such a diet is a low energy density (MJ/kg) or expressed in practical terms: the large amount or volume of such a diet that has to be taken to cover energy needs. While a low-fibre diet can have a total weight of less than 0.5 kg per 10 MJ a fibre-rich (40–50 g) diet can weigh 1.5–2.5 kg/10 MJ. This will for example affect time for consumption of a meal.

A high-fibre diet with natural foods will also often have a low fat content and will therefore have beneficial effects on other diseases than obesity. That is not necessarily the case when isolated fibre preparations are added to any type of diet.

Chapter 16

Dietary Fibre in the Prevention and Treatment of Diabetes Mellitus

M. Berger and A. Venhaus

Introduction

During the past 15 years a number of attempts have been made to suggest a crucial role for dietary fibre in the prevention and treatment of diabetes mellitus. However, with regard to prevention, only type 2 (non-insulin-dependent) diabetes mellitus may be a matter of discussion, while the autoimmune nature of type 1 (insulin-dependent) diabetes mellitus appears to leave little room for any nutritive prevention.

Earlier reports by Trowell and Burkitt (Trowell, 1975; Burkitt and Trowell, 1975) had suggested that average dietary fibre intakes might be associated with the prevalence of type 2 diabetes for a given population. Their experience with "geographical medicine" and its developmental aspects in Africa did, at first sight, point to an inverse causal relationship between dietary fibre intake and incidence rates for type 2 diabetes.

However, since (apart from the decrease in dietary fibre intake) so many other potentially more relevant environmental factors (and especially life expectancy) have changed in parallel with the dramatic increase in incidence and prevalence of type 2 diabetes around the world, the hypothesis of a primary aetiological role of low dietary fibre intake for type 2 diabetes has to be discarded. Hence, at present there remains no reason for discussing the *prevention* of type 2 diabetes by focusing nutritional recommendations on dietary fibre intake modification.

As a consequence, this review attempts to discuss the possibilities and potentials of dietary fibre in the treatment of type 1 and type 2 diabetic patients. Relevant studies concerned with this type of dietary treatment will be analysed with particular reference to the amount and type of fibre used, the short- and long-term efficacy on metabolic control as well as its acceptability by the patients.

Different Glycaemic Responses of Foods

The general objectives of any dietary treatment in diabetic patients are directed at overcoming the relative insulin deficiencies and/or perturbations of insulin secretion during and after carbohydrate consumption.

Wishnofski and Kane showed in 1935 that equivalent amounts of isolated starch and glucose resulted in identical blood glucose responses: suggesting that the chain length of a carbohydrate does not have an impact on the blood glucose response. This was confirmed by Wahlqvist et al. (1978). Yet different carbohydrate-rich foods cause different glycaemic responses. The first systematic investigations of glycaemic responses to carbohydrate foods were described by Külz (1899) and later became well known through the work of Jenkins et al. under the term "Glycaemic Index" (Jenkins et al., 1981, 1984).

A lot of studies were conducted not only to investigate the different glycaemic indices of different carbohydrate foods but also to find a plausible and possibly predictable cause for their different glycaemic responses. Dietary fibre seemed to be a potential candidate to explain the different metabolic effects after the consumption of foods with different glycaemic indices.

Metabolic Effects of Fibre

The term "fibre" covers a wide variety of substances and there are different methods of analysis which may give different values for the same fibre source (Fig. 16.1). Thus, fibre data from different countries, even different food tables of the same country, offer different information which may not be comparable. Thus, for comparative purposes it is of importance to cite the method of analysis used (Eastwood, 1986; Feldheim, 1989).

However, in relation to diabetes one convenient differentiation among fibres is of unequivocal importance: water-soluble fibres and water-insoluble fibres.

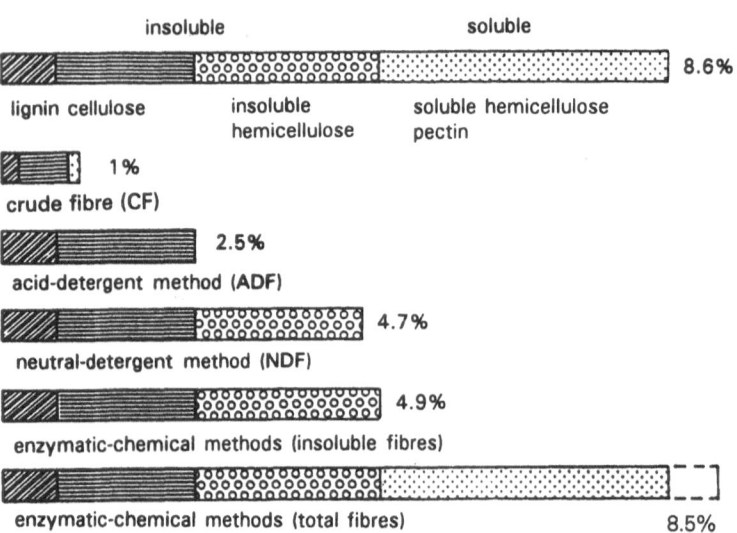

Fig. 16.1. Comparison of different methods of dietary fibre analysis on a wholemeal rye bread (g fibre/100 g bread). From Feldheim, 1989, with permission.

Studies with Soluble Fibre

Soluble fibres, such as guar, pectin, carrageenan, locust bean gum or tragacanth, have a reproducible effect on glycaemia. The delay of gastric emptying was regarded as an important mechanism of action for postprandial blood glucose reduction by soluble fibres (Schwartz et al., 1988). However, studies by Torsdottir et al. (1989), Blackburn et al. (1984) and Edwards et al. (1987) have suggested that gastric emptying does not seem to be related to the blood glucose reducing effects of some fibres. A high degree of viscosity which acts by reducing glucose absorption in the small intestine is regarded as the main mechanism (Blackburn et al., 1984; Edwards et al., 1987).

Most studies with water-soluble fibres in diabetic patients were performed with guar gum and pectin. Jenkins et al. (1976) reported that rather large amounts of guar and pectin (16 g and 10 g) resulted in lowered postprandial blood glucose (by approximately 50%) and insulin levels (by approximately 50%) in meal studies in eight type 2 diabetic patients. The same authors also carried out long-term studies with 14–26 g guar daily over six months in 11 insulin-treated diabetic patients (Jenkins et al., 1980). However, these patients showed a statistically significant weight loss of 2.2 kg after 6 months. Since weight reduction by itself will improve glucose metabolism in such patients (Hockaday et al., 1978; Atkinson and Kaiser, 1985; Beattie et al., 1988) the reported beneficial metabolic effects of this study can not be attributed to the increased fibre consumption.

Guar gum, a galactomannan, is obtained from the seeds of the guar bean (*Cyamopsis tetragonoloba*) which is found in the tropical regions of Asia. Thus, in Europe and North America guar is not a common part of the daily food and would therefore have to be added to the diet.

Guar gum has to be consumed thoroughly mixed into the meals, and it seems to work best only when stirred into fluids. Other obstacles for a daily supply of such an isolated fibre are its palatability and the frequently occurring side effects, such as diarrhoea, flatulence, or nausea (Mann and Simpson, 1980; Beattie et al., 1988), not to mention obstructions of the oesophagus (Ranft and Imhoff, 1983; Henry et al., 1986). Furthermore, the observed blood glucose lowering effects of guar are of a magnitude which can also be achieved by "lente" (or low-glycaemic) carbohydrate foods.

Insoluble Fibre and High-Carbohydrate, High-Fibre Studies

The prevailing dietary fibres in Western countries are insoluble fibres, since naturally occurring soluble fibres make up only about one-quarter or one-third of the total fibre intake (Story et al., 1985). In general, insoluble fibres affect glucose metabolism to only a minor degree compared with soluble fibres, as they do not increase luminal viscosity in the small intestine. Instead, they increase faecal bulking, stool frequency, and reduce intestinal passage time (Thomas and Elchazly, 1976; Wyman et al., 1976; Cummings et al., 1978; Spiller et al., 1986; Stevens et al., 1988).

Most studies on the influence of fibre on post-prandial glucose metabolism cover time intervals of only two to three hours after the meals. Therefore, much of the serum glucose or insulin responses after slowly absorbed foods is underestimated, especially in diabetic patients (Krezowski et al., 1987), because fasting values are commonly reattained only *after* two to three hours (Gannon and Nuttall, 1987).

Since fibre which is added to a food in an isolated form (e.g. as bran) has less effect than fibre which is still naturally incorporated into the food (Jenkins et al., 1983b) studies were conducted using diets which are naturally high in fibre.

Increasing the natural amount of dietary fibre in a diet usually increases also the carbohydrate content of the diet. Such an increase of the carbohydrate content of the diet is bound to exert a substantial effect on glucose metabolism by itself. Himsworth (1935) showed that a high percentage of carbohydrate in the diet has a beneficial effect on glucose homeostasis. Several studies confirmed this finding in diabetic patients using diets with carbohydrate contents of up to 80% of total energy (Weinsier et al., 1974; Kiehm et al., 1976; Simpson et al., 1979a, b; Anderson and Bryant, 1986). However, increasing the carbohydrate content (especially of starch plus dietary fibre) of the diabetes diet to around 50%–60%, a recommendation which has been adopted by leading national diabetes and nutrition societies over the past 10 years (Canadian Diabetes Association, Special Report Committee, 1981; British Diabetes Association's Medical Advisory Committee, Nutrition Sub-Committee, 1982; American Diabetes Association, 1987; Diabetes and Nutrition Study Group of the European Association for the Study of Diabetes, 1988), has recently met with outspoken scepticism (Reaven, 1980, 1988).

Studies with extreme nutrient compositions – particularly from Anderson's group – became popular under the term "high-carbohydrate, high-fibre" (HCF) diet (Anderson, 1977; Anderson and Ward, 1978, 1979). Twenty type 2 diabetics on insulin or sulphonylureas received a "weight-maintaining diet" with 70% of energy as carbohydrates and about 65 g of fibres (8.6 g/MJ) daily. After 16 days, insulin and sulphonylurea doses could be substantially reduced or even discontinued (Anderson and Ward, 1979). Fasting and postprandial blood glucose levels remained more or less constant. After 15 months on a maintenance diet with 55%–60% of energy as carbohydrate and $\geq$ 40 g of fibre daily, seven out of 10 patients had continued their diabetes treatment without using insulin or sulphonylureas. But these patients had lost approximately 5 kg body weight which by itself should be an explanation for the reduction in antidiabetic drug treatment.

A study with even higher fibre intakes was conducted by Simpson et al. (1981). They treated diabetic patients with 97 g fibre daily and 60% of energy as carbohydrate. After six weeks pre- and postprandial blood glucose values were improved with insignificant insulin dose reductions. Again, the non-insulin-dependent group of patients showed a significant weight loss (0.9 kg) along with improved glycosylated haemoglobin values. Thus, the increased fibre consumption by itself can not account for the observed improvement in diabetes control.

That fibre may have a beneficial effect on diabetes control via weight loss still has to be proven. Some studies on the effect of fibre actually showed a weight loss in patients (Mickelsen et al., 1979; Simpson et al., 1981; Weinsier et al., 1983; Thornton et al., 1983), others showed no change in weight (Kahaner et al., 1976; Anderson and Ward, 1979; Hylander and Rössner, 1983; Liebman et al.,

1983; Harold et al., 1985; Russ and Atkinson, 1985; Hollenbeck et al., 1986; Beattie et al., 1988; Venhaus and Chantelau, 1988), and a few studies even showed an increase in body weight after a high-fibre diet (Rivellese et al., 1980; in rats: Nygren et al., 1985). This was confirmed by a recent review from Stevens (1988).

Things may be different in diabetic patients in unsatisfactory metabolic control. Scott et al. (1988) showed in poorly controlled type 2 diabetic patients a deterioration of blood glucose and HbA_{1c} levels after six months of increased fibre intake (from 19 g to 35 g fibre per day) along with an increase of carbohydrate consumption from 35% to 40% of total energy intake. On the other hand, an improved insulin sensitivity in poorly controlled overweight diabetic patients on a fibre-rich diet was observed by Pedersen et al. (1980) and Ward et al. (1982).

As with soluble fibres, meal studies usually showed a more substantial benefit on glucose metabolism than long-term studies, and fibre was more potent in type 2 then in type 1 diabetic patients.

Acceptability of High-Carbohydrate, High-Fibre Diets

In order to influence blood glucose values or insulin needs in diabetic patients, fibre intake was increased to amounts of up to 97 g fibre a day. Reports about the average fibre intake in Europe (whatever fibre analysis is used) range between 21 g/day and 45 g/day (Bright-See, 1985; Rutishauser, 1985) with habitual fibre consumption being higher in Mediterranean countries. Recent calculations for the average intake in the USA even report only 13 g/day (Lanza et al., 1987). In the above cited study of Simpson et al. (1981) with a daily fibre consumption of about 100 g, the authors report that these high intakes were accomplished through a consumption of beans at nearly every meal. It is more than doubtful if diabetic patients are willing, in general, to eat beans several times daily lifelong and to change their life style in order extensively to increase their fibre and carbohydrate intake in response to dietary recommendations the efficacy of which is still not fully proven (Tattersall and McCulloch, 1985; Nuttall, 1983). Children flatly refused to eat several bean meals a day, anyway (Baumer et al. 1982).

High intakes of dietary fibre as mentioned above can be achieved only with very substantial changes in food habits. Even for study purposes (i.e. for limited time periods) intensive counselling, including practical training courses, is necessary (Mann et al., 1981; McCulloch et al., 1985), as well as enthusiasm from the counsellor (Geekie et al., 1986), motivation of the patients (Ney et al., 1982), and sometimes even behaviour modification (Kahaner et al., 1976).

No Direct Effects of Fibre in Diabetes Treatment?

Since about 1980, some authors questioned whether fibre itself does have any effect on the blood glucose response of carbohydrate foods (Mann and Simpson,

1980). Crapo et al. (Crapo et al., 1980, 1981) concluded from studies they performed with potatoes, rice, corn, and bread that the fibre content of these foods has no relation to postprandial blood glucose responses. Simpson et al. (1982) confirmed these findings in studies on diets which differed in carbohydrate content but were constant in fibre. Varying postprandial blood glucose responses independently of the fibre amount in carbohydrate-rich foods were described by Jenkins et al. (1983a) for white bread, wholemeal bread, and spaghetti; by d'Emden et al. (1987) for the same foods and wholemeal spaghetti; by O'Dea et al. (1980) for brown and white rice; and by Björck et al. (1984) for different types of flour.

The question still remains what causes the different glycaemic responses of different carbohydrate foods which are comparable in carbohydrate and fibre content.

Evidence Suggesting Starch as the Responsible Factor for Different Glycaemic Responses

Because neither the type of fibre nor its amount in a food could explain satisfactorily the differences in blood glucose responses to different carbo-hydrate-rich foods, the nature of starch and its processing might actually be the responsible factor. In the following, a brief review over different starch characteristics and the influence of thermal and mechanical processing on starch resulting in different glucose responses shall be given as a hint to future research concerning dietary treatment of diabetes.

Effects of Thermal Processing and Starch Characteristics

In 1929, Rosenthal and Ziegler showed that raw starch (of potatoes and chestnuts) caused less postprandial blood glucose elevations than did the boiled form of such foods, a finding which was later confirmed by Collings et al. in 1981.

Starch consists of amylose and amylopectin. A high amount of amylose (of special rice or corn varieties) led to low blood glucose responses and, above all, insulin responses (Goddard et al., 1984; Behall et al., 1988, 1989). The authors explain this with a more rigid gel which is produced by amylose (Behall et al., 1988), or a lipid–starch complex which occurs in amylose-rich rice varieties and which hinders starch hydrolysis (Goddard et al., 1984). Bornet et al. (1989) suggest that the amount of amylose becomes important as soon as the food is processed.

Starch is hydrolysed by amylase. Amylase cannot act efficiently on the surface of raw starch granules. In general, heating allows the starch to be attacked more easily by enzymes. Here, gelatinisation of the starch plays an important role.

Gelatinisation depends on a variety of factors: starch and starch granules themselves, temperature, water availability, pH, electrolytes, or sugar content. In general, starch rich in amylose gelatinises more slowly than starch high in amylopectin; small-sized starch granules gelatinise more slowly than large ones; the tighter the surrounding tissue is and the more lipids, proteins or fibres that surround the starch granules the more limited is starch swelling (Blanshard 1979; Greenwood and Munro, 1979a, b; Würsch et al., 1986). A comprehensive overview on starch and the properties influencing starch digestion and metabolic responses was published by Würsch in 1989.

Mechanical Processing and "Antinutrients"

Mechanical processing such as finely chopping or grinding of carbohydrate-rich foods also has effects on postprandial blood sugar and insulin levels. Ground rice caused faster blood sugar increases and higher insulin responses in non-diabetic and type 2 diabetic volunteers than unground rice of the same kind (O'Dea et al., 1980; Collier and O'Dea, 1982). In vitro hydrolysis studies with starch confirm the findings that starch is hydrolysed faster in ground rice (O'Dea et al., 1981). Legumes ground before cooking also resulted in increased glucose and insulin areas under the curve in type 2 diabetics compared with unground legumes (Golay et al., 1986).

The particle size after grinding also plays a role: small particles of wheat or corn cause higher glucose or insulin responses than larger ones such as whole kernels (Heaton et al., 1988; Jenkins et al., 1988; O'Donnell et al., 1989).

However, the effects of thermal processing seem to have a greater impact on glucose metabolism for diabetic patients than differences in mechanical processing (Sichert-Oevermann et al., 1987).

Besides fibre, heating, and grinding, other factors also may have an effect on postprandial blood glucose and insulin: so-called "antinutrients" like enzyme inhibitors, lectins, saponins, phytic acid, tannins, and oxalates. Enzyme inhibitors occur naturally in food, particularly in wheat and legumes. It is controversial as to whether they are able to diminish the amylase action as was demonstrated in a study by Levitt et al. (1984), but challenged by others like Tappy et al. (1986) and Würsch et al. (1986). Enzyme inhibitors are also employed as antidiabetic drugs in the treatment of diabetes, but the overall benefit of such drugs is controversial (Anonymous, 1985, 1988).

Dietary fibres are also affected by thermal, chemical or mechanical processing. Cooked bran had fewer gastro-intestinal effects than raw bran (Wyman et al., 1976), and fine-ground bran had fewer effects than coarse-ground bran (Heller et al., 1980). Drying and cooking obviously lead to a collapse of the matrix structure of the fibre and, thus, to a loss of the ability to hydrate (Eastwood and Brydon, 1985). Wet heat diluted pectic substances and destroyed them thereafter, dry heat increased Maillard browning products, which were later isolated with the lignin fraction, whereas hemicellulose and cellulose fractions remained virtually unchanged (Anderson and Clydesdale, 1980).

Studies Including Fibre and the Effect of Processing

Since meal studies showed that diets high in fibre and unrefined food caused diminished insulin responses in diabetic patients, it is often stated in the literature that with this kind of food diabetics need less insulin.

This hypothesis was addressed in a study with 10 diabetic patients on continuous subcutaneous insulin infusion therapy (CSII) who were in good metabolic control (HbA$_{1c}$: 6.4%). They were randomly assigned to either follow a diet high in fibre and unrefined food (URD), or to follow a diet low in fibre but rich in refined food for six weeks each (RD)(Venhaus and Chantelau, 1988; Venhaus, 1990). After six weeks the groups changed following a cross-over design. Using seven-day-food records the patients' diet was surveyed, additional to weekly phone calls and bi-weekly visits by the patients to the outpatient clinic. The patients followed the diet instructions very well according to their food records and self-reported stool frequencies. Their fibre intake nearly doubled during the unrefined period (URD: 35 g/day or 3.5 g/MJ; RD: 18 g/day or 1.6 g/MJ; total fibre intake: $P = 0.013$, fibre density : $P = 0.001$; source for fibre values: Paul and Southgate, 1978). The semi-quantitative assessment of the intake of refined or unrefined food was statistically significantly different in the two study periods and according to the recommendations. Stool frequency increased significantly during URD (URD: 1.9 times/day, RD: 1.0 times/day; $P = 0.008$). Body weight and metabolic control remained constant throughout the study. Self-selected daily insulin doses (Fig. 16.2) of the patients decreased slightly but insignificantly during URD (total insulin in URD: 40 IU/day, RD: 43 IU/day; NS). This study demonstrates that the degree of refinement of carbohydrate foods has little or no impact on metabolic control and insulin therapy in near-normoglycaemic type 1 diabetic patients on CSII. Likewise, any

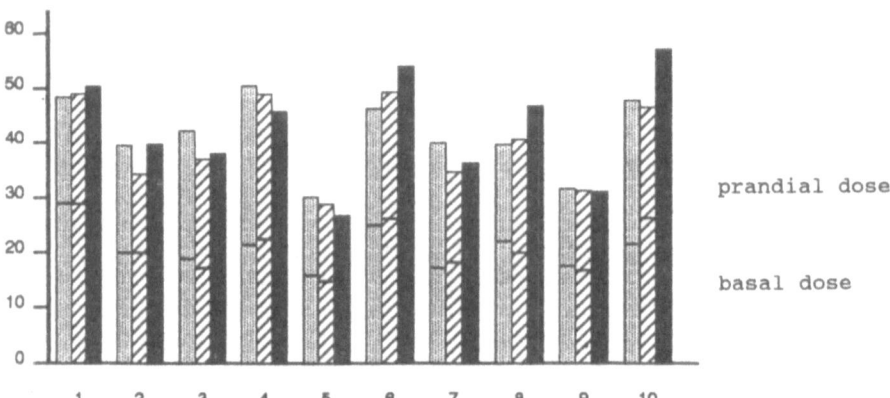

Fig. 16.2. Insulin doses of 10 diabetic patients on CSII during three six-week study periods. Dotted columns, run-in; hatched columns, high-fibre unrefined-food diet (URD); solid columns, low-fibre refined food diet (RD). (From Venhaus, 1990, with permission.)

potential benefit of an unrefined diet is negligible, if diabetic control is poor due to insufficient insulin replacement (Lindsay et al., 1984; Weyman-Daum et al., 1987). In patients on intensive insulin therapy any potential insulin sparing effect of such a diet may be overruled by other factors requiring insulin dosage adaptation during type 1 diabetes treatment.

Recent studies confirmed our findings (Venhaus and Chantelau, 1988): Lafrance et al. (1989) found no changes in insulin dosages in type-1-diabetics on CSII in good metabolic control after a diet with 55 g fibre/day Capani et al. (1988) and Lafrance et al. (1990) concluded from nearly identical studies with type 1 diabetic patients in good metabolic control that meals with identical carbohydrate content but different glycaemic indexes are subject to such a high variability in insulin needs that attempts to adapt insulin dosages on the basis of differences in "glycaemic indexes" are of little value for the establishment of appropriate insulin therapy.

In a comparable, as yet unpublished study we have recently prescribed high-fibre, unrefined food (URD) diets to elderly type 2 diabetic patients. These patients were followed up after six weeks and, again after one year. Seven-day food records and stool frequency at both times showed that patients did not follow diet instructions although on questioning they maintained that they did. In our experience, it seems to be impracticable and probably unjustified to switch elderly patients from their lifelong food habits to predominant consumption of unrefined high-fibre foods.

Conclusions and Areas for Future Research

The history of dietary recommendations and therapies for patients with diabetes mellitus must be regarded as a continuous chain of failure, scientific incompetence and unethical propagation of false hopes (West, 1973; Oyen et al., 1985) – most often put forward by medical authorities, opinion leaders and scientific associations. One of the principal duties of contemporary diabetology should be to protect diabetic patients from unjustified dietary recommendations and other such substantial interventions into their personal life style. It is in this context, that every proposal for a dietary treatment of diabetic patients needs to be most thoroughly scrutinised before such therapeutic advice can be brought forward into clinical medicine. In accordance with recent review articles by Tattersall and Mansell (1990) and Heaton (1990), we conclude from published evidence and from our own clinical experience that dietary fibre plays, if anything, a minor role concerning the postprandial glycaemic and insulinaemic responses following the ingestion of mixed (carbohydrate-rich) meals. The relevance of dietary fibre in the long-term management of metabolic control in type 1 or type 2 diabetic patients appears to be negligible. There is no evidence that dietary fibre may play an independent role in the prevention of either type of diabetes mellitus.

In the future, nutrition research will have to focus upon the possibility of changing the glycaemic and insulinaemic responses of foodstuffs and meals by altering the degree of food processing and, in particular, the processing of starch.

References

American Diabetes Association (1987) Nutritional recommendations and principles for individuals with diabetes mellitus: 1986. Diabetes Care 10:126–132

Anderson JW (1977) Therapeutic effectiveness of high carbohydrate, high-fibre, weight-maintaining diets for lean, insulin-treated diabetic men. Clin Res 25:619A

Anderson JW, Bryant CA (1986) Dietary fiber: diabetes and obesity. Am J Gastroenterol 81:898–906

Anderson JW, Ward K (1978) Long-term effects of high-carbohydrate, high-fiber diets on glucose and lipid metabolism: a preliminary report on patients with diabetes. Diabetes Care 1:77–82

Anderson JW, Ward K (1979) High-carbohydrate, high-fiber diets for insulin-treated men with diabetes mellitus. Am J Clin Nutr 32:2312–2321

Anderson NE, Clydesdale FM (1980) Effects of processing on the dietary fiber content of wheat bran, pureed green beans, and carrots. J Food Science 45:1533–1537

Anonymous (1985) Starch blockers do not block starch digestion. Nutr Rev 43:46–48

Anonymous (1988) Absorptionsverzögerung von Kohlenhydraten – langfristig ohne Vorteil für Diabetiker. Arznei-Telegramm 5:44

Atkinson RL, Kaiser DL (1985) Effects of calorie restriction and weight loss on glucose and insulin levels in obese humans. J Am Coll Nutr 4:411–419

Baumer JH, Drakeford JA, Wadsworth J, Savage DCL (1982) Effects of dietary fibre and exercise on mid-morning diabetic control – a controlled trial. Arch Dis Child 57: 905–909

Beattie VA, Edwards CA, Hosker JP, Cullen DR, Ward JD, Read NW (1988) Does adding fibre to a low energy, high carbohydrate, low fat diet confer any benefit to the management of newly diagnosed overweight type II diabetics? Br Med J 296:1147–1149

Behall KM, Scholfield DJ, Canary J (1988) Effect of starch structure on glucose and insulin responses in adults. Am J Clin Nutr 47:428–432

Behall KM, Scholfield DJ, Yuhaniak I, Canary J (1989) Diets containing high amylose vs. amylopectin starch: effects on metabolic variables in human subjects. Am J Clin Nutr 49:337–344

Björck J, Asp N-G, Birkhed D, Lundquist J (1984) Effects of processing on availability of starch for digestion in vitro and in vivo. J. Cereal Sci 2:91–103

Blackburn NA, Redfern JS, Jarjis H et al. (1984) The mechanism of action of guar gum in improving glucose tolerance in man. Clin Sci 66:329–336

Blanshard JMV (1979) Physicochemical aspects of starch gelatinization. In: Blanshard JMV, Mitchell JR (eds) Polysaccharides in food. Butterworth, London, pp 139–152

Bornet FRJ, Fontvieille AM, Rizkalla S et al. (1989) Insulin and glycemic responses in healthy humans to native starches processed in different ways: correlation with in vitro alpha-amylase hydrolysis. Am J Clin Nutr 50:315–323

Bright-See E (1985) Reply to letter to the Editor: Rutishauser 1985, Estimation of dietary fiber supply. Am J Clin Nutr 41:825–826

British Diabetes Association's Medical Advisory Committee, Nutrition Subcommittee (1982) Dietary recommendations for the 1980s – a policy statement by the British Diabetes Association. Hum Nutr Appl Nutr 36A:378–394

Burkitt DP, Trowell HC (eds) (1975) Refined carbohydrate foods and disease: some implications of dietary fibre. Academic Press, London

Canadian Diabetes Association, Special Report Committee (1981) 1980. Guidelines for the nutritional management of diabetes mellitus. J Can Diabetes Assoc 42:110–118

Capani F, Casalini G, D'Emilio A et al. (1988) Insulin requirement of simple and complex carbohydrate meals in type 1 (insulin-dependent) continuous subcutaneous insulin infusion-treated diabetic patients. Correlation with glycaemic index. Diabetologia 31:477A

Collier G, O'Dea K (1982) Effect of physical form of carbohydrate on the postprandial glucose, insulin, and gastric inhibitory polypeptide responses in type 2 diabetes. Am J Clin Nutr 36:10–14

Collings P, Williams C, MacDonald I (1981) Effects of cooking on serum glucose and insulin responses to starch. Br Med J 282:1032

Crapo PA, Kolterman OG, Waldeck N, Reaven GM, Olefsky JM (1980) Postprandial hormonal responses to different types of complex carbohydrate individuals with impaired glucose tolerance. Am J Clin Nutr 33:1723–1728

Crapo PA, Insel J, Sperling M, Kolterman OG (1981) Comparison of serum glucose, insulin, and glucagon responses to different types of complex carbohydrate in non-insulin-dependent diabetic patients. Am J Clin Nutr 34:184–190

Cummings JH, Branch W, Jenkins DJA, Southgate DAT, Houston H, James WPT (1978) Colonic response to dietary fibre from carrot, cabbage, apple, bran, and guar gum. Lancet i:5–8

d'Emden MC, Marwick TH, Dreghorn J, Howlett VL, Cameron DP (1987) Postprandial glucose and insulin responses to different types of spaghetti and bread. Diabetes Res Clin Prac 3:221–226

Diabetes and Nutrition Study Group of the European Association for the Study of Diabetes (1988) Nutritional recommendations for individuals with diabetes mellitus. Diabetes Nutr Metab 1:145–149

Eastwood MA (1986) What does the measurement of dietary fibre mean? Lancet i:1487–1488

Eastwood MA, Brydon G (1985) Physiological effects of dietary fibre on the alimentary tract. In: Trowell H et al. (eds) Dietary fibre, fibre-depleted foods and disease. Academic Press, London, pp 105–131

Edwards CA, Blackburn NA, Craigen L et al. (1987) Viscosity of food gums determined in vitro related to their hypoglycemic actions. Am J Clin Nutr 46:72–77

Feldheim W (1989) Verwertbare und nicht verwertbare Kohlenhydrate – Definition und chemische Bestimmungsverfahren. Ernähr Umschau 36:40–44

Gannon MC, Nuttall FQ (1987) Factors affecting interpretation of postprandial glucose and insulin areas. Diabetes Care 10:759–763

Geekie MA, Porteous J, Hockaday TDR, Mann JI (1986) Acceptability of high-fibre diets in diabetic patients. Diabetic Med 3:65–68

Goddard MS, Young G, Marcus R (1984) The effect of amylose content on insulin and glucose responses to ingested rice. Am J Clin Nutr 39:388–392

Golay A, Coulston AM, Hollenbeck CB, Kaiser LL, Würsch P, Reaven GM (1986) Comparison of metabolic effects of white beans processed into two different physical forms. Diabetes Care 9:260–266

Greenwood CT, Munro DN (1979a) Carbohydrates: some heat-dependent properties of polysaccharides. In: Priestley RJ (ed) Effects of heating on foodstuffs. Applied Science Publishers, London, pp 72–76

Greenwood CT, Munro DN (1979b) Cereals, roots and other starch-based products. In: Priestly RJ (ed) Effects of heating on foodstuffs. Applied Science Publishers, London, pp 373–402

Harold MR, Reeves RD, Bolze S, Guthrie RW, Guthrie DW (1985) Effect of dietary fiber in insulin-dependent diabetics: insulin requirements and serum lipids. J Am Diet Assoc 85:1455–1460

Heaton KW (1990) Dietary fibre: after 21 years of study the verdict remains one of fruition and frustration. Br Med J 300:1479–1480

Heaton KW, Marcus SN, Emmett PM, Bolton CH (1988) Particle size of wheat, maize, and oat test meals: effects on plasma glucose and insulin responses and on the rate of starch digestion in vitro. Am J Clin Nutr 47:675–682

Heller SN, Hackler LR, Rivers JM et al. (1980) Dietary fiber: the effect of particle size of wheat bran on colonic function in young men. Am J Clin Nutr 33: 1734–1744

Henry DA, Mitchell AS, Aylward J (1986) Glucomannan and risk of oesophageal obstruction. Br Med J 292:591–592

Himsworth HP (1935) The dietetic factor determining the glucose tolerance and sensitivity to insulin of healthy men. Clin Sci 2:67–94

Hockaday TDR, Hockaday JM, Mann JI, Turner RC (1978) Prospective comparison of modified-fat, high-carbohydrate with standard low-carbohydrate dietary advice in the treatment of diabetes: one year follow-up study. Br J Nutr 39:357–362

Hollenbeck CB, Couston AM, Reaven GM (1986) To what extent does increased dietary fiber improve glucose and lipid metabolism in patients with non-insulin-dependent diabetes mellitus? Am J Clin Nutr 43:16–24

Hylander B, Rössner S (1983) Effects of dietary fiber intake before meals on weight loss and hunger in a weight-reducing club. Acta Med Scand 213:217–220

Jenkins DJA, Goff DV, Leeds AR et al. (1976) Unabsorbable carbohydrates and diabetes: decreased postprandial hyperglycaemia. Lancet ii:172–174

Jenkins DJA, Wolever TMS, Taylor H, Reynolds D, Nineham R, Hockaday TDR (1980) Diabetic glucose control, lipids, and trace elements on long-term guar. Br Med J 280:1353–1354

Jenkins DJA, Wolever TMS, Taylor RH et al. (1981) Glycemic index of foods: a physiological basis for carbohydrate exchange. Am J Clin Nutr 34:362–366

Jenkins DJA, Wolever TMS, Jenkins AL, Lee R, Wong GS, Josse R (1983a) Glycemic response to wheat products: reduced response to pasta but no effect of fiber. Diabetes Care 6:155–159

Jenkins DJA, Wolever TMS, Jenkins AL et al. (1983b) The glycaemic index of foods tested in diabetic patients: a new basis for carbohydrate exchange favouring the use of legumes. Diabetologia 24:257–264

Jenkins DJA, Wolever TMS, Jenkins AL, Josse RG, Wong GS (1984) The glycaemic response to carbohydrate foods. Lancet ii:388–391

Jenkins DJA, Wesson V, Wolever TMS et al. (1988) Wholemeal versus wholegrain breads: proportion of whole or cracked grain and the glycaemic response. Br Med J 297:958–960

Kahaner N, Fuchs HM, Floch MH (1976) The effect of dietary fiber supplementation in man. I. modification of eating habits. Am J Clin Nutr 29:1437–1442

Kiehm TG, Anderson JW, Ward K (1976) Beneficial effects of a high carbohydrate, high-fiber diet on hyperglycemic diabetic men. Am J Clin Nutr 29:895–899

Krezowski PA, Nuttall FQ, Gannon MC, Billington CJ, Parner S (1987) Insulin and glucose responses to various starch-containing foods in type 2 diabetic subjects. Diabetes Care 10:205–212

Külz E (1899) Klinische Erfahrungen über Diabetes mellitus, bearbeitet von Th Rumpf. Jena

Lafrance L, Ducros F, Chiasson JL (1989) Les fibres alimentaires et l'insulinothérapie intensive. Diabète Metab 15:XV

Lafrance L, Poisson D, Ducros F, Chiasson JL (1990) L'effet de l'indice glycémique de la diète sur les besoins en insuline lors de l'insulinothérapie intensive. Diabète Metab 16:XVI

Lanza E, Jones DY, Block G, Kessler L (1987) Dietary fiber intake in the US population. Am J Clin Nutr 46:790–797

Levitt MD, Ellis CJ, Fetzer CP, Bond JH, Levine AS (1984) Causes of malabsorption of flour. Gastroenterology 86:1162

Liebman M, Smith MC, Iverson J et al. (1983) Effects of coarse wheat bran fiber and exercise on plasma lipids and lipoproteins in moderately overweight men. Am J Clin Nutr 37:71–81

Lindsay AN, Hardy S, Jarrett L, Rallison ML (1984) High-carbohydrate, high-fibre diet in children with type 1 diabetes mellitus. Diabetes Care 7:63–67

Mann JI, Simpson HCR (1980) Fibre, diabetes, and hyperlipidaemia. Lancet i:44–45

Mann JI, Kinmonth AL, Todd E, Angus RM, Simpson HCR, Hockaday TDR (1981) High-fibre diets and diabetes. Lancet i:731–732

McCulloch DK, Mitchell RD, Ambler J, Tattersall RB (1985) A prospective comparison of "conventional" and high carbohydrate/high fibre/low fat diets in adults with established type 1 (insulin-dependent) diabetes. Diabetologia 28:208–212

Mickelsen O, Makdani DD, Cotton RH, Titcomb ST, Colmey JC, Gatty R (1979) Effects of a high fiber bread diet on weight loss in college-age males. Am J Clin Nutr 32:1703–1709

Ney D, Hollingsworth DR, Cousins L (1982) Decreased insulin requirement and improved control of diabetes in pregnant women given a high-carbohydrate, high-fiber, low-fat diet. Diabetes Care 5:529–533

Nuttall FQ (1983) Diet and the diabetic patient. Diabetes Care 6:197–207

Nygren C, Hallmans G, Johnsson L (1985) Effects of various brans on energy intake and glucose metabolism in alloxan diabetic rats. Diabete Metab 11:205–209

O'Dea K, Nestel PJ, Antionoff L (1980) Physical factors influencing postprandial glucose and insulin responses to starch. Am J Clin Nutr 33:760–765

O'Dea K, Snow P, Nestel PJ (1981) Rate of starch hydrolysis in vitro as a predictor of metabolic responses to complex carbohydrate in vivo. Am J Clin Nutr 34:1991–1993

O'Donnell LJD, Emmett PM, Heaton KW (1989) Size of flour particles and its relation to glycaemia, insulinaemia, and colonic disease. Br Med J 298:1616–1617

Oyen D, Chantelau EA, Berger M (1985) Zur Geschichte der Diabetesdiät. Springer, Berlin Heidelberg New York

Paul AA, Southgate DAT (1978) McCance and Widdowson's The composition of foods, 4th edn. HMSO, London

Pedersen O, Hjollund E, Lindskov HO, Sorensen HS (1980) Increased insulin receptors on monocytes from insulin-dependent diabetics after a high-starch, high-fibre diet. Diabetologia 19:306

Ranft K, Imhof W (1983) Bolusobstruktion des distalen Oesophagus durch pflanzliche Quellstoffe (Guarmehl). Dtsch Med Wochenschr 108:1968–1969

Reaven GM (1980) How high the carbohydrate? Diabetologia 19:409–413

Reaven GM (1988) Dietary therapy for non-insulin-dependent diabetes mellitus. N Engl J Med 319:862–864

Rivellese A, Riccardie G, Giacco A et al. (1980) Effect of dietary fibre on glucose control and serum lipoproteins in diabetic patients. Lancet ii:447–449

Rosenthal SM, Ziegler EE (1929) The effect of uncooked starches on the blood sugar of normal and of diabetic subjects. Arch Intern Med 44:344–350

Russ CS, Atkinson RL (1985) Use of high-fiber diets for the outpatient treatment of obesity. Nutr Rep Int 32:193–198

Rutishauser IHE (1985) Estimation of dietary fiber supply. Am J Clin Nutr 41:824–826

Schwartz SE, Levine RA, Weinstock RS, Petokas S, Mills CA, Thomas FD (1988) Sustained pectin ingestion: effect on gastric emptying and glucose tolerance in non-insulin-dependent diabetic patients. Am J Clin Nutr 48:1413–1417

Scott AR, Attenborough Y, Peacock I, Fletcher E, Jeffcoate W, Tattersall RB (1988) Comparison of high-fibre diets, basal insulin supplements, and flexible insulin treatment for non-insulin-dependent (type II) diabetics poorly controlled with sulphonylureas. Br Med J 297:707–710

Sichert-Oevermann W, Koerber VK, Bretthauer B, Leitzmann C, Laube H (1987) Blutglucose- und Insulinverlauf bei Gesunden und Diabetikern nach Gabe roher Vollkornzubereitungen, insbesondere Frischkornmüsli. Dtsch Med Wochenschr 112:1977–1983

Simpson RW, Mann JI, Eaton J, Carter RD, Hockaday TDR (1979a) High-carbohydrate diets and insulin-dependent diabetes. Br Med J ii:523–525

Simpson RW, Mann JI, Eaton J, Moore RA, Carter R, Hockaday TDR (1979b) Improved glucose control in maturity-onset diabetes treated with high-carbohydrate, modified fat diet. Br Med J i:1753–1756

Simpson HCR, Simpson RW, Lousley S et al. (1981) A high-carbohydrate leguminous fibre diet improves all aspects of diabetic control. Lancet i:1–5

Simpson HCR, Carter RD, Lousley S, Mann JI (1982) Digestible carbohydrate – an independent effect on diabetic control in type 2 (non-insulin dependent) diabetic patients? Diabetologia 23:235–239

Spiller GA, Story JA, Wong LG et al. (1986) Effect of increasing levels of hard wheat fiber on fecal weight, minerals and steroids and gastrointestinal transit time in healthy young women. J Nutr 116:778–785

Stevens J (1988) Does dietary fiber affect food intake and body weight? J Am Diet Assoc 88:939–945

Stevens J, Van Soest PJ, Robertson JB, Levitsky DA (1988) Comparison of the effects of psyllium and wheat bran on gastrointestinal transit time and stool characteristics. J Am Diet Assoc 88:323–326

Story L, Anderson JW, Chen WJL, Karounos D, Jefferson B (1985) Adherence to high-carbohydrate, high-fiber diets: long-term studies of non-obese diabetic men. J Am Diet Assoc 85:1105–1110

Tappy L, Würsch P, Randin JP, Felber JP, Jequier E (1986) Metabolic effect of pre-cooked instant preparation of bean and potato in normal and diabetics subjects. Am J Clin Nutr 43:30–36

Tattersall RB, Mansell P (1990) Fibre in the management of diabetes: benefits of fibre itself are uncertain. Br Med J 300:1336

Tattersall RB, McCulloch DK (1985) Reply from authors to Letter to the Editor: "Conventional" and high carbohydrate/high-fibre/low-fat diets in adults with established type 1 (insulin-dependent) diabetes. Diabetologia 28:793–794

Thomas B, Elchazly M (1976) Functionelle Wirkungen und Veränderungen der Ballaststoffe des Weizens während des Verdauungsablaufes. Qual Plant: Plant Foods Hum Nutr 26:211–226

Thornton JR, Emmett PM, Heaton KW (1983) Diet and gall stones: effect of refined and unrefined carbohydrate diets on bile cholesterol saturation and bile acid metabolism. Gut 24:2–6

Torsdottir I, Alpsten M, Andersson H, Einarsson S (1989) Dietary guar gum effects on postprandial blood glucose insulin and hydroxyproline in humans. J Nutr 119:1925–1931

Trowell H (1975) Dietary fiber hypothesis of the etiology of diabetes mellitus. Diabetes 24:762–765

Venhaus A (1990) Einfluß von Ballaststoffgehalt und Verarbeitungsgrad der Lebensmittel auf den Stoffwechsel von Patienten mit Typ-1-Diabetes mellitus. Wissenschaftlicher Fachverlag, Gießen

Venhaus A, Chantelau EA (1988) Self-selected unrefined and refined carbohydrate diets do not affect metabolic control in pump-treated diabetic patients. Diabetologia 31:153–157

Wahlqvist ML, Wilmshurst EG, Murton CR, Richardson EN (1978) The effect of chain length on glucose absorption and the related metabolic response. Am J Clin Nutr 31:1998–2001

Ward GM, Simpson RW, Simpson HCR, Naylor BA, Mann JI, Turner RC (1982) Insulin receptor binding increased by high carbohydrate low fat diet in noninsulin dependent diabetics. Eur J Clin Invest 12:93–96

Weinsier RL, Seeman A, Herrera MG, Assal J-P, Soeldner JS, Gleason RE (1974) High- and low-carbohydrate diets in diabetes mellitus. Study of effects on diabetic control, insulin secretion, and blood lipids. Ann Intern Med 80:332–341

Weinsier RL, Johnston MH, Doleys DM, Bacon JA (1983) Dietary management of obesity: evaluation of the time–energy displacement diet in terms of its efficacy and nutritional adequacy for long-term weight control. Br J Nutr 47:367–379

West KM (1973) Diet therapy of diabetes: an analysis of failure. Ann Int Med 79:425–434

Weyman-Daum M, Fort P, Recker B, Lanes R, Lifshitz F (1987) Glycemic response in children with insulin-dependent diabetes mellitus after high- or low-glycemic index breakfasts. Am J Clin Nutr 46:798–803

Wishnofsky M, Kane AP (1935) The effect of equivalent amounts of dextrose and starch on glycemia and glycosuria in diabetics. Am J Med Sci 189:545–550

Würsch P (1989) Starch in human nutrition. In: Bourne GH (ed) Nutritional value of cereal products, beans and starches. Karger, Basel, pp 199–256 (World Rev Nutr Diet, vol 60)

Würsch P, Del Vedovo S, Koellreutter B (1986) Cell structure and starch nature as key determinant of the digestion rate of starch in legumes. Am J Clin Nutr 43:25–29

Wyman JB, Heaton KW, Manning AP, Wicks ACB (1976) The effect on intestinal transit and the feces of raw and cooked bran in different doses. Am J Clin Nutr 29:1474–1479

Commentary

Morris: Although the crucial distinction between soluble and insoluble fibre is clearly stated under the heading "Metabolic Effects of Fibre", no attempt has been made to relate it to the "negative evidence" quoted later on.

Guar gum originated, indeed, in tropical regions of Asia, but it is now widely available in the West as a major industrial hydrocolloid, and North American production is probably greater than (or at least comparable to) the amounts grown in Asia.

Edwards: Oesophageal obstruction after consumption of fibre preparations is probably rare, and due to inadequate formulation or instruction of use.

Flourié: Weight reduction by itself can improve diabetic control, and increased consumption of fibre may be involved in weight loss by acting on satiety and energy intake. Thus, some beneficial effects of dietary fibre on diabetic control might be directly related to fibre consumption via its effect on weight loss.

Southgate: This paper provides a good review of the role of dietary fibre in the management of diabetes mellitus. The author's decision to restrict the discussion to NIDDM is sound but I think that the possible role of dietary fibre-poor diets in the aetiology of NIDDM is dismissed too briefly. The dietary fibre hypothesis relates to a type of diet, i.e. the amounts and *types* of foods consumed and this needs to be considered in relation to the changes in incidence of NIDDM in different communities with time. I would have expected to see evidence that changes in life expectancy could account for the changes in incidence. The dietary changes that have occurred could be argued to be *one* of the environmental changes.

Heaton: Overall this is an excellent summary with a thoughtful discussion and challenging conclusions. However, I wonder if the authors do not put too much emphasis on the very slight weight loss, 0.9 kg, of the patients in the study of Simpson et al. (1981). This may have been statistically significant but it is hard to believe that it is biologically significant and contributed importantly to the improved diabetic control.

The authors quote me as having concluded in a recent review (Heaton, 1990) that dietary fibre plays a minor role in postprandial glycaemic and insulinaemic responses. Actually that article does not refer to this aspect of dietary fibre. However, our study with wheat and maize of different particle sizes (Heaton et al., 1988) would tend to support this view.

The authors suggest that drying of a foodstuff will tend to make it more digestible (by causing the matrix to collapse). However, drying of fruit makes the texture more cohesive and can reduce the insulin response. In our studies with fresh grapes (Bolton et al., 1981) and dried grapes, i.e. raisins (Oettlé et al., 1987) the fresh grapes produced a considerably larger insulin response than the raisins.

References

Bolton RP, Heaton KW, Burroughs LF (1981) The role of dietary fiber in satiety, glucose, and insulin: studies with fruit and fruit juice. Am J Clin Nutr 34:211–217

Oettlé GJ, Emmett PM, Heaton KW (1987) Glucose and insulin responses to manufactured and whole-food snacks. Am J Clin Nutr 45:86–91

(Other references are in the chapter.)

Chapter 17

Dietary Fibre and Plasma Lipids: Potential for Prevention and Treatment of Hyperlipidaemias

A.S. Truswell and A.C. Beynen

Introduction

One of the major postulates of the dietary fibre hypothesis (Trowell, 1972) was that coronary heart disease (CHD) is associated with diets low in fibre and a high-fibre diet may protect against CHD. The most obvious *direct* mechanism for such an effect is by reduction of plasma total and LDL-cholesterol, presumably by some interference with sterol metabolism which would have to start in the gastro-intestinal tract, since fibre is by definition indigestible (by human enzymes) and so not absorbable as such. It is difficult to visualise how any *other direct* mechanism could work, such as a reduced tendency to thrombosis, reduced blood pressure or reduced liability to dangerous cardiac arrhythmias, from eating more dietary fibre.

Whether or not there is a significant direct effect, it has always been likely that *indirect* effects can explain, at least partly, the negative association of dietary fibre with CHD. A high fibre intake, if obtained from foods, must come from high intakes of whole grain cereals and/or vegetables, including legumes, and/or fruits. These could displace fatty foods in the diet and so reduce saturated fat, calorie and cholesterol intakes. Alternatively they might provide extra amounts of protective substances other than fibre. Speculative possibilities here include potassium, magnesium, vitamin C, carotenoids, etc. Indirect effects of dietary fibre will be discussed later but first we will review the evidence about dietary fibre and plasma lipids. There are five questions:

(1) Can dietary fibre lower plasma lipid concentration(s) in man; if so which lipids?
(2) Which type(s) of dietary fibre has/have this effect?
(3) How much fibre is needed?
(4) What is/are the physiological and biochemical mechanism(s)?
(5) Are there undesirable effects of the lipid-lowering amount of fibre?

We have reviewed this subject at intervals (Truswell and Kay, 1976; Truswell, 1977, 1984; Kay et al., 1978; Kay and Truswell, 1980; Judd and Truswell, 1985a). The number of papers has grown and the picture becomes clearer by the method of meta-analysis. We can also recommend a recent comprehensive survey by Anderson et al. (1990a) and a useful review on guar (Gatenby, 1990).

Wheat Fibre

For researchers setting out to test the dietary fibre hypothesis in the early 1970s this was the obvious type of dietary fibre to experiment with. Trowell (1975) had reasoned that it would lower plasma cholesterol. It is available in concentrated, fairly reproducible yet natural food form as bran, or whole grain wheat breads can be readily compared with low-fibre white bread.

When we tested wheat fibre experimentally, in rats under a variety of conditions, and in hamsters, we were surprised to find no effect on the plasma cholesterol. Our results were received with polite disbelief when presented at the (British) Nutrition Society (Kay and Truswell, 1975) but a similar lack of effect was reported in rats before and after (Ranhotra, 1973; Tsai et al., 1976; Van Beresteijn et al., 1979).

In healthy human adults who ate all their meals in the metabolic unit, enough wheat fibre to almost double faecal weight had no effect on plasma cholesterol or triglycerides. We concluded our preliminary report (Truswell and Kay, 1975): "These results do not mean that all dietary fibre is without effect on plasma-lipid concentration in man. Many different substances come under this general heading and they are likely to vary qualitatively and quantitatively in different foods". The search would have to start for types of fibre that could affect plasma cholesterol, and pectin appeared very promising. This was the first paper to make it clear that different types of dietary fibre vary in their effect on plasma lipids. Ancel Keys and colleagues had, however, reported 15 years earlier (Keys et al. 1961) that cellulose did not lower plasma cholesterol in men but pectin did.

The position with wheat fibre is summarised in Table 17.1. There are now 34 reports of controlled human experiments. In 27 of them plasma cholesterol did not go down – it even rose significantly in two trials (van Dokkum, 1978; Stasse-Wolthuis et al., 1979). Most of these 27 experiments were well designed, with control–test–control (e.g. Kay and Truswell, 1977a) or crossover design (Liebman et al., 1983) or parallel control groups (Heaton et al., 1976; Stasse-Wolthuis et al., 1980) and some were of long duration (Heaton et al., 1976; Tarpila et al., 1978; Brodribb and Humphreys, 1976). In some studies all food was provided for the subjects in a metabolic unit (Jenkins et al., 1975b; Kay and Truswell, 1977a; Raymond et al., 1977; Stasse-Wolthuis et al., 1980). In the best of these negative reports frequent estimations were made of plasma cholesterol levels. Several of the research groups that could not demonstrate an effect with wheat fibre did find a cholesterol-lowering effect of pectin, using similar methods (Jenkins et al., 1975a; Durrington et al., 1975; Kay and Truswell, 1977b; Miettinen and Tarpila, 1977; Stasse-Wolthuis et al., 1980).

By contrast, in the seven papers reporting lower plasma cholesterol on wheat fibre the subjects total less than one-quarter of those in the 27 negative reports. One noted a lower cholesterol intake in the bran period; several used only one-way designs, i.e. control period followed by test period, and only one plasma cholesterol per period (Persson et al., 1975; Mathur et al., 1977; Farrell et al., 1978; Letchford et al., 1978; Van Berge-Henegouwen et al., 1979). In some cases the cholesterols were measured in the routine hospital biochemistry laboratory (Farrell et al., 1978). All the subjects were outpatients and in some cases ate *ad libitum* (Van Berge-Henegouwen et al., 1979; Mathur et al., 1977). In one interesting paper in this group, Munoz et al. (1979) reported reduction in

Table 17.1. Wheat fibre and plasma total cholesterol

Reference	Effects	Notes
Eastwood (1969)	0	28 monks; 14 g bran; 2 weeks
Eastwood et al. (1973)	0	8 men; 16 g bran; 3 weeks
Heaton and Pomare (1974)	0	6 normal, 8 cholelithiasis; 38 g bran; 5 weeks
Connell et al. (1975)	0	23 students; 28–57 g bran; 11 weeks
Truswell and Kay (1975); Kay and Truswell (1977a)	0	6 normals; 23 g bran + 167 g whole wheat bread; 3 weeks
Jenkins et al. (1975a, b)	0	6 men; 30 g bran, 77 g bran products, WW bread; 3 weeks
Durrington et al. (1975)	0	12 men; 30 g bread; 6 weeks
Bremner et al. (1975)	0	5 men hypertriglyceridaemia; 50 g bran; 12 weeks
Persson et al. (1975, 1976)	−7%	14 elderly; 20 g bran; 12 weeks
Brodribb and Humphreys (1976)	0	40 with diverticulosis; 24 g bran; 52 weeks
Heaton et al. (1976)	0	19 students; 180 g WW bread; 19 weeks
Weinreich et al. (1977)	0	25 nurses; 24 g bran; 5 weeks
Mathur et al. (1977)	↓	20 normal, 10 HL; 40 g bran; 4 weeks
Rhodes et al. (1977/8)	0	
Avgerinos et al. (1977)	−20%	6 normal; 90 g All Bran; 3 weeks (abstract only)
Raymond et al. (1977)	0	12 subjects; 72 g bran; 4 weeks metabolic ward
McDougall et al. (1978)	0	9 normal, 9 cholelithiasis; 50 g bran; 4 weeks
Letchford et al. (1978)	↓	17 subjects, no dietary control (abstract only)
Farrell et al. (1978)	↓	Same group; 14 males; short experiment
O'Moore et al. (1978)	0	12 irritable bowel; bran; 4 weeks
Tarpila et al. (1978)	0	22 diverticulosis; 25 g bran; 26–52 weeks
Dixon (1978)	0	16 normal; bran + WW bread; 13 weeks
Henry et al. (1978)	0	Bran-enriched bread
Angelico et al. (1978)	0	
Van Dokkum (1978)	↑ Sig	8 normal, metabolic ward; bread + bran cf white bread
Watts et al. (1978)	0	11 normal; 30 g bran; 8 weeks
Munoz et al. (1979)	0	6 normal; soft white bran; 4 weeks
Munoz et al. (1979)	↓	9 normal; hard red spring wheat bran; 4 weeks
Van Berge-Henegouwen et al. (1979)	−10%	7 males; 35 g bran; 4 weeks
Stasse-Wolthuis et al. (1979, 1980)	↑	Significantly ↑ 16 subjects, all food provided; 38 g bran; 5 weeks
Flanagan et al. (1980)	0	16 irritable bowel; bran; 12 weeks
Liebman et al. (1983)	0	20 overweight men; 0.5 g bran/kg; 6 weeks
Lindgärde and Larsson (1984)	0	12 men HC; 11 g conc wheat fibre; 8 weeks
Gariot et al. (1986)	0	4 normal; 20 g bran; 7 weeks
Kestin et al. (1990)	0	24 men, mild HC; 35 g bran; 4 weeks

WW, whole wheat; HL, hyperlipidaemia; HC, hypercholesterolaemia.

plasma cholesterol when subjects ate bran from hard red spring wheat but not with ordinary soft white wheat bran.

Except for the possibility this raises – that there might be some reproducible "super-bran" – it is clear that wheat fibre does not have a cholesterol-lowering effect. In recent years wheat bran has been used as the placebo control in trials on guar (Vaaler et al., 1986; Bremner et al., 1986; Fuessl et al., 1987) and on oat bran (Storch et al., 1984).

The possibility remains that wheat fibre might raise HDL-cholesterol (Trowell, 1978), even if it does not lower plasma total cholesterol. This was reported by O'Moore et al. (1978) and Lindgärde and Larsson (1984). In the earlier trials of wheat fibre only total cholesterol was measured, not lipoprotein fractions. However, in most papers that do report HDL-cholesterol it was not changed significantly by wheat fibre (McDougall et al., 1978; Dixon, 1978; Stasse-Wolthuis et al., 1979; Flanagan et al., 1980; Gariot et al., 1986; Kestin et al., 1990). Wheat fibre has no consistent effect on fasting plasma triglycerides (Truswell and Kay, 1976).

Pectin

Pectin is one component of the dietary fibre in all fruits and vegetables, averaging around 1% of wet weight. It is not fibrous but forms a viscous solution; it is used as a gelling agent, e.g. for jams, and is a by-product of the apple and citrus juice industry. It is therefore available as a concentrated form of one chemical type of dietary fibre (polygalacturonic acid, with variable degrees of esterification by methoxyl groups). Because it is very viscous it has to be handled in experiments differently from wheat bran. We gave it mixed with raspberries and a little sugar, as a sort of superjam (Kay and Truswell, 1977b) or with blackcurrant juice (Judd and Truswell, 1982), and taken with meals. The human experiments with pectin are summarised in Table 17.2. This shows a very different picture from the results with wheat fibre. Sixteen of the 19 authors report some fall of plasma total cholesterol, 10 of them statistically significant. Though some of the papers report outpatient trials, several are very well controlled experiments (Keys et al., 1961; Kay and Truswell, 1977b; Miettinen and Tarpila, 1977; Stasse-Wolthuis et al., 1979; Judd and Truswell, 1982).

Only three papers report no change. These represent less than one-fifth of the number of subjects in the 16 that report cholesterol reduction, and these three papers used an unreliable one-way design: control, then test, with only one blood sample for each period.

Citrus pectin was used in at least nine trials; apple pectin in three. The usual dose of purified pectin has been 15 g per day (given as 5 g with each of the three main meals) but doses have ranged from 2 g to nearly 50 g per day. The average plasma cholesterol reduction was about −10% (i.e. *not* mg per dl) but it was often over 10%. Cholesterol reductions were no greater when the dose was more than 15 g/day. Below this dose cholesterol reductions tended to be less. In 1977 we published a graph (Kay and Truswell, 1977b) based on the literature to that time, suggesting a linear response up to about 15 g/day but little further effect beyond this. The data in Table 17.2 seem to support this but there is a shortage of well-designed experiments with low dosages of pectin.

Pectin appears to be more effective taken as a gel with meals than in biscuits (Keys et al., 1961) or capsules (Palmer and Dixon, 1966). Its effect is on LDL-cholesterol, and probably apo-B lipoprotein (Durrington et al., 1976), not on HDL or triglycerides. Plasma cholesterol is lowered by about the same percentage in normals and in people with hypercholesterolaemia and this effect is well established by one week (Judd and Truswell, 1982). Pectin was fully effective when given to patients with familial hypercholesterolaemia already

Table 17.2. Pectin

Reference	Subjects	Pectin	Design	Effect on plasma cholesterol (total)	Remarks
Keys et al. (1961), USA	24 male mental patients. NL	15 g/day in biscuit (3 for 3 weeks). Pectin NF (citrus)	In metabolic ward; Strictly controlled diet; 8 groups multiple crossover and placebo-controlled	−4.7%, Sig	Mean of 4.8% and 4.6% on 2 different basal diets (Italian or American types). No effect of cellulose in same series
Fahrenbach et al. (1965), USA	23 normals	6 g/day for 66 days and 12 g/day for 52 days		No change	
Fisher et al. (1965), USA	Not given. Normocholesterolaemic	Not given	Diets with and without 2 eggs per day	When dietary cholesterol 0, NS When dietary cholesterol +, −15%	Letter to the editor, they suggest pectin only lowers cholesterol when it is in the diet
Palmer and Dixon (1966), USA	16 subjects	Pectin NF (citrus) in capsules: 2 or 4 or 6 or 8 or 10 g/day taken bd	6 four-week pectin periods, different doses randomised. Outpatients; placebo-controlled	−2% to −6% with increasing dose	See plot in Kay and Truswell (1977b)
Hopson (1967), USA Lopez et al. (1968), USA	3 subjects	20–23 g/day for 5 weeks		−13%	↑ faecal bile acids
Weinand and Sack (1970), Germany	94 middle-aged people with PI cholesterol > 300 mg/dl	Pectin granulate. Dose and method of taking not described	Started with 128 outpatients. 34 did not return or otherwise unsuitable	↓ in 73/94 (Sig)	Reduction of plasma cholesterol 1%–10% in 19 patients 10%–20% in 30 patients 20%–30% in 20 patients over 30% in 4 patients

Continued on next page

Table 17.2. Continued

Reference	Subjects	Pectin	Design	Effect on plasma cholesterol (total)	Remarks
Jenkins et al. (1975a), UK	7 healthy men	Pectin (Bulmers) 36 g/day in powder form taken in water or orange juice just before meals for 2 weeks	Baseline then pectin for 2 weeks. Blood before and at end of the period	−13%	36 g of guar produced 16% reduction of plasma cholesterol. Jenkins et al. (Clin. Sci., 1976, 51:8) ↑ faecal bile acids
Durrington et al. (1976), UK	12 healthy men, 22–45 years	12 g/day Bulmers pectin powder in water or juice tid before meals for 3 weeks	Continued their usual diets. 2 cholesterols before then 4, (2 days, 7 days, 14 days, 21 days) on pectin	−8%, Sig	Stool wet weight 150 → 186 g/day. No clear change in TGs. Apo-B ↓
Kay and Truswell (1977b), UK	9 healthy adults (4 male, 5 female); postgrads or staff in nutrition	Citrus pectin (Bulmers) 15 g/day, taken tid in fruit gel with meals	2-week control period before and after 3-week pectin period. Bloods last 3 mornings of each period. Controlled diet in metabolic unit	−13%, Sig	Faecal bile acids ↑ 33%, neutral steroids ↑ 17%. TGs NC
Delbarre et al. (1977), France	23 with different types of moderate HC	Lemon pectin 6 g/day or apple pectin 6 g/day. Both given tid and for 6 weeks	10 given lemon pectin, 13 different patients given apple pectin. 1 blood before and after 6 weeks on pectin	+5 lemon pectin, NS −4 apple pectin, NS	Lemon pectin 6.3% methyl groups; apple pectin 10.5%
Langley and Thye (1977), USA	33 healthy men	10 g/day citrus pectin for 4 weeks (Sunkist). Groups 3 and 4 wheat bran, group 5 some pectin only	OP fasting blood sample collected 3 weeks before, 4 weeks during and 2 weeks after the experimental period	Gps 3, 4 and 5 ↓ cf 2 and 1, Sig	Group 1: 45 g bran/day Group 2: 90 g bran/day Group 3: 10 g pectin + 45 g bran Group 4: 10 g pectin + 90 g bran Group 5: 10 g pectin (only)/day

Miettinen and Tarpila (1977), Finland	9 HL and 2 N	40 to 50 g/day "Firmagel", starting 20 g/day working up for 2 weeks	7 in metabolic ward. Controlled diet. 2 weeks control then 2 weeks pectin	−13%, Sig	Faecal bile acids ↑ +51% ($P<0.005$); neutral sterols +10%. Increased serum methyl sterols (suggests ↑ chol synthesis). TGs NC. But ↑ faecal steroids less than on cholestyramine
Ginter et al. (1979), Czechoslovakia	21 HC, mild to moderate (mean 278 mg/dl) = men and women. 11 HL, some type IV some type II	15 g/day for 6 weeks + ascorbic acid (AA)	Outpatients, self-controlled; one month control, then 6 weeks on pectin + ascorbic. Blood at start, 3 and 6 weeks	−9% Sig −19% Sig	Subjects also given 450 mg/day ascorbic acid (AA) -HDL and TG NS They suggest AA potentiates pectin by stimulating cholesterol → bile acids
Stasse-Wolthuis et al. (1980), The Netherlands	15 normals	9 g/day for 5 weeks Citrus pectin (Bulmers)	Self-controlled; parallel. Diets well controlled. Prior control and parallel. 2 bloods end control and pectin	−7% Sig (more at 2 weeks)	HDL NS. Increased faecal bile acids (0.77→1.16 mmol/day) Sig
Richter et al. (1981), Germany	10 older stable patients with HC, type IIa, mean cholesterol 374 mg/dl	Apple pectin granulate 18 g/day (12% methoxy taken with main meals for 4 weeks)	On lipid lowering diet as before. Medications stopped 2 months before. 1 month control, then 1 month pectin. 1 blood before cf 1 blood on pectin (not randomised). Outpatients	−3%	But 7 of the 10 responded and their cholesterol fell by mean −11%
Schwandt et al. (1982), Germany	6 men, familial hypercholesterolaemia, 5 with tendon xanthomata. Serum cholesterols Ave 11.4 mmol on diet alone	Pectin 12g/day as granulate for 8 weeks (12% methoxy) supplied by Merck. Apple pectin	Outpatients. Off other treatments; stabilised on 30% fat diet (P/S = 1). Then cholestyramine (48 g/day) for 2 months. Then pectin added	−19% Sig	Pectin effective; additional effect when added to maximally tolerated dose of cholestyramine; LDL ↓ 12%; HDL ↓ 12% (latter NS) TG up on cholestyramine; no change on pectin

Continued on next page

Table 17.2. Continued

Reference	Subjects	Pectin	Design	Effect on plasma cholesterol (total)	Remarks
Judd and Truswell (1982), UK	10 normals, nutrition postgraduates or staff (5 men, 5 women)	Pectin, 15 g/day, taken tid in jelly with blackcurrant juice, with meals for 2 weeks (LMP) and 2 weeks (HMP). Citrus (Bulmers) LMP 37% methoxy; HMP usual methoxy 70%	Carefully controlled normal diet. 1 week control, then 2 weeks low methoxy → 2 weeks high methoxy pectin or (randomised) vice versa. Bloods for cholesterol last 3 days (F) of each week. Faeces doubly marked	−16% Sig on LMP −18% Sig on HMP LMP cf HMP NS	Pl cholesterol down after 1 week (L&H-MP). No difference in faecal steroids between L and HMP (mean 888 mg per day on HMP; 811 mg per day on LMP)
Hillman et al. (1985), NZ	10 normals (2 male medical students and 8 female postgraduate nurses)	12 g/day pectin for 4 weeks (9.3% methoxyl content on dry basis from Yahkin Canning, Tel Aviv), to be taken tid with meals	Outpatients, self-controlled crossover. Usual diets, no pectin in the other 4 weeks. ½ control 1st; ½ pectin 1st. Only one blood at end of each period (F)	No change (slight rise NS)	No change in HDL or TG "Subjects experienced great difficulty in taking the full amount of pectin because of its gelling properties". Authors couldn't explain discrepancy between these results and the effects reported by others.
Vargo et al. (1985)	10 normals, volunteers	15 g/day for 3 weeks, taken with meals with fruit and sugar as gel; citrus pectin	Outpatients. 1st 7 days control then 3 weeks on pectin. Blood for 6 subjects after 14 days and for 9 subjects after 21 days. Food intake diaries 28 days	−18% Sig at 2 weeks −10% NS at 3 weeks	No change in HDL or TG

HC, hypercholesterolaemia; HDL, high-density lipoprotein; LDL, low-density lipoprotein; NC, no change; NF (pectin), National Formulary; Nl, normal (plasma) lipids; NS, not significant; Sig, (statistically) significant; OP, outpatient(s); Pl, plasma; P/S, polyunsaturated/saturated ratio (fatty acids); TG, triglyceride; tid, three times a day; bd, twice a day.

taking large doses of the bile acid-binding resin, cholestyramine (Schwandt et al., 1982).

Accepting that large amounts of purified pectin lower plasma LDL and total cholesterol, what is the mechanism? There are two main hypotheses. One, first proposed for humans by Kay and Truswell (1977b) is interference with reabsorption of bile acids in the small intestine, either by chemical binding or as a direct result of viscous entrapment. This leads to a negative sterol balance. The alternative hypothesis (Anderson and Chen, 1979) is that fermentation of pectin in the large bowel produces volatile fatty acids, which are absorbed into the portal vein and could suppress hepatic cholesterol synthesis. Propionate inhibits cholesterol synthesis from [^{14}C]acetate in isolated rat liver cells (Anderson and Bridges, 1981).

In all of the six sets of experiments (Table 17.2) in which faecal bile acids were measured they were significantly higher in the pectin periods (Lopez et al., 1968; Jenkins et al., 1976; Kay and Truswell, 1977b; Miettinen and Tarpila, 1977; Stasse-Wolthuis et al., 1980; Nakamura et al., 1982). For comparison faecal bile acids are not usually increased when extra wheat bran is given (Kay and Truswell, 1980). Increased bile acids were excreted by ileostomy patients given pectin (Bosaeus et al., 1986). The same occurs in rats (Leveille and Sauberlich, 1966) and mice (Komai and Kimura, 1987). The cause of the faecal loss of bile acids is more likely entrapment from viscosity than chemical binding because pectin is acidic. Guar, which does not have carboxyl groups has a similar effect (see below), and there is little difference between the cholesterol-lowering effect of low and high methoxy pectins in man (Judd and Truswell, 1982b). The intestinal contents of rats that were given pectin are very different from control animals. When centrifuged a supernatant liquid does not usually separate and the pellet is sticky (Judd and Truswell, 1985b). The small intestines are fuller and larger. NMR spectroscopy indicates that interactions of pectin and bile acids are not the result of chemical reactions but probably due to viscosity effects (Pfeffer et al., 1981). The extra loss of bile acids in the faeces is, however, only about a quarter of that seen with cholestyramine (Miettinen and Tarpila, 1977).

The fermentation and volatile fatty acid inhibition hypothesis has not been directly demonstrated. Pectin still lowers plasma cholesterol in germ-free mice (Komai and Kimura, 1987) and in rats given oral succinylsulphathiazole to inhibit colonic bacteria (Leveille and Sauberlich, 1966; Vahouny, 1982). It is ineffective when administered intra-caecally in minipigs (Ahrens et al., 1986). Hepatic cholesterol synthesis was reported as *increased* in pectin-fed rats (Mokady, 1974; Nishina et al., 1991). Propionate feeding does lower plasma cholesterol in pigs but the reduction is only of HDL (Thacker and Bowland, 1981). Illman et al. (1988) found that in experiments with rats and pigs hepatic cholesterol synthesis was not reduced when propionate was fed and the concentration attainable in the hepatic vein after oral propionate, and after feeding pectin (Illman et al., 1982), is less than that needed to suppress cholesterol synthesis in perfused liver preparations.

Guar

Guar gum is used in the food industry as a thickening agent, a natural product from the seed of the leguminous plant *Cyamopsis tetragonoloba*. The active

Table 17.3. Guar

Reference	Subjects	Dose, type, duration	Design	Pl cholesterol (total)	Other effects
Fahrenbach et al. (1965), USA	Normals and HC	6, 12 and 18 g/day before meals. 66 and 45 days	Inpatients	−5% ↓ Sig	
Jenkins et al. (1975), UK	Normals	'Norgine' powder just before or during meals with water or as a gel. 2 weeks, 36 g/day	Free-living	↓	Not with wheat fibre Guar more effect than pectin
Jenkins et al. (1976), UK	HC (type II), $n = 7$	15 g/day guar gum, soup or powder mixed with foods start of each meal, 2 weeks		↓	
Jenkins et al. (1979a), UK	10 HC whose Pl cholesterols had been stable	15 g/day (5 g tid) before meals in special soup or mixed with food, 2 weeks, H. J. Heinz	Outpatients	−11% ↓ Sig	TC fell in 3 who stayed on cholestyramine −18%. TG NC
Jenkins et al. (1979b), UK	22 normals, hospital staff or students; 3 actually took guar	20 g/day guar (or other fibres) for 3 weeks	Controlled diets. Lived in or near students res, Central Middlesex Hospital, London	−13% ↓	Wheat fibre −ve no change HDL 31 g pectin also ↓ TC by 13%
Jenkins et al. (1980), UK	11 HL	Ave 13 g/day in guar crispbreads for 2 to 8 weeks		−13% ↓	Not HDL or TG
Tuomilehto et al. (1980), Finland	Middle-aged females HC	Guar gum 15 g/day	Double-blind, controlled trial	No change	
Botha et al. (1981), South Africa	10 IDDs	Guar gum in buttermilk rusks (Ave 22 g/day) for 3 months		−17% ↓ Sig	No improvement in glycosylated Hb
Khan et al. (1981), USA	24 normal volunteers	Guar gum in capsule form, total 9 g/day for 4 weeks	Double-blind, glucose in placebo caps	−17% ↓ Sig	
Aro et al. (1981), Finland	9 NIDDs	Granulated guar gum, 3 doses, at main meals. Total 21 g/day 3 months	Double-blind, cross-over	−14% ↓	LDL ↓ not HDL

Reference	Subjects	Treatment	Design	% change	Effects
Carroll et al. (1981), NZ	6 IDDs	Guar in biscuits, 6–60 g/day for 4–6 weeks	In general practice	Small reduction	Little improvement in diabetic control
Johansen (1981)	10 NIDDs on sulphonylureas	Granulated guar, 18 g/day for 4 weeks		↓ Sig	Urine glucose fell
Kyllästinen and Lahikainen (1981), Finland	41 elderly NIDDs	Granulated guar, 16 g/day for 2 months		−12% ↓	Little change in diabetic control. No change HDL
Rasmussen et al. (1981), Denmark	10 NIDDs	Guar gum granulate (Sloose) in water, 4 g before meals for 3 months, 12 g/day	Double-blind cross-over trial	NS	Did not appear to improve diabetes
Wirth et al. (1982), Germany	12 HC (type IIa)	Guar 15.6 g/day	Crossover: guar + bezafibrate compared with bezafibrate alone	−7% ↓.	Apo B ↓. HDL, VLDL and TGs normal
Simons et al. (1982), Australia	17 HC	New guar formulation, 6 g tid with meals for 3 months (Wellcome preparation)	Placebo-controlled single-blind study	−15% ↓ Sig	LDL ↓ 20%. No change in HDL
Smith and Holm (1982), Sweden	6 normals, 6 IDDs, 11 NIDDs	Specially processed palatable guar gum 10 g bd immediately before meals. Total 20 g/day for 1–3 weeks (or longer)		−14% ↓	HDL NS TG NC
Tuomilehto et al. (1983), Finland	12 obese HC males	'Guarem', 5 g in water just before meals. Total 15 g/day for 3 months	Double-blind cross-over	−5% ↓	NC HDLs TG slightly higher
Catenazzo et al. (1983), Italy	10 normals	Test meal of pasta, egg, bacon and cheese or guar	Test meal		↓ postprandial TGs and glucose
Tagliaferro et al. (1985), Italy	8 newly diagnosed NIDDs (mild)	Guar gum, 8 g/day (4 g guar flour in 200 ml water) for 6 weeks		−11% ↓	HDL NS
Gatti et al. (1984), Italy	Small numbers of normal HL and NIDD	Guar-enriched pasta 'Cesalpinia'		↓	

Continued on next page

Table 17.3. Continued

Reference	Subjects	Dose, type, duration	Design	Pl cholesterol (total)	Other effects
Bosello et al. (1984) and Cominacini et al. (1985), Italy	12 familial combined HL	16 g guar gum/day for 60 days. Made by Guidotti (gels easily)	Outpatients	↓ Sig	HDL NC ↓ LDL and TG ↓ apo c-III o
Aro et al. (1984), Finland	14 HC males	5 g 'Guarem' tid (15 g/day) in water (before gelling) immediately before meals, for 12 weeks	Double-blind cross-over	−12% ↓ Sig	Not HDL. Total cholesterol Sig at 6 weeks, less low at 12 weeks and then NS
Najemnik et al. (1984)	Diabetics 38 IDDs, 41 on sulphonylureas	Guar minitablets, 5 g tid (= 15 g/day). 2 weeks	2 weeks treatment with pre- and post-controls. Crossover design	−25% ↓ Sig	Sig lowering 1 hour postprandial blood glucose
Uusitupa et al. (1984), Finland	17 NIDDS	Guar gum with meals tid. Dose gradually increased to 21 g/day for 18 weeks	Double-blind, placebo-controlled trial	−11% ↓	Not HDL. Slight but NS improvement in diabetic control
Peterson et al. (1984), UK	12 NIDDs (4 on diet alone, 8 on tablets)	Guar bread (6 g) or guar granulate (10 g) for 6 weeks	Randomised crossover of 3 × 6 week periods; control was bread without guar	−10% ↓	Improved FBG and HbA1c and TGs
Krotkiewski (1984), Sweden	9 obese non-diabetics	Granulated guar ('Lejguar') 20 g/day for 8 weeks		−8% ↓	Not HDL or TG
Penagini et al. (1986), Italy	6 normal males	Guar 5.7 g bd in crispbread (12 g/day) for 2 weeks		−16% ↓ Sig	No Sig change in transit times
McNaughton et al. (1985), USA	28 female diabetics, 13 diabetics	2.5 g Guar gum baked in rolls 2/day (total 5 g/day) 12 weeks	Free-living	−5% ↓ −14%	2 experiments one after the other
Dalzell et al. (1985), N. Ireland	11 NIDDs poorly controlled on diet though complaint	20 g guar/day as tablets in divided doses for 6 weeks	Trial with control periods	↓ −20%	↓ urine glucose
Jones et al. (1985), England	20 diabetics (12 NIDD, 8 IDD)	Boehringer guar granules 5 g bd (total 10 g/day) for 2 months	Outpatients Trial with control periods before and after	NS	Glycosylated Hb ↓ Urine glucose NC

Reference	Subjects	Treatment	Design	Result	Comments
Dodson et al. (1981), UK	6 IDDs	Granulated guar 20 g/day for 3 months mixed with orange juice		NS	
Ray et al. (1983), USA	12 obese NIDDs, poorly controlled	Granulated guar, 20 g/day sprinkled over food, for 2 months	Outpatients but admitted for special studies	−30% ↓ Sig	HDL, NS; TG NS; 10 g wheat bran as well
Vaaler et al. (1986), Norway	28 IDDs	Guar gum 29 g/day in bread spread through the day for 3 months	3 periods of 3 months: randomised crossover cf wheat bran bread and lower fibre period	→	Diabetic control seemed to improve about as much on bran but not Pl cholesterol
Tognarelli et al. (1986), Italy	10 obese females (not diabetic)	Guar pasta, 10 g guar per day, for 7 days	Compared with wheat pasta	→	Lower glucose and insulin response as well
Bremer et al. (1986), NZ	12 poorly controlled NIDDs	Guar bread compared with wheat bran bread (each 5 g fibre/day for 1 month each)	Crossover trial	−11% ↓	No worthwhile reductions in BG (only lower peak postprandial BG)
McIvor et al. (1986), USA	16 obese NIDDs	Granola bars with 6.5 g guar, 4–6 bars/day for 6 months	Outpatients	NS slight rise	↓ LDL in males. Beneficial effect on the CH_2O metabolism
Atkins et al. (1987), UK	7 NIDDs	Granulated guar (5 g in 200 ml water) before each meal for 1 month		NS, but lower	
Fuessl et al. (1987), UK	18 NIDDs	'Guarem' 5 g sprinkled over food at each meal (= 15 g/day) for 4 weeks	Double-blind cross-over trial. Control 5 g wheat bran (2 weeks washout between)	−10% ↓	↓ LDL, not HDL; Improved FBG, glycosylated Hb and postprandial BG
Holman et al. (1987), UK	29 NIDDs (near normal FBG)	5 g guar minitablets tid with meals for 8 weeks	Compared with placebo in random crossover	LDL ↓ −10%	No improvement of diabetic control; HDL NC
Superko et al. (1988), USA	50 men moderate HC	3 forms of guar (all 15 g/day): a) medium viscosity solid b) medium viscosity liquid c) high viscosity liquid 4 weeks	Compared with placebo 2 × 4 weeks trial outpatients single-blind crossover	−10% ↓ medium viscosity; −14% ↓ high viscosity	

Continued on next page

Table 17.3. Continued

Reference	Subjects	Dose, type, duration	Design	Pl cholesterol (total)	Other effects
Ebeling et al. (1988), Finland	9 IDDs on continuous subcutaneous insulin	'Guarem' with meals 4 times/day (= 20 g/day) for 4 weeks	Crossover, with placebo	−21% ↓ Sig	Insulin requirements lower. Postprandial glucose lower; but not FBG or glycosylated Hb
Tuomilehto et al. (1988), Finland	29 HC (23 finished) Pl cholesterol >9 mmol/l	15 g/day rising to 30 g/day as 'Guarem' (tid) for 1 year	Open plan trial 1 month placebo start and finish	−10% ↓	LDL ↓ 15% and apo B. HDL and TG NS
Tuomilehto et al. (1989), Finland	29 HC whose cholesterol > 6.25 on bezafibrate	'Guarem' 5 g tid mixed with food at meals (= 15 g/day) for 3 months	Double-blind crossover. Patients continued bezafibrate	−13% ↓ Sig	LDL ↓ HDL NS TG NC
Uusitupa et al. (1989), Finland	39 NIDDs, poorly controlled on diet or oral agents	'Guarem' 5 g tid before meal, premixed with juice, milk or water (= 15 g/day) for 3 months	3 month crossover cf placebo, then 10-month open trial (placebo granules wheat flour)	−13% ↓ Sig	No consistent changes HDL and TG. No clear improvement of diabetic control

HC, hypercholesterolaemia; HL, hyperlipidaemia; TG(s), triglyceride(s); IDD, insulin-dependent diabetic; NIDD, non-insulin-dependent diabetic; tid, three times a day; bd, twice a day; Pl, plasma; TC, total cholesterol; Hb, haemoglobin; Sig, statistically significant reduction; NS, not significant; NC, no change; BG, blood glucose; FBG, fasting blood glucose; HDL, high density lipoprotein; LDL, low density lipoprotein; res, residence.

substance is a galactomannan. Guar appears to be a good model with which to examine the effect of increased luminal viscosity on small intestinal function (Garcia et al., 1988) The published human experiments and trials on guar and plasma lipids are summarised in Table 17.3. There are over 100 reports on guar; those not reviewed here do not report plasma lipids or are in inaccessible publications.

There have been more trials with guar than other forms of dietary fibre because in large dosage it lowers the plasma glucose response to meals and has become a second-line drug for diabetes mellitus in some clinics. In 23 of the papers in Table 17.3 the subjects were diabetics; in 20 they were either normals or people with hyperlipidaemia (not diabetics) and two papers report on diabetics and non-diabetics. The dose of guar has usually been 5 g thrice daily (15 g/day) but in a few experiments it was as low as 8 or as high as 36 g/day. Catenazzo et al. (1983) report only on postprandial plasma (triglycerides were lower). In the other reports plasma (total) cholesterols were lower in 39 out of 44 papers. Many of these trials with guar had good designs, e.g. double-blind crossovers. Over 750 subjects participated. Where the percentage change is available, the average in diabetics (15 papers) was −15% and in non-diabetics −11%. When guar and pectin have been compared in the same laboratory guar had a rather greater cholesterol-lowering action (Jenkins et al., 1976).

Incidentally, pectin also reduces glycaemia after meals (Jenkins et al., 1977) but unlike guar its use has not been taken up as a treatment for diabetes. Several pharmaceutical companies have provided preparations of guar targeted at the diabetic market. As with pectin, plasma total cholesterol and LDL-cholesterol are reduced by guar; HDL-cholesterol and triglyceride are not changed consistently. In some papers a dissociation can be seen between the plasma glucose-lowering and cholesterol-lowering actions. Guar is more likely to be effective in lowering cholesterol than in controlling diabetes (Botha et al., 1981; Kyllastinen and Lahikainen, 1981; Peterson and Mann, 1985; Bremer et al., 1986; Holman et al., 1987; Uusitupa et al., 1989). Increased viscosity of small intestinal contents evidently has more effect on sterol metabolism than on glucose absorption.

It is important that guar is taken with food (Peterson and Mann, 1985). It is viscous and rather unpalatable. Some patients have found it unacceptable. As well as several pharmaceutical preparations taken in water or sprinkled on food, different workers have incorporated it in soups, crispbreads, rusks, biscuits, pasta or bread. Guar products vary in physico-chemical properties (Ellis et al., 1986).

Guar slows the rate of diffusion of cholesterol mixed micelles in vitro at concentrations as low as 0.25% (Phillips, 1986). It appears to inhibit convection effects of intestinal movements (Edwards et al., 1988). In vivo it binds or entraps bile acids (Gallaher and Schneeman, 1986). There are two reports of increased bile acid excretion with guar gum (Jenkins et al., 1976; Miettinen, 1980).

Oat Fibre

We started human experiments on rolled oats in 1977 (Judd and Truswell, 1981). Wheat fibre did not appear to lower plasma cholesterol and we were looking for another major food that might. An early letter in *The Lancet* by de Groot et al. (1963) describing a 10% reduction of plasma cholesterol by people who took 140 g rolled oats daily had not been followed up. There were a couple of animal experiments in chicks with similar results and it was known that the carbohydrate of oats includes a sticky gum. This might have an effect like pectin.

Hugh Trowell wrote to Truswell on 30 December 1976 "I am very thrilled that you are starting soon to evaluate oatmeal. I am pretty certain that it is very different from the fibre of whole wheat. For many months now I take a very large helping of oatmeal every morning, about 140 g/day . . . ". He wrote that in January 1977 he would be visiting Professor Anderson at Lexington. We found that the effects of rolled oats are intermediate between those of wheat fibre and those of pectin (Judd and Truswell, 1981). Plasma cholesterol fell by 8% but this was only approaching statistical significance. J.W. Anderson reported just before us rather more enthusiastically about oat bran (Anderson, 1980) and in the late 1980s oat bran became fashionable and expensive following the popular book by Kowalski *The 8 Week Cholesterol Cure*, which dramatised the publications by Anderson's group. Consequently many doctors found that their patients were "eating quantities of oat bran with definite effects on the bowel but with unknown effects on the plasma cholesterol level" (Connor, 1990). Many foods with added oat bran appeared on the market. The pendulum, has, however swung back since Swain et al. (1990) reported no significant effect of oat fibre in *The New England Journal of Medicine*.

Table 17.4 summarises the published experiments on oat meal or oat bran. The first two questions to be settled are: does oat fibre directly lower plasma cholesterol? And is there a difference in biological effect between oat bran and whole ground oats (rolled oats)? Of the 21 trials, as many as seven report no worthwhile percentage reduction of plasma cholesterol (3% reduction or less), some after substantial consumption of oats (Kretsch et al., 1979; Roth and Leitzmann, 1985; Van Horn et al., 1986, 1988; Birkeland et al., 1990; Swain et al., 1990; Leadbetter et al., 1991). But in the most publicised of the papers with negative results, by Swain et al. (1990), the subjects had plasma total cholesterols averaging only 4.44 mmol/l (170 mg/dl); their fat and energy intakes were higher in the oat bran period, and although total cholesterols were only 3% less on oat bran than on the comparison low-fibre diet, the ratio of LDL/HDL was actually 9% less (the statistical significance of this latter number was not reported) on oat bran than in the low-fibre comparison period.

The most encouraging results are those by Anderson's group in 1984 (Anderson et al., 1984a, b; Storch et al., 1984). It comes as some surprise to find that the first two of these had very small numbers of subjects and a one-way design (control–oat bran). The third was only published in abstract. Except for the trial by Demark-Wahnefried et al. (1990) (in which less fat was consumed in the oat meal periods), all the other papers reported plasma cholesterol reductions of 10% or less and most nearer 5% on substantial intakes of oats or oat bran.

There are two further questions. One is whether the polyunsaturated oil of oats (7 to 10 g/100 g) influenced any of the results. Our experiment was the only one in which a simulated oat oil was given in the control periods (Judd and Truswell, 1981). The other question is that oat bran is not a clearly separable fraction like wheat bran and until recently authors have not tested the product they used for its β-glucan content. The American Association of Cereal

Table 17.4. Oat bran and oat meal

Reference	Oats preparation and diet	Subjects	Dose	Design	Initial Pl cholesterol (TC)	Change of TC	Change of LDL/HDL/TG	Remarks
de Groot et al. (1963), Netherlands	Rolled oats in bread	21 healthy volunteers, male, 30–35 years	140 g/day 3 weeks	Free-living EC Control bread	251	251 246 223 −10%		In parallel rat experiments extracted oat lipid appeared to have about the same cholesterol-lowering effect as defatted rolled oats
Luyken et al. (1965), Netherlands	Rolled oats in bread	95 adults 76 male, 19 female	50 g/day	4-week periods, free-living ECC CEE	248 in men 237 in women	NS after 4 weeks; −6% after 8 weeks		They did further experiments with some subjects on high, some on medium, some on low fat diets. Least oats effect on low fat
Kretsch et al. (1979), USA	Oatbran, untoasted or toasted. Dietary cholesterol 250 mg/day	6 healthy American males	0.6 g/kg BW 15 days	4 diets compared egg-formula (EF); EF + untoasted oat bran (OB); EF + toasted OB; Guatemalan rural		NC	NS	Faecal wet weight almost double on OB diets but little change in transit time. Faecal bile acids ↑ 20% on toasted OB and less than this on untoasted
Judd and Truswell (1981), England	Rolled oats 37% fat, strictly controlled in metabolic unit	10 Nutrition graduates, 6 male, 4 female, 24–37 years	Mean 125 g/day (range 110–160) incorporated into each meal 3 weeks	CEC Bloods taken last 3 mornings (F) of each period	5.26 mmol/l	−8% $0.05 < P < 0.1$	0 0	In control periods an imitation oat oil was given, so this experiment tested only the fibre effect. Faecal bile acids increased 35% in oat periods (not neutral steroids)

Continued on the next page

Table 17.4. Continued

Reference	Oats preparation and diet	Subjects	Dose	Design	Initial Pl cholesterol (TC)	Change of TC	Change of LDL/HDL/TG	Remarks
Kirby et al. (1981), USA	Oat bran preparation (Quaker Oats)	In metabolic ward constant fat and cholesterol, 8 males, 35–62 years "Hypercholesterolaemia"	100 g/day 10 days	CE EC Randomised	263 mg/dl (150–354)	-13%	-13% 0 -2%	Faecal bile acids increased 54% on oat bran (neutral steroids did not)
Anderson et al. (1984a), USA	Oat bran Metabolic ward, strictly controlled	10/20 men (34–66 years) "Hypercholesterolaemic" (10 given beans; 10 given oat bran)	100 g/day	7 days control, then 3 weeks experiment C-OB (n = 10) C-beans (n = 10)	(6) 257 with normal TGs (4) 313 with raised TGs	-19%	-23% (calc) slightly lower (more in those who lost weight)	Note short control period and only before. Subjects lost weight on OB. On beans (pinto + navy, also 100 g) TC also appeared to fall by 19% OB increased faecal bile acids
Anderson et al. (1984b), USA	Oat bran Metabolic ward, strictly controlled	4/10 men (46–66 years) Hypercholesterolaemia	100 g/day	7 days control, then 3 weeks experiment C-OB (n = 4) C-beans (n = 6)	309 mg	-23%	-23% -20% -21%	Loss of weight in hospital 1.8kg Note: not 10 but only 4 men on OB Follow-up all 10 men 24 and 99 weeks on OB + bean supplement (50 g OB prescribed) and pl TC remained down
Storch et al. (1984), USA	Oat bran Outpatients Self-controlled	12 normal subjects maintaining their usual diets and activities	53 g/day 6 weeks	Crossover Placebo wheat bran washout between		-12%	No change	Only reported in abstract TC minus 6 on wheat bran
Roth and Leitzmann (1985), Germany	Rolled oats Outpatients Self-controlled	18 normal subjects	19 g/day 12 weeks	Placebo		+2	NC +23% HDL NC	

Study	Regimen	Subjects	Dose	Design	Baseline	TC change	Lipid change	Comments
Van Horn et al. (1986), USA	Oat bran or oatmeal Background AHA fat-modified diet Outpatients	208 healthy adult male and female volunteers (30–65 years)	Oat bran prescription 60 g/day but consumption averaged 39 g. Estimated 35 g of oatmeal	6-week periods C-C C-OB C-oatmeal	208 mg/dl	−3% on oat bran −3% on oatmeal	−3 (OB) −3 (OM) NC +5 (OB)	There would have been a larger intake of oat oil in the oatmeal group
Turnbull and Leeds (1987), England	Rolled oats Outpatients Self-controlled	17 normal subjects TC above 6.0	150 g/day 4 weeks	Crossover, randomly assigned; wheat fibre control diet		−5% (P < 0.02)	−14% +17 +18	Quoted by Anderson et al. (1990)
Gold and Davidson (1988), USA	Oat bran Free-living	72 medical students 19 had oat bran 53 controls (mean age 26 years)	2 oat bran muffins = 17 g oat bran/day 4 weeks	Randomly assigned. Initial blood, then wheat muffins, oat/wheat muffins or oat bran muffins	179 mg/dl	−5%	−9% (calc) NC −8%	Two blood samples only, at beginning and end of 28-day period
Van Horn et al. (1988), USA	Oat meal Free-living AHA fat controlled	Adult volunteers from a bank 113 had oatmeal 123 were controls	56 g (2 oz) prescribed/day	4 weeks AHA diet, then 4 weeks and 4 weeks on oatmeal (for other carbohydrate foods) or control CEE CCC	205 mg/dl	−3%	−2% NC NS	Cholesterol reduction a little more in those who started with TC above the median Table 2 not adequately captioned
Hamilton et al. (1989), USA	Oat bran cereal (Quaker oats) Inpatient controlled diet in metabolic ward	12 hypercholesterolaemic males	30 g oat bran per day in ready to eat cereal (taken twice in day) 2 weeks	Crossover Placebo-controlled Diet cornflakes	265 mg/dl	−7%	−11% NC NC	Abstract, but we also have copy of full paper
Reynolds et al. (1989), USA	Oat bran cereal ("Cheerios") Outpatients	43 with "mild to moderate hypercholesterolaemia" (M = F)	24 g oat bran from 3 oz of the breakfast cereal/day 4 weeks	Randomised, double-blind, placebo-controlled (Cornflakes)	229 mg/dl	−4%	−5% NS NS	Patients seen at 2-week intervals

Continued on next page

Table 17.4. Continued

Reference	Oats preparation and diet	Subjects	Dose	Design	Initial Pl cholesterol (TC)	Change of TC	Change of LDL/HDL/TG	Remarks
Birkeland et al. (1990), Norway	Oat bran in bread and muffins Outpatients (general practice)	54 hyper-cholesterolaemia They had previously been advised to adhere to a low-fat diet	5 weeks	Double-blind Control was wheat, bread and muffins	7.7 mmol/l	0		Brief report in letter to N Engl J Med
Swain et al. (1990), USA	High-fibre oat bran Usual diets continued. Outpatients	20 healthy subjects: dieticians, etc. 16 female, 4 male	87 g/day 6 weeks	One week baseline, then 6 weeks oat or wheat, 2 weeks wash out, 6 weeks wheat or oats. (Low-fibre wheat control) Subjects not blind	4.80 mmol/l	0%	−3% +6% NC	The women began each treatment period at the same point in their menstrual cycle. Bloods taken the last 2 days of oat or LF wheat periods. On both experimental diets pl cholesterol lower than at the start. Subjects ate less saturated fat and cholesterol and more PUF
Demark-Wahnefried et al. (1990), USA	Oat bran or processed, ready to eat oat bran cereal (POB) Outpatients	71 males and females with hypercholesterol-aemia	50 g/day oat bran or 43 g/day POB 12 weeks	4 diets compared low fat and low cholesterol LFLC + OB OB POB	7.35 mmol/l	−12% OB −10% POB	HDL small rise on POB Small fall on OB	Subjects on OB or POB consumed 14% less far and 24% less saturated fat than at baseline. Pl cholesterol lower on low-fat diet than on low fat + OB
Hegsted et al. (1990), USA	Oat bran or rice bran	11 subjects	100 g/day prescribed 3 weeks	Crossover design. Two 3-week periods with 2 weeks no bran before each (total 10 weeks)	227 mg/dl	−7% (P < 0.05)	−10% NC +8% (NS)	There was about the same reduction of TC and LDL-C on rice bran

Reference	Design	Subjects	Dose	Protocol	TC	TC change	Lipoprotein change	Comments
Kestin et al. (1990), Australia	Oat bran in bread and muffins Low fibre basal diet Outpatients with dietetic advice	24 male volunteers, mild hypercholesterol-aemia No metabolic disorders	95 g oat bran (11.8 g fibre) 4 weeks	3 week control, then 4 week periods on oat, rice or wheat fibre Double-blind crossover	6.34 mmol/l	−5.6%	−6.5% +4%	% change on oats the difference between oats and wheat fibre periods. If compared baseline result would be similar. No change of apo-A but apo-B lower on oats
Leadbetter et al. (1991), New Zealand	Oat bran Outpatients on usual diet	40 hyper-cholesterolaemic 20 male, 20 female (25–64 years)	Prescribed 30 g, 60 g, 90 g/day	4 weeks each Blood at end of each month 4 × 4 Latin square design Randomised Each sequence 1 month Each subject's bloods for all periods analysed together	7.21 (6.5–9.0) mmol/l	NC	NC NC	Oat bran used had 3.7% to 4.4% β-glucan
Van Horn et al. (1991), USA	Instant oats (Quaker oats)	Healthy volunteers in Chicago, with TC above 5.2 42 intervention 38 controls	2 servings per day (2 ounces) or 56 g for 8 weeks	1 blood at start, another at 4 weeks, another at 8 weeks. Parallel randomised control group. Rest of diet free but recorded	6.56 mmol/l	−3% Sig	Lower LDL NC of HDL	No change in bodyweight

TC, total cholesterol; AHA, American Heart Association; LDL, low density lipoprotein; HDL, high density lipoprotein; TG, triglyceride; OB, oat bran; NC, no change; NS, not significant; POB, processed oat bran.
In design column: C, control period; E, experimental period.

Chemists, in response to the confusion, recently suggested that oat bran should be defined to be not more than 50% of the starting material and to contain (dry weight basis) at least 5.5% β-glucan, and 16% total dietary fibre, one-third of which is soluble fibre. We shall never know how many of the trials in Table 17.4 used oat bran that would meet these criteria.

There is little doubt that the gum of oats is the part of its total dietary fibre responsible for whatever plasma cholesterol-lowering property it has. This has been shown in animals by testing different fractions (Chenoweth and Bennink, 1976; Welch et al., 1988). In an ingenious experiment Tietyen et al. (1990) treated oat bran with a β-glucanase. Its free sugars increased and viscosity decreased and so did its plasma and liver cholesterol-lowering action in cholesterol-fed rats. On the other hand it may be important that hot extrusion of oat bran and high-fibre oat flour appears to increase the solubility of its β-glucan (Shinnick et al., 1988). This may explain the 7% and 4% plasma cholesterol falls, in well-controlled experiments, from oat bran "breakfast" cereals taken two or three times a day (Hamilton et al., 1989; Reynolds et al., 1989).

On balance we conclude that oat fibre (i.e. gum) has a small cholesterol-lowering effect and this is on LDL not HDL or triglycerides. Because the effect is small it may be missed, obscured by other influences affecting variability of plasma cholesterol; it can be seen, however, in most of the well-designed trials in Table 17.4 (Judd and Truswell, 1981; Turnbull and Leeds, 1987; Hamilton et al., 1989; Hegsted et al., 1990; Kestin et al., 1990). Increased faecal bile acids (but not neutral sterols) were found by Judd and Truswell (1981) and Kirby et al. (1981) in man and have been reported in rat experiments as well (Illman and Topping, 1985).

Cellulose

To assess the impact of cellulose on plasma cholesterol concentrations, this particulate fibre should be supplemental to the diet. If cellulose is compared with hypocholesterolaemic fibres such as pectin or guar gum, cellulose may by definition be hypercholesterolaemic. Cellulose addition to the diet has been studied in six trials. In two well-controlled trials it did not influence plasma total cholesterol. Keys et al. (1961) fed 12 and 13 middle-aged men two types of diets of natural foods with and without 15 g cellulose supplements daily, incorporated into biscuits. During control periods, the men ate placebo biscuits equivalent in calories. The dietary periods lasted three weeks each, the order of the periods being designed so that possible time-trends were taken into account. With both basal diets, cellulose did not alter plasma cholesterol. Likewise, Behall et al. (1984) in a well-designed experiment found that about 22.5 g cellulose per day did not significantly affect plasma total cholesterol concentrations in 12 men. However, it did appear to increase LDL-cholesterol significantly (by 8%) without changing HDL-cholesterol. In two studies with a one-way design 16 g (Eastwood et al., 1973) or 60 g cellulose per day (Huth and Fettel, 1975) left plasma total cholesterol unchanged. Prather (1964) showed that a supplement of 13 g cellulose per day lowered plasma cholesterol in five young women by 10% but possible drifts of plasma cholesterol with time were not taken into account.

In a study with 10 Indian girls aged 10–12 years, 4 g of cholesterol per day was given for 10 days with or without 100 g cellulose per day (Shurpalekar et al., 1971). Cellulose reduced plasma cholesterol. However, the large cellulose intake altered the composition of the diet, which may have contributed to the observed cholesterol lowering.

In rats fed a high-cholesterol diet, the addition of 5%–10% (w/w) cellulose to the diet at the expense of an identical weight of the carbohydrate source generally elevates plasma and liver cholesterol concentrations (Kiriyama et al., 1969; Tsai et al., 1976; Van Beresteijn et al., 1979; Story et al., 1981; Mueller et al., 1983). Thus, the insoluble cellulose can be considered hypercholesterolaemic in rats.

Lignin

There are two conflicting reports on the effect of lignin on plasma cholesterol in humans. Thiffault et al. (1970) using a one-way design found a reduction of plasma total cholesterol by 21% when six hypercholesterolaemic patients ingested 4 g of lignin per day. Lindner and Möller (1973) gave 2 g of lignin per day to seven hypercholesterolaemic patients in a control–test–control design and found a statistically significant increase in plasma cholesterol (by 9%) as induced by lignin.

Judd et al. (1976) fed rats cholesterol-free diets containing either 6% (w/w) of cellulose or 3% of cellulose plus 3% of lignin. The rats fed the diet containing lignin displayed serum cholesterol concentrations 15% lower than the animals fed cellulose as the sole fibre.

Other Types of Dietary Fibre

There are single reports of lower plasma cholesterol with five different gums that are used as thickeners in the food or pharmaceutical industry.

Ross et al. (1983) gave 25 g/day gum arabic to five subjects and found plasma cholesterol 6% less.

Osilesi et al. (1985) gave 12 g/day xanthan gum to nine diabetic subjects and plasma cholesterol averaged 7% less.

Sharma (1985) gave 30 g/day of gum acacia to seven hypercholesterolaemic subjects: plasma cholesterol fell by 10%.

Behall et al. (1984) gave 18 g/day of karaya gum to 12 subjects and plasma cholesterol was 12% less.

Zavoral et al. (1983) gave 10 g/day of locust bean gum to 18 subjects and plasma cholesterol was 11% lower.

These reported effects all require confirmation. Some trials used only the unreliable control–test design and very few subjects. Presumably they owe what effect they have to increased viscosity of small intestinal contents. This may not be the same as their relative viscosity in vitro (Edwards et al., 1987). They were tested in the search for alternatives to guar, which is rather unpalatable. Of course no food would normally provide 10 to 30 g/day of any of these gums.

The most tested alternative to guar, however, appears to be the mucilage psyllium, a polysaccharide based on arabinose, xylose and galacturonic acid units which comes from *Plantago ovata* (or ispaghula). It is well known in medicine under the trade names "Metamucil" and "Isogel" as a bulk laxative. Between 1965 and 1988 there have been 10 reports on its effect on plasma cholesterol in man, usually in doses of 10 g/day. These are summarised in a table by Anderson et al. (1990a). Participating subjects numbered 159, some normals, some diabetics and some with hypercholesterolaemia. Mean plasma total cholesterol fell in 10/10 reports by percentages from −8 to −20. One of the trials was a well-designed double-blind, placebo-controlled parallel study (Anderson et al., 1988). Plasma cholesterol fell 15% after eight weeks on psyllium (which is what the authors claim for its effect) but it fell 4% from the initial control period in the cellulose placebo group (15% − 4% = 11%). Gastro-intestinal side effects were mild and Anderson et al. (1988) suggest that psyllium should be an additional, quite palatable medicine for hypercholesterolaemia. It may also be possible to incorporate it into dietetic foods but there have been two cases of intestinal obstruction and six case reports of IgE allergic reactions, including bronchospasm and anaphylaxis (Anderson et al., 1988).

Legumes

Eleven trials with legumes other than soya are summarised in Table 17.5. A much quoted trial in diabetics by Simpson et al. (1981) is not in the table because the patients on the very high legume prescription (190 g/day) had a very low total fat intake of 18% energy while fat in the control low-fibre diet was 40%. Mean changes of plasma cholesterol in the table range from 0% to −19%. To evaluate which of these results may have been partly affected by other variables and which are most likely to show a direct effect, we can put these 11 reports in four groups.

Mathur et al. (1968) used a one-way design and appear to have had small control of their subjects' diets. The decline of plasma cholesterol was surprisingly late and eventually much larger than in the other reports.

Four papers report controlled diets but one-way designs: Anderson et al., (1984a, 1990b); Shutler et al., (1989), and Nervi et al., (1989). With such designs it is possible that part of the difference in plasma cholesterol may be due to seasonal change or continuing adjustment from usual to the basal experimental diet. It is noticeable that reported percentage changes in mean plasma cholesterol in these four articles, of −19, −11, −12 and −9, are larger than in the other reports.

Two papers report well-designed studies without dietary control: the classic article by Luyken et al. (1962) and that by Gormley et al. (1979). Luyken et al. used a crossover design, had long periods, repeated bloods and an adequate number of subjects. Gormley et al. had more subjects, a parallel placebo group and adequate six-week periods. But neither controlled nor monitored their subjects' diets, so it is possible that some of the plasma cholesterol reduction may have been due to subjects eating less fat when they increased legume intake. These two authors reported plasma cholesterol reductions of 5% and 6% respectively.

We can best estimate the direct effect of legumes from the remaining four experiments: the rest of the diets were controlled and experimental design was good. Grande et al. (1965) gave their subjects all their food in metabolic units. Five hundred kcal carbohydrate from equal amounts of three legumes (Phaseolus vulgaris, Phaseolus lunatus and Pisum sativum) were compared with sucrose plus soy protein in a randomised crossover design. In 24 middle-aged chronic mental patients, with three-week periods, plasma cholesterols were 6% lower on the legumes. But in 12 male university students and with two-week periods no differences were found between legumes and sucrose/soy protein or wheat flour or chick peas (Grande et al., 1974).

Jenkins et al. (1983) and Cobiac et al. (1990) had their subjects eat at home but the legumes were provided and the rest of their diets were closely supervised and monitored. Jenkins' patients' mean plasma cholesterols, measured five times over the bean supplemented period, were 7% less than the mean of the five measurements before legumes. Plasma triglycerides fell by 25%. Small reductions in dietary cholesterol and fat were not significant (Jenkins et al., 1983). Cobiac et al. (1990) compared canned baked beans in tomato sauce with canned spaghetti in tomato and cheese sauce in a 4/4 week crossover experiment. The beans added 12 g/day non-starch polysaccharides to the diet (low fat milk in the spaghetti period balanced the protein in the beans). Food diaries on eight random days showed no significant differences in fat or fatty acids. Plasma total cholesterol and triglycerides were indistinguishable between the baked beans and spaghetti periods.

Thus it would seem that substantial regular intakes of these legumes are associated with reductions of plasma cholesterol. This is partly an indirect effect: when the rest of the diet was well controlled the average fall of plasma cholesterol was only 3.4% (i.e. in the experiments of Grande et al. (1965), Grande et al. (1974), Jenkins et al. (1983) and Cobiac et al. (1990).

In *soya beans* both the protein (Sirtori et al. 1979; Descovich et al., 1980; Van Raaij et al., 1982) and the fibre have been reported to lower plasma cholesterol. The method of processing appears to be important both for the protein (Van Raaij et al., 1982) and for the fibre effects. A soya bean "crude fibre" preparation, containing 33% dietary fibre did not lower plasma cholesterol in subjects with mildly elevated cholesterol (Sasaki et al., 1985). In 1983 two groups reported on different concentrated soya cotyledon fibre preparations (Schweizer et al, 1983; Tsai et al., 1983). Neither lowered plasma cholesterol in normal subjects at daily intakes of 20–25 g polysaccharide.

Subsequently a similar soybean polysaccharide preparation at 25 g/day lowered plasma total cholesterol significantly by an average of 8% in 31 subjects with mild or moderate hypercholesterolaemia (Shorey et al., 1985). In a second paper (Lo et al., 1986) the same product again produced an 8% fall of plasma cholesterol in subjects with primary hypertriglyceridaemia (moderate type IV hyperlipidaemia) but in patients with familial hypercholesterolaemia plasma cholesterol fell by only 3%.

Table 17.5. Beans and other legumes

Reference	Legume(s)	Design	Plasma cholesterol	Comments
Luyken et al. (1962)	100 g beans/day mainly brown weighed dry 14 weeks	Crossover, with controls before and after n = 20 Repeated bloods	−5% Sig	Rest of diet not controlled or monitored
Grande et al. (1965)	500 kcal of carbohydrate from *Phaseolus vulgaris*, *Phaseolus lunatus* and *Pisum sativum* compared with sucrose + soy protein 3 weeks	Metabolic unit Randomised crossover n = 24	−6% Sig	Chronic mental patients at Hastings State Hospital, Minnesota
Mathur et al. (1968)	Bengal gram (*Cicer arietinum*) replacing cereals	One-way design Outpatients Long trial n = 16	Declined from 4 to 20 weeks	Diets not closely monitored Subjects started on high butter diet 10 weeks before legume started
Grande et al. (1974)	Same legumes as above cf sucrose + soy protein *and* wheat flour and chick peas 2 weeks	Metabolic unit Randomised crossover (no wash outs) n = 12	0	Male university students
Gormley et al. (1979)	30 g/day freeze-dried peas added to usual diets	Placebo-controlled (20 g corn flakes) Free-living rest of diet n = 28 + 28	−6% Sig	56 apparently healthy subjects, 30–50 years, (50 men, 6 women) Half took peas, half took placebo

Reference	Intervention	Design	Result	Notes
Jenkins et al. (1983)	140 g/day dried legumes (kidney and pinto beans, chick peas and lentils) 16 weeks	Control → test design. Legumes replaced starchy foods. Repeated bloods. $n = 7$	−7% Sig	Although one-way design subjects stable and 5 repeat bloods before legumes. Subjects: 3 different types of hyperlipidaemia
Anderson et al. (1984a)	115 g "dried beans" per day 3 weeks	7 days control then 21 days experiment. Rest of diet controlled. $n = 10$	−19% Sig	One-way design. Subjects lost weight. Type of beans not stated
Shutler et al. (1989)	440 g/day canned beans in tomato sauce 2 weeks	Canned beans 14 days, then wash out, then 440 g spaghetti in same sauce	−12% Sig	Healthy male students. No effect on plasma TGs. HDLs fell too
Nervi et al. (1989)	120 g dry legumes per day (beans, peas and lentils) for 30 days	25 days control diet then 30 days added legumes. Diets controlled, provided in research institution. 6 day/week. $n = 20$	−9% Sig	Volunteers serving in the army. From Table 2, fall of cholesterol −10%
Anderson et al. (1990b)	Canned beans in tomato sauce: (A) 227 g (total) once/day (B) 227 g/day divided doses (C) More beans, less tomato sauce	One-way design. 7 days control, then 21 days on beans. $n = 6, 9, 9$ for groups A, B, C	−10.4% −10.8%	227 g canned beans + tomato sauce contained 120 g beans (groups A and B). Group C took 162 g beans and 20 g tomato sauce
Cobiac et al. (1990)	6 × 440 g canned baked beans/week. Compared with same weight canned spaghetti 4 weeks	Crossover; two 4-week periods after 2.5 weeks baseline. $n = 20$	−1.4% NS	Mildly hypercholesterolaemic men

While soy protein isolates seem to be most effective in people with hypercholesterolaemia (Sirtori, 1980), this has not been the experience with soy polysaccharide concentrates. Soya bean hulls, as distinct from polysaccharides from the cotyledon, are not usually eaten and did not lower plasma cholesterol at 25 or 50 g fibre per day (Mahalko et al., 1984).

Whole Foods

There have been a few reports of the effect on plasma cholesterol of increased intake of single vegetable or fruit foods. Robertson et al. (1979) reported a cholesterol-lowering effect of carrots but this was not confirmed by another group (Jenkins et al., 1979b). This illustrates that a single report is not enough. Results depend on what foods were displaced from the diet by the test food, and are susceptible to natural variations in plasma cholesterol.

With high intakes of another pectin-containing food, apples, there are three reports of lower plasma cholesterols (Canella et al., 1962; Sicart et al., 1974; Gormley et al., 1977). In the trial by Gormley et al. 16 free-living men in Dublin agricultural research centres were paired. For 4 months in the season when fresh apples were available one group ate 17 Irish Golden Delicious apples a week; the control group ate not more than three apples a week. No other dietary control was exerted. Mean serum cholesterols were lower in the (+) apple group at four of the monthly blood tests but not before or after the experiment. The mean monthly difference was −4.5%; the largest monthly difference was −8% (the figure given in the abstract). One can only speculate, as Gormley did, how much of this small but nicely demonstrated difference was due to displacement of fatty foods and how much directly due to the pectin – perhaps 3 or 4 g/day – in the apples.

It is monotonous to eat large amounts of apples, beans or any other single vegetable food day after day. But generous intakes of a variety of vegetables and fruits are an integral part of some highly developed and widely enjoyed cuisines, such as the Italian or the Japanese. Ancel Keys (1955) observed that about 0.5 mmol/l (20 mg/dl) of the difference in men's mean plasma cholesterols between Naples (Italy) and Minnesota (USA) could not be explained by their pattern of fatty acid and cholesterol intake. Later, in the metabolic ward in Minnesota, Keys et al. (1960) demonstrated a direct effect (fats constant) of diets high in cereals, vegetables, legumes and fruits of (average) 17 mg/dl (0.44 mmol/l) lower plasma cholesterol.

There are three other well-controlled demonstrations of a direct cholesterol-lowering effect of mixed fibre-containing foods with fats and calorie intakes held constant. Stasse-Wolthuis et al. (1980) compared four diets: low fibre; added vegetable/fruits; added pectins and added wheat bran. Under strictly controlled conditions, with all food provided to healthy volunteers, the vegetable/fruit group ate 400 g of cooked vegetables (made up of green cabbage, sliced beans, carrots, endive and beetroot), 170 g/day of tomatoes and 600 g/day of apples (with skin). These provided an additional 26 g of total dietary fibre including 7 g of pectin. In this group total cholesterol declined 4%. This was statistically significant at two weeks, not after five weeks. There was no change in

HDL-cholesterol. Faecal steroids increased in the vegetable/fruit and pectin groups by about the same amount. Stasse-Wolthuis et al. imply in their discussion that much of the cholesterol-lowering effect of the vegetable/fruit diet was due to the pectin it contained.

With the dedicated cooperation of monks at an abbey in the Netherlands, Lewis et al. (1981) compared four diets. Each of 12 men ate each diet for five weeks in different order. Total cholesterol on the fat-modified diet with 27% fat, (polyunsaturated/saturated = 1) was 21.6% lower than on the typical 40% fat Western diet. But the same fat-modified diet with three to four times the dietary fibre (as apples, oranges, bananas, wheat fibre, beans and vegetables) resulted in plasma cholesterol 29.2% lower than the "Western" control diets; i.e. increasing fibre from a mixture of vegetable sources produced a 7.6% further fall of plasma total cholesterol, all as LDL-cholesterol. There was also a larger proportion of vegetable protein on the high-fibre diet but the authors in their discussion implied that the effect of the high-fibre diet was mostly due to its pectin and hemicellulose.

Kesäniemi et al. (1990) report a mean 4.5% reduction of plasma cholesterol in 34 50-year-old men, half of whom increased their dietary fibre intake from 11 to 26 g/day from a combination of whole grain cereals, vegetables, fruits, berries and salads. With dietetic supervision they kept their fat and cholesterol intakes, polyunsaturated/saturated ratio and body weight constant.

Discussion

Three groups of people have different interests in the area we have reviewed:

1. People who believe in whole and natural foods and who would like as little processing of their food as possible will be supported in their beliefs by the few well-designed experiments with mixtures of vegetables and fruits. But the four groups that carried out the experiments we have quoted also tested pectin and other components. If we know which components of vegetables and fruits do and which do not lower plasma cholesterol, and by what mechanism, we have the best chance of predicting combinations of plant foods that should lower plasma cholesterol. Whole grain wheat is a natural whole plant food but we can now be fairly sure it will not lower plasma cholesterol.

2. The pharmaceutical industry and some physicians are interested in finding purified non-starch polysaccharides which will lower plasma cholesterol. Guar products have been used for this purpose. They are more likely to be acceptable for diabetics because they reduce the rise of blood glucose after meals as well as the fasting blood cholesterol. Almost all the trials with guar have been short-term and reduced absorption of some drugs, taken at the same time, is possible (Vinik and Jenkins, 1988). Guar is not easy to take and the emphasis in therapeutic dietetics for diabetes is now less on fibre, more on the combined factors (of which viscous fibre is only one) that can reduce glycaemic index. For treatment of hypercholesterolaemia guar looks less useful now that the HMGCoA reductase inhibitors are proving so efficient.

3. The food industry is interested in modifying foods in ways which make them more marketable. One of these is to make them contribute to a healthy

diet, e.g. by tending to lower plasma cholesterol more than the standard, or a competitor's product. This is why we have seen a lot of products recently "with added oat bran". From our review of oat fibre, we can see that oat bran has been rather over-sold. Breakfast cereals made largely from oat bran may make a modest contribution to a lower plasma cholesterol but a few grams of oat bran here and a few grams there cannot have any measurable effect. There may be a backlash to the overenthusiasm about oat bran and there is a real need for biologically meaningful standardisation of this product. Some of the newer viscous polysaccharides, such as psyllium, may have a place for cholesterol-lowering dietetic foods if we can be sure that allergic reactions would be very rare and not very serious.

Conclusion

Is there a place for either purified fibre preparations or fibre-containing foods in the prevention and treatment of hypercholesterolaemia? Pectin and other viscous polysaccharides lower cholesterol whereas cellulose does not. In order to lower plasma cholesterol directly by 5%–10% pectin in amounts of approximately 10 g per day should be ingested. If this is to be obtained using regular foodstuffs, about 1 kg of fruits and/or vegetables must be consumed per day. On the other hand cellulose does not lower plasma cholesterol and increased consumption of wheat bran or whole wheat will not lower cholesterol directly.

Increased consumption of cellulose-containing foods and wheat fibre can nevertheless contribute to plasma cholesterol lowering by displacing foods rich in saturated fatty acids and cholesterol. Pectin-containing foods by contrast have both direct and indirect effects.

Where dietary fibre does lower plasma cholesterol, it is the total cholesterol and LDL that are affected. No consistent effects on HDL or triglycerides have been seen.

Acknowledgements. We thank Isa Hopwood, Marianne Sylvada de Soza, Marie Jansen, Riekie Janssen, Marcel van Leuteren, and Ineke Zaalmink for typing.

References

Ahrens F, Hagemeister H, Pfeuffer M, Barth CA (1986) Effects of oral and intracaecal pectin administration on blood lipids in minipigs. J Nutr 116:70–76

Anderson JW (1980) Oat bran ingestion selectively lowers serum low-density lipoprotein concentration in man. Am J Clin Nutr 33:915

Anderson JW, Bridges SR (1981) Plant fiber metabolites alter hepatic glucose and lipid metabolism. Diabetes 30(suppl 1):133A

Anderson JW, Chen W-JL (1979) Plant fibre, carbohydrate and lipid metabolism. Am J Clin Nutr 32:346–363

Anderson JW, Story L, Sieling B, Chen W-JL, Petro MS, Story J (1984a) Hypercholesterolemic effects of oat bran or bean intake for hypercholesterolemic men. Am J Clin Nutr 40:1146–1155

Anderson JW, Story L, Sieling B, Chen W-JL (1984b) Hypercholesterolemic effects of high-fibre diets rich in water-soluble plant fibres. J Can Diet Assoc 45:140–148

Anderson JW, Zettwock N, Feldman T, Tietyen-Clark J, Oeltgen P, Bishop CW (1988) Cholesterol-lowering effects of psyllium hydrophilic mucilloid for hypercholesterolemic men. Arch Int Med 148:292–296

Anderson JW, Deakins DA, Floore TL, Smith BM, Whitis SE (1990a) Dietary fiber and coronary heart disease. Crit Rev Food Sci Nutr 29:95–146

Anderson JW, Gustafson NJ, Spencer DB, Tietyen J, Bryant CA (1990b) Serum lipid response of hypercholesterolemic men to single and divided doses of canned beans. Am J Clin Nutr 51:1013–1019

Angelico F, Clements P, Menotti A, Ricci G, Urbinati G (1978) Bran and changes in serum lipids: observations during a project of primary prevention of coronary heart disease. In: Carlson LA (ed) International conference on atherosclerosis. Raven Press, New York, p 205

Aro A, Uusitupa M, Voultilainen E, Hersio K, Korhonen T, Siitonen O (1981) Improved diabetic control and hypocholesterolaemic effect induced by long-term dietary supplementation with guar gum in type 2 (insulin-independent) diabetes. Diabetologia 21:29–33

Aro A, Uusitupa M, Voutilainen E, Korhonen T (1984) Effects of guar gum in male subjects with hypercholesterolemia. Am J Clin Nutr 39:911–916

Atkins TW, Al-Hussary NAJ, Taylor KG (1987) The treatment of poorly controlled non-insulin-dependent diabetic subjects with granulated guar gum. Diabetes Res Clin Pract 3:153–159

Avgerinos GC, Fuchs HM, Flock MH (1977) Increased cholesterol and bile acid excretion during a high fibre diet. Gastroenterology 72:1026

Behall KM, Lee KH, Moser PB (1984) Blood lipids and lipoproteins in adult men fed four refined fibres. Am J Clin Nutr 39:209–214

Birkeland KI, Gullestad L, Falch D, Torsvik H (1990) Oat bran and serum cholesterol. N Engl J Med 322:1748–1749

Bosaeus I, Carlsson N-G, Sandberg A-S, Andersson H (1986) Effect of wheat bran and pectin on bile acid and cholesterol excretion in ileostomy patients. Hum Nutr Clin Nutr 40C:429–440

Bosello O, Cominacini I, Zocca I, Garbin U, Ferrari F, Davioli A (1984) Effects of guar gum on plasma lipoproteins and apolipoproteins CII and CIII in patients affected by familial combined hyperlipoproteinemia. Am J Clin Nutr 40:1165–1174

Botha APJ, Steyn AF, Esterhuysen AJ, Slabbert M (1981) Glycosylated haemoglobin, blood glucose and serum cholesterol levels in diabetics treated with guar gum. S Afr Med J 59:333–334

Bremner JM, McElrea R, Scott RS (1986) Treatment of non-insulin-dependent diabetes with high fibre diets: comparison of guar and bran. J N Z Diet Assoc 40:29–37

Bremner WF, Brooks PM, Third JL, Lawrie TDV (1975) Bran in hypertriglyceridaemia: a failure of response. Br Med J iii:574

Brodribb AJM, Humphreys DM (1976) Diverticular disease. Three studies. Br Med J i:424–430

Canella C, Golinelli G, Melli A (1962) Influenza sui valori colestrerolemici della polpa de mela aggiunta al normale alimentazione. Arch S Anna de Ferrara 15:803–814

Carroll DG, Dykes V, Hodgson W (1981) Guar gum is not a panacea in diabetes management. NZ Med J 93:292–294

Catenazzo C, Torri A, Camisasca E et al. (1983) Effeti del guar sulle variazione della triglicerdemia dopo un pasto di provo e dopo omministrazione acido di MCT. Minerva Dietol Gastroenterol 29:307

Chenoweth WL, Bennink MR (1976) Hypocholesterolemic effect of oat fiber. Fed Proc 35:495

Cobiac L, McArthur R, Nestel PJ (1990) Can eating baked beans lower plasma cholesterol? Eur J Clin Nutr 44:819–822

Connell AM, Smith CL, Somsel M (1975) Absence of effect of bran on blood lipids. Lancet i:496–497

Connor WE (1990) Dietary fiber – nostrum or critical nutrient? N Engl J Med 322:193–195

Dalzell GW, McNeill AJ, Hadden DR (1985) Effect of guar in poorly controlled non-insulin-dependent diabetes mellitus. Autumn meeting of British Diabetic Association, Belfast, 5–7 Sept, p 34

de Groot AP, Luyken R, Pikaar NA (1963) Cholesterol-lowering effect of rolled oats. Lancet ii:303–304

Delbarre F, Rondier J, de Géry A (1977) Lack of effect of two pectins in idiopathic or gout-associated hyperdyslipidemia hypercholesterolemia. Am J Clin Nutr 30:463–465

Demark-Wahnefried W, Bowering J, Cohen PS (1990) Reduced serum cholesterol with dietary change using fat-modified and oat bran supplemented diet. J Am Diet Assoc 90:223–229

Descovich GC, Sirtori CR et al. (1980) Multicentre study of soybean protein diet for outpatient hypercholesterolaemic patients. Lancet ii:709–712

Dixon M (1978) Bran and HDL cholesterol. Lancet i:578

Dodson PM, Stocks J, Holdsworth G, Galton DJ (1981) High-fibre and low-fat diets in diabetes mellitus. Br J Nutr 46:289–294

Durrington P, Wicks ACB, Heaton KW (1975) Effect of bran on blood lipids. Lancet ii:133

Durrington PN, Manning AP, Bolton CH, Hartog M (1976) Effect of pectin on serum lipids and lipoproteins, whole-gut transit-time, and stool weight. Lancet ii:394–396

Eastwood M (1969) Dietary fibre and serum lipids. Lancet ii:1222–1225

Eastwood MA, Kirkpatrick JR, Mitchell WD, Bone A, Hamilton T (1973) Effects of dietary supplements of wheat bran and cellulose on faeces and bowel function. Br Med J iv:392–394

Ebeling P, Hannele YJ, Aro A, Helve E, Sinisalo M, Koivisto VA (1988) Glucose and lipid metabolism and insulin sensitivity in type I diabetes: the effect of guar gum. Am J Clin Nutr 48:98–103

Edwards CA, Blackburn NA, Craigen L et al. (1987) Viscosity of food gums determined in vitro related to their hypoglycemic actions. Am J Clin Nutr 38:72–77

Edwards CA, Johnson IT, Read NW (1988) Do viscous polysaccharides slow absorption by inhibiting diffusion or convection? Eur J Clin Nutr 42:307–312

Ellis PR, Morris ER, Low AG (1986) Guar gum: the importance of reporting data on its physico-chemical properties. Diabetic Med 3:490–491

Fahrenbach MH, Riccardi BA, Saunders JC, Lourie N, Heider JC (1965) Comparative effects of guar gum and pectin on human serum cholesterol levels. Circulation 31 & 32 (Suppl II):11

Farrell DJ, Girle L, Arthur J (1978) Effects of dietary fibre on the apparent digestibility of major food components and blood lipids in man. Aus J Exp Biol Med Sci 56:469–479

Fisher H, Griminger P, Sostman ER, Brush MK (1965) Dietary pectin and plasma cholesterol. J Nutr 86:113

Flanagan M, Little C, Milliken J et al. (1980) The effects of diet on high density lipoprotein. J Hum Nutr 34:43–45

Fuessl HS, Williams G, Adrian TE, Bloom SR (1987) Guar sprinkled on food: effect on glycaemic control, plasma lipids and gut hormones in NIDDM. Diabetic Med 4:463–468

Gallaher D, Schneeman BO (1986) Intestinal interaction of bile acids, phospholipids, dietary fibers and cholestyramine. Am J Physiol 250:G420–426

Garcia MJ, Charlez M, Fauli C, delPozo Carrascosa A, Ghirardi PE (1988) Physicochemical comparison of the dietary fibers glucomannan, galactomannan, carboxymethylcellulose, pectin, and wheat bran. Curr Ther Res 43:1010–1013

Gariot P, Digby JP, Genton P, Lambert D, Bau RMH, Debry G (1986) Long-term effect of bran ingestion on lipid metabolism in healthy men. Ann Nutr Metab 30:369–373

Gatenby JJ (1990) Guar gum and hyperlipidaemia – a review of the literature. In: Leeds AR, Burley VJ (eds) Dietary fibre perspectives, reviews and bibliography, vol 2. John Libbey, London, pp 100–115

Gatti E, Catenazzo G, Camisasca E, Torri A, Denegri E, Sirtori CR (1984) Effects of guar-enriched pasta in the treatment of diabetes and hyperlipidaemia. Nutr Metab 28:1–10

Ginter E, Kubec FJ, Vozar J, Bobek P (1979) Natural hypercholesterolemic agent: pectin plus ascorbic acid. Int J Vitam Nutr Res 49:406–412

Gold KV, Davidson DM (1988) Oat bran as a cholesterol-reducing dietary adjunct in a young, healthy population. West J Med 148:299–302

Gormley TR, Kevany J, Egan JP, McFarlane R (1977) Effects of apples on serum cholesterol levels in humans. Irish J Food Sci Technol 1:117–128

Gormley TR, Kevany J, O'Donnell B, McFarlane R (1979) Effect of peas on serum cholesterol levels in humans. Irish J Food Sci Technol 3:101–109

Grande F, Anderson JT, Keys A (1965) Effect of carbohydrates of leguminous seeds, wheat and potatoes on serum cholesterol concentrations in man. J Nutr 86:313–317

Grande F, Anderson JT, Keys A (1974) Sucrose and various carbohydrate-containing foods and serum lipids in man. Am J Clin Nutr 27:1043–1051

Groen JJ, Tijong KB, Koster M, Willebrands AF, Verdonck G, Pierloot M (1962) The influence of nutrition and ways of life on blood cholesterol and the prevalence of hypertension and coronary heart disease among Trappist and Benedictine monks. Am J Clin Nutr 10:456–470

Hamilton CC, Tietyen J, Spencer BA, Anderson JW (1989) Serum lipid responses of hypercholesterolemic men to a ready to eat oat bran cereal. J Am Diet Assoc 89 (Suppl):A1

Heaton KW, Pomare EW (1974) Effect of bran on blood lipids and calcium. Lancet i:49–50

Heaton KW, Manning AP, Hartog M (1976) Lack of effect on blood lipid and calcium concentrations of young men on changing from white to whole meal bread. Br J Nutr 35:55–60

Hegsted M, Windhauser MM, Lester SB, Morris SK (1990) Stabilized rice bran and oat bran lower cholesterol in humans. FASEB J 4:A368

Henry RW, Stout RW, Love HG (1978) Lack of effect of bran enriched bread on plasma lipids, calcium, glucose and body weight. Irish J Med Sci 147:249–251

Hillman LC, Peters SG, Fisher CA, Pomare EW (1985) The effects of the fibre components pectin, cellulose and lignin on serum cholesterol levels. Am J Clin Nutr 42:207–213

Holman RR, Steenson J, Darling P, Turner RC (1987) No glycemic benefit from guar administration in NIDDM. Diabetes Care 10:68–71

Hopson JJ (1967) Studies on the effect of dietary pectin on plasma and fecal lipids. MSc thesis, University of Iowa, quoted by Chenoweth WL, Leveille GA: Metabolism and physiological effects of food pectins. In: Jeanes A, Hodge J (eds) Physiological effects of food carbohydrates, pp 312–334

Huth K, Fettel M (1975) Bran and blood-lipids. Lancet ii:456

Illman RJ, Topping DL (1985) Effects of dietary oat bran on faecal steroid excretion, plasma volatile fatty acids and lipid synthesis in rats. Nutr Res 5:839

Illman RJ, Trimble RP, Snowsell AM, Topping DL (1982) Daily variations in the concentrations of volatile fatty acids in the splanchnic blood vessels of rats fed diets high in pectin and bran. Nutr Rep Int 26:439–446

Illman RJ, Topping DL, McIntosh GH et al. (1988) Hypocholesterolemic effects of dietary propionate: studies in whole animals and perfused rat liver. Ann Nutr Metab 32:97–107

Jenkins DJA, Leeds AR, Newton C, Cummings JH (1975a) Effect of pectin guar gum and wheat fibre on serum cholesterol. Lancet i:1116–1117

Jenkins DJA, Hill MS, Cummings JH (1975b) Effect of wheat fiber on blood lipids, fecal steroid excretion and serum iron. Am J Clin Nutr 28:1408–1411

Jenkins DJA, Leeds AR, Gassull HH, Houston MA, Goff DV, Hill MJ (1976) The cholesterol lowering properties of guar and pectin. Clin Sci Mol Med 51:8

Jenkins DJA, Leeds AR, Gassull MA, Cochet B, Alberti KGMM (1977) Decrease in postprandial insulin and glucose concentrations from guar and pectin. Ann Intern Med 86:20–23

Jenkins DJA, Leeds AR, Slavin B, Mann J, Jepson EM (1979a) Dietary fiber and blood lipids: reduction of serum cholesterol in type II hyperlipidaemia by guar gum. Am J Clin Nutr 32:16–18

Jenkins DJA, Reynolds D, Leeds AR, Waller AL, Cummings JH (1979b) Hypocholesterolemic action of dietary fiber unrelated to fecal bulking effect. Am J Clin Nutr 32:2430–2435

Jenkins DJA, Reynolds D, Slavin B, Leeds AR, Jenkins AL, Jepson EM (1980) Dietary fibre and blood lipids: treatment of hypercholesterolaemia with guar crispbread. Am J Clin Nutr 33:575–581

Jenkins DJA, Wong GS, Patten R et al. (1983) Leguminous seeds in the dietary management of hyperlipidaemia. Am J Clin Nutr 38:567–573

Johansen K (1981) Decreased urinary glucose excretion and plasma cholesterol level in non-insulin-dependent diabetic patients with guar. Diabète Métab 7:87–90

Jones DB, Slaughter P, Lousley S, Carter JD, Jelfs R, Mann JI (1985) Low dose guar improves diabetic control. J R Soc Med 78:546–548

Judd PA, Truswell AS (1981) The effect of rolled oats on blood lipids and fecal steroid excretion in man. Am J Clin Nutr 34:2061–2067

Judd PA, Truswell AS (1982) Comparison of the effects of high and low-methoxyl pectins on blood and faecal lipids in men. Br J Nutr 48:451–458

Judd PA, Truswell AS (1985a) Dietary fibre and blood lipids in man. In: Leeds AR (ed) Dietary fibre perspectives, vol 1. John Libbey, London, pp 23–39

Judd PA, Truswell AS (1985b) The hypocholesterolaemic effects of pectins in rats. Br J Nutr 53:409–425

Judd PA, Kay RM, Truswell AS (1976) Cholesterol-lowering effect of lignin in rats. Proc Nutr Soc 35:73A

Kay RM, Truswell AS (1975) The effect of wheat fibre on the plasma cholesterol in rats. Proc Nutr Soc 34:17A

Kay RM, Truswell AS (1977a) The effect of wheat fibre on plasma lipids and faecal steroid excretion in man. Br J Nutr 37:227–235

Kay RM, Truswell AS (1977b) Effect of citrus pectin on blood lipids and fecal steroids in men. Am J Clin Nutr 30:171–175

Kay RM, Truswell AS (1980) Dietary fiber: effects on plasma and biliary lipids in man. In: Spiller GA, Kay RM (eds) Medical aspects of dietary fiber. Plenum Press, New York, pp 153–173

Kay RM, Judd PA, Truswell AS (1978) The effect of pectin on serum cholesterol. Am J Clin Nutr 31:562–563

Kesäniemi YA, Tarpila S, Miettinen TA (1990) Low vs. high dietary fiber and serum, biliary, and fecal lipids in middle-aged men. Am J Clin Nutr 51:1007–1012

Kestin M, Moss R, Clifton PM, Nestel PJ (1990) Comparative effects of three cereal brans on plasma lipids, blood pressure and glucose metabolism in mildly hypercholesterolemic men. Am J Clin Nutr 52:661–666

Keys A, Fidanza F, Keys MH (1955) Further studies on serum cholesterol of clinically healthy men in Italy. Voeding 16:492–497

Keys A, Anderson JT, Grande F (1960) Diet-type (fats constant) and blood lipids in man. J Nutr 70:257–266

Keys A, Grande F, Anderson JT (1961) Fiber and pectin in the diet and serum cholesterol concentration in man. Proc Soc Exp Biol Med 106:555–558

Khan AR, Khan GY, Mitchel A, Qadeer MA (1981) Effect of guar gum on blood lipids. Am J Clin Nutr 34:2446–2449

Kirby RW, Anderson JW, Sieling B et al. (1981) Oat-bran intake selectively lowers serum low-density lipoprotein cholesterol concentrations of hypercholesterolemic men. Am J Clin Nutr 34:824–829

Kiriyama S, Okazaki Y, Yoshida A (1969) Hypocholesterolemic effect of polysaccharides and polysaccharide-rich foodstuffs in cholesterol-fed rats. J Nutr 97:382–388

Komai M, Kimura S (1987) Effect of dietary fiber on fecal steroid profiles in germfree and conventional mice. Nutr Rep Int 36:365–375

Kretsch MJ, Crawford L, Calloway DH (1979) Some aspects of bile acid and urobilinogen excretion and fecal elimination in men given a rural Guatemalan diet and egg formulas with and without oat bran. Am J Clin Nutr 32:1492–1496

Krotkiewski M (1984) Effect of guar gum on body weight, hunger ratings and metabolism in obese subjects. Br J Nutr 52:97–105

Kyllastinen M, Lahikainen T (1981) Long-term dietary supplementation with a fibre product (guar gum) in elderly diabetics. Curr Ther Res 30:872–879

Langley NJ, Thye FW (1977) The effect of wheat bran and/or citrus pectin on serum cholesterol and triglycerides in middle aged men. Fed Proc 36:1118

Leadbetter J, Ball MJ, Mann JI (1991) Effect of increasing quantities of oat bran in hypercholesterolemic people? Am J Clin Nutr 54:841–845

Letchford P, Zabroja R, Arthur J, Farrell D (1978) Manipulation of plasma cholesterol in man and its suppression. Proc Nutrition Soc Australia 3:97

Leveille GA, Sauberlich HE (1966) Mechanisms of the cholesterol depressing effect of pectin in the cholesterol-fed rat. J Nutr 88:209–214

Lewis B, Katan M, Merkx I et al. (1981) Towards an improved lipid-lowering diet; additive effects of changes in nutrient intake. Lancet ii:1310–1313

Liebman M, Smith MC, Iverson J et al. (1983) Effects of coarse wheat bran fiber and exercise on plasma lipids and lipoproteins in moderately overweight men. Am J Clin Nutr 37:71–81

Lindgärde F, Larsson L (1984) Effects of a concentrated bran fibre preparation on HDL-cholesterol in hypercholesterolaemic men. Human Nutr Clin Nutr 38C:39–45

Lindner P, Möller B (1973) Lignin: a cholesterol-lowering agent? Lancet ii:1259–1260

Lo GS, Goldberg AP, Lim A, Grundhauser JJ, Anderson C, Schonfeld G (1986) Soy fiber improves lipid and carbohydrate metabolism in primary hyperlipidemic subjects. Atherosclerosis 62:239–248

Lopez A, Hopson J, Krehl WA (1968) Effects of dietary pectin on plasma and fecal lipids. Fed Proc 27:485

Luyken R, Pikaar NA, Polman H, Schippers FA (1962) The influence of legumes on the serum cholesterol level. Voeding 23:447–453

Luyken R, de Wijn JF, Pikaar NA, van der Meer R (1965) De invloed van havermout op het serum-cholesterolgehalte van het bloed. Voeding 26:229–244

Mahalko JR, Sandstead HH, Johnson LAK et al. (1984) Effect of consuming fiber from corn bran, soy hulls, or apple powder on glucose tolerance and plasma lipids in type II diabetes. Am J Clin Nutr 39:25–34

Mathur KS, Khan MA, Sharma RD (1968) Hypocholesterolaemic effect of Bengal gram: a long-term study in man. Br Med J i:30–31

Mathur MS, Singh F, Chadda VS (1977) Effect of bran on blood lipids. J Assoc Physicians India 25:275–278

McDougall RM, Yakymyshyn L, Walker K, Thurston OG (1978) Effect of wheat bran on serum lipoproteins and biliary lipids. Can J Surg 21:433–435

McIvor ME, Cummings CC, Duyn MA et al. (1986) Long-term effects of guar gum on blood lipids. Atherosclerosis 60:7–13

McNaughton JP, Morrison DD, Huhner LJ, Earnest MM, Ellis MA, Howell GL (1985) Changes in total serum cholesterol levels of diabetics fed 5 g guar gum daily. Nutr Rep Int 31:505–520

Miettinen TA (1980) Effects of dietary fibre on serum lipids and cholesterol metabolism in man. In: Gotto AM, Smith LC, Allen NB (eds) Atherosclerosis V. Springer, Berlin Heidelberg New York, pp 311–315

Miettinen TA, Tarpila S (1977) Effect of pectin on serum cholesterol fecal bile acids and biliary lipids in normolipidemic and hyperlipidemic individuals. Clin Chim Acta 79:471–477

Mokady S (1974) Effect of dietary pectin and algin on the biosynthesis of hepatic lipids in growing rats. Nutr Metab 16:203–207

Mueller MA, Cleary MP, Kritchevsky D (1983) Influence of dietary fibre on lipid metabolism in meal-fed rats. J Nutr 113:2229–2238

Munoz JM, Sandstead HH, Jacob RA (1979) Effects of some cereal brans and TVP on plasma lipids. Am J Clin Nutr 32:508–592

Najemnik C, Kritz H, Irsiglier K et al. (1984) Guar and its effect on metabolic control in type II diabetic subjects. Diabetes Care 7:215–220

Nakamura H, Ishikawa T, Tada N et al. (1982) Effect of several kinds of dietary fibres on serum and lipoprotein lipids. Nutr Rep Int 26:215–221

Nervi F, Covarrubias C, Bravo P et al. (1989) Influence of legume intake on biliary lipids and cholesterol saturation in young Chilean men. Gastroenterology 96:825–830

Nishina PM, Schneeman BO, Freedland RA (1991) Effects of dietary fibers on nonfasting plasma lipoprotein and apolipoprotein levels in rats. J Nutr 121:431–437

O'Moore RR, Flanagan M, McGill AR, Wright EA, Little C, Weir DG (1978) Diet and heart disease. Br Med J i:1213

Osilesi O, Trout DL, Gover EE et al. (1985) Use of xanthan gum in dietary management of diabetes mellitus. Am J Clin Nutr 42:597–603

Palmer GH, Dixon DG (1966) Effects of pectin dose on serum cholesterol levels. Am J Clin Nutr 18:437–442

Penagini R, Veilio P, Vigorelli R et al. (1986) The effect of dietary guar on serum cholesterol, intestinal transit, and fecal output in man. Am J Gastroenterol 81:123–125

Persson I, Ruby K, Fønns-Beck P, Jensen E (1975) Bran and blood lipids. Lancet ii:1208

Persson I, Ruby K, Fønss-Beck P, Jensen E (1976) Effects of prolonged bran administration on serum levels of cholesterol, ionized calcium and iron in the elderly. J Am Geriatr Soc 24:334–335

Peterson DB, Mann JI (1985) Guar: pharmacological fibre or food fibre? Diabetic Med 2:345–347

Peterson DB, Ellis PR, Baylis JM, Frost PG, Leeds AR, Jepson EM (1984) Effects of guar on diabetes and lipids – food and pharmacology compared. Diabetologia 27:319A

Pfeffer PE, Doner LW, Hoagland PD, McDonald GG (1981) Molecular interactions with dietary fiber components. Investigation of the possible association of pectin and bile acids. J Agric Food Chem 29:455–461

Phillips DR (1986) The effect of guar gum in solution on diffusion of cholesterol mixed micelles. J Sci Food Agric 37:548–552

Prather ES (1964) Effect of cellulose on serum lipids in young women. J Am Diet Assoc 45:230–233

Ranhotra GS (1973) Effect of cellulose and wheat millfractions on plasma and liver cholesterol levels in cholesterol-fed rats. Cereal Chem 50:358–363

Rasmussen LP, Damsgaard EM, Iversen S (1981) Granuleret guargummi (Slocose) til ikke-insulinkraevende diabetikere. Ugeskr Laeger 143:1267–1270

Ray TK, Mansell KM, Knight LC, Malmud LS, Owen OE, Boden G (1983) Long-term effects of dietary fibre on glucose tolerance and gastric emptying in non-insulin-dependent diabetic patients. Am J Clin Nutr 37:376–381

Raymond TL, Connor WE, Lin DS, Warner S, Fry MM, Connor SL (1977) The interaction of dietary fibres and cholesterol upon the plasma lipids and lipoproteins, sterol balance and bowel function in human subjects. J Clin Invest 60:1429–1437

Reynolds HR, Lindeke E, Hunninghake DB (1989) Effect of oat bran on serum lipids. J Am Diet Assoc 89 (suppl):A112

Rhodes J, Jones GR, Newcombe RG, Davies D (1977/8) Effect of dietary bran on serum lipids in patients with previous myocardial infarction, with gallstones and in normal subjects. Curr Med Res Opin 5:310–314

Richter WO, Weisweiler P, Schwandt P (1981) Therapie der Hypercholesterinemie mit Apfelpektin. Deutsch Med Wochenschr 106:628

Robertson J, Brydon WG, Tadesse K, Wenham P, Walls A, Eastwood MA (1979) The effect of raw carrot on serum lipids and colon function. Am J Clin Nutr 32:1889–1892

Ross AH, Eastwood MA, Brydon WG, Anderson JR, Anderson DMW (1983) A study of the effects of dietary gum arabic in humans. Am J Clin Nutr 37:368–375

Roth G, Leitzmann C (1985) Langzeiteinfluss ballaststoffreicher Frühstückscerealien auf die Blutlipide beim Menschen. Akt Ernahr 10:106

Sasaki J, Funakoshi M, Arakawa K (1985) Effect of soybean crude fiber on the concentrations of serum lipids and apolipoproteins in hyperlipidemic subjects. Ann Nutr Metab 29:274–278

Schwandt P, Richter WO, Weisweiler P, Neurenther G (1982) Cholestyramine plus pectin in treatment of patients with familial hypercholesterolemia. Atherosclerosis 44:379–383

Schweizer TF, Bekhechi AR, Koellreutter B, Reimann S, Pometta D, Bron BA (1983) Metabolic effects of dietary fiber from dehulled soybeans in humans. Am J Clin Nutr 38:1–11

Sharma RD (1985) Hypocholesterolemic effect of gum acacia in men. Nutr Res 5:1321

Shinnick FL, Longacre MJ, Ink SL, Marlett JA (1988) Oat fiber: composition versus physiological function in rats. J Nutr 118:144–151

Shorey RAL, Day PJ, Willis RA, Lo GS, Steinke FH (1985) Effects of soybean polysaccharide on plasma lipids. J Am Diet Assoc 85:1461–1465

Shurpalekar KS, Doraiswamy TR, Sundaravalli OE, Narayana Rao M (1971) Effect of inclusion of cellulose in an "atherogenic" diet on the blood lipids of children. Nature 232:554–555

Shutler SM, Bircher GM, Tredger JS, Morgan LM, Walker AF, Low AG (1989) The effect of daily baked bean (*Phaseolus vulgaris*) consumption on the plasma lipid levels of young normocholestrolaemic men. Br J Nutr 61:257–265

Sicart R, Sable-Amplis R, Agid R (1974) Diminution de cholesterol sanguin et hepatique induite chez le hamster pas un regime alimentaire complemente en pommes. Essais chez l'homme. Comte Rend Sean Societ Biol 173:937–943

Simons LA, Gayst S, Balsubramanian S, Ruys J (1982) Long-term treatment of hypercholesterol-aemia with a new palatable formulation of guar gum. Atherosclerosis 45:101–108

Simpson HCR, Simpson RW, Lousley S (1981) A high carbohydrate leguminous fibre diet improves all aspects of diabetic control. Lancet i:1–5

Sirtori CR, Gatti E, Mantero O et al. (1979) Clinical experience with the soybean protein diet in the treatment of hypercholesterolemia. Am J Clin Nutr 32:1645–1658

Sirtori CR, Descovich G, Noseda (1980) Textured soy protein and serum cholesterol level. Lancet i:149

Smith U, Holm G (1982) Effect of a modified guar gum preparation on glucose and lipid levels in diabetics and healthy volunteers. Atherosclerosis 45:1–10

Stanley MM, Paul D, Gacke D, Murphy J (1973) Effect of cholestyramine, metamucil and cellulose on fecal bile acid excretion in man. Gastroenterology 65:889–894

Stasse-Wolthuis M, Katan MB, Hermus RJJ, Hautvast JGAJ (1979) Increase of serum cholesterol in man fed a bran diet. Atherosclerosis 45:87–91

Stasse-Wolthuis M, Albers HFF, van Jeveren JGC et al. (1980) Influence of dietary fiber from vegetables and fruits, bran or citrus pectin on serum lipids, fecal lipids and colonic function. Am J Clin Nutr 33:1745–1756

Storch K, Anderson JW, Young VR (1984) Oat-bran muffins low serum cholesterol of healthy young people. Clin Res 34:740A

Story JA, Baldino A, Czarnecki SK, Kritchevsky D (1981) Modification of liver cholesterol accumulation of cholesterol-fed rats. Nutr Rep Int 24:1213–1219

Superko HK, Haskell WL, Sawrey-Kubicek L, Farquhar JW (1988) Effects of solid and liquid guar gum on plasma cholesterol and triglyceride concentrations in moderate hypercholesterolemia. Am J Cardiol 62:51–55

Swain JF, Rouse IL, Curley CB, Sacks FM (1990) Comparison of the effects of oat bran and low-fibre wheat on serum lipoprotein levels and blood pressure. N Engl J Med 322:147–152

Tagliaferro V, Cassader M, Bozzo C et al. (1985) Moderate guar gum addition to usual diet improved peripheral sensitivity to insulin and lipaemic profile in NIDD. Diabète Métab 11:380–385

Tarpila S, Miettinen TA, Metsaranto L (1978) Effects of bran on serum cholesterol, faecal mass, fat, bile acids and neutral steroids and biliary lipids in patients with diverticular disease of the colon. Gut 19:137–145

Thacker PA, Bowland JP (1981) Effects of dietary propionic acid on serum lipids and lipoproteins of pigs fed diets supplemented with soybean meal or canola meal. Can J Anim Sci 61:439–448

Thiffault C, Belanger M, Pouliot M (1970) Traitement de l'hyperlipoproteinemie essentielle de type II par un nouvel agent therapeutique, la Celluline. Can Med Assoc J 103: 165–166

Tietyen JL, Nevins DJ, Schneeman BO (1990) Characterization of the hypcholesterolemic potential of oat bran. FASEB J 4:A527

Tognarelli M, Niccoli R, Giampietro O, Cerri M, Navalesi R (1986) Guar pasta: a new diet for obese subjects. Acta Diabetol Lat 23:77

Trowell HC (1972) Ischaemic heart disease and dietary fiber. Am J Clin Nutr 25:926–932

Trowell HC (1975) Ischaemic heart disease, atheroma and fibrinolysis. In: Burkitt DP, Trowell HC (eds) Refined carbohydrate foods and disease: Some implications of dietary fibre. Academic Press, London, pp 195–226

Trowell HC (1978) Diet and heart disease. Br Med J i:120–121

Truswell AS (1977) Food fibre and blood lipids. Nutr Revs 35:51–54

Truswell AS (1984) Dietary fiber and lipid metabolism. In: Tanphaichitr V, Dahlan W, Suphakara V, Valyasevi A (eds) Human nutrition: Better nutrition, better life. Proceedings of 4th Asian Congress of Nutrition. Aksornsmai Press, Bangkok, pp 478–487

Truswell AS, Kay RM (1975) Absence of effect of bran on blood lipids. Lancet i:922–923

Truswell AS, Kay RM (1976) Bran and blood lipids. Lancet i:367

Tsai AC, Elias J, Kelley JJ, Lin RSC, Robson JRK (1976) Influence of certain dietary fibres on serum and tissue cholesterol levels in rats. J Nutr 106:118–123

Tsai AC, Mott EL, Owen GM, Bennick MR, Lo GS, Steinke FH (1983) Effects of soy polysaccharide on gastrointestinal functions, nutrient balance, steroid excretions, glucose tolerance, serum lipids, and other parameters in humans. Am J Clin Nutr 38:504–511

Tuomilehto J, Voutilainen E, Huttunen J, Vinni S, Homan K (1980) Effect of guar gum on body weight and serum lipids in hypercholesterolaemic females. Acta Med Scand 280:45–48

Tuomilehto J, Karttunen P, Vinni S, Kostiainen E, Uusitupa M (1983) A double-blind evaluation of guar gum in patients with dyslipidaemia. Hum Nutr Clin Nutr 37C:109–116

Tuomilehto J, Silvasti M, Aro A et al. (1988) Long-term treatment of severe hypercholesterolaemia with guar gum. Atherosclerosis 72:157–162

Tuomilehto J, Silvasti M, Marrvinen V, Uusitupa M, Aro A (1989) Guar gum and gemfibrozil: an effective combination in the treatment of hypercholesterolaemia. Atherosclerosis 76:71–77

Turnbull WH, Leeds AR (1987) Reduction of total and LDL-cholesterol in plasma by rolled oats. J Clin Nutr Gastroenterol 2:177–181

Uusitupa M, Tuomilehto J, Karttunen P, Wolf E (1984) Long-term effects of guar gum on metabolic control, serum cholesterol and blood pressure in type 2 (NID) diabetic patients with high blood pressure. Ann Clin Res 16 (Suppl 43):126–131

Uusitupa M, Siituone O, Savolainen K, Silvasti M, Penttila M, Parvioinen M (1989) Metabolic and nutritional effects of long-term use of guar gum in the treatment of non-insulin-dependent diabetes of poor metabolic control. Am J Clin Nutr 49:345–351

Vaaler S, Hanssen KF, Dahl-Jorgensson K et al. (1986) Diabetic control is improved by guar gum and wheat bran supplementation. Diabetic Med 3:230–233

Vahouny GV (1982) Dietary fibers and intestinal absorption of lipids. In: Vahouny GV, Kritchevsky D (eds) Dietary fiber in health and disease. Plenum Press, New York, pp 203–227

Van Beresteijn ECH, Van Schaik M, Mogot MFK (1979) Effect of bran and cellulose on lipid metabolism in obese female Zucker rats. J Nutr 109:2085–2097

Van Berge-Henegouwen GP, Huybregts AW, de Werf S, Demacker P, Schade RW (1979) Effect of a standardized wheat bran preparation on serum lipids in young healthy males. Am J Clin Nutr 32:794–798

Van Dokkum W (1978) Zemelen in brood: verteerbaarheid en invloed op het defaecatiepatroon, de mineralen-balans en de serumlipidenconcentraties bij de mens. Voedingsmiddelentechnologie 11:(41)18–21

Van Horn L, Liu K, Parker D et al. (1986) Serum lipid response to oat product intake with a fat-modified diet. J Am Diet Assoc 86:759–764

Van Horn L, Emidy LA, Liu K et al. (1988) Serum lipid responses to fat-modified oatmeal-enhanced diet. Prev Med 17:377–386

Van Horn L, Moag-Stahlberg A, Lui K et al. (1991) Effects on serum lipids of adding instant oats to usual American diets. Am J Public Health 81:183–188

Van Raaij JMA, Katan MB, West CE, Hautvast JGAJ (1982) Influence of diets containing casein, soy isolate and soy concentrate on serum cholesterol and lipoproteins in middle-aged volunteers. Am J Clin Nutr 35:925–934

Vargo D, Doyle R, Floch MH (1985) Colonic bacterial flora and serum cholesterol: alterations induced by dietary citrus pectin. Am J Gastroenterol 80:361–364

Vinik AI, Jenkins DJA (1988) Dietary fibre in management of diabetes. Diabetes Care 11:236–249

Watts JM, Jablonski P, Toouli J (1978) The effect of added bran to the diet on the saturation of bile in people without gallstones. Am J Surg 135:321–324

Weinand HA, Sack H (1970) Beinflussung des Cholesterinstoffwechsels durch Pektin. Med Welt 23:1426–1427

Weinreich J, Pedersen O, Dinesen K (1977) Role of bran in normals. Acta Med Scand 202:125–130

Welch RW, Peterson DM, Schramka N (1988) Hypocholesterolemic and gastrointestinal effects of oat bran fractions in chicks. Nutr Rep Int 38:551–561

Wirth A, Middlehoff G, Braeunuig C, Schlierf G (1982) Treatment of familial hypercholesterol-aemia with a combination of bezafibrate and guar. Atherosclerosis 45:291–297

Zavoral JH, Hannan P, Fields DJ et al. (1983) The hypolipidemic effect of locust bean gum food products in familial hypercholesterolemic adults and children. Am J Clin Nutr 38:285–294

Commentary

Southgate: Isolated pectin has substantial differences from the pectic substances present in plant cell walls. It has a lower molecular weight and has lost most of the sidechains present in the native pectic substances. Cellulose preparations are also very different to cellulose as it occurs in the plant cell wall. This is even more true for isolated lignins which have had their carbohydrate matrix removed, and it is difficult to extrapolate from studies with isolated lignins to lignin as it occurs in plants.

General Discussion

The principal aim of this final workshop discussion was to review some of the practical considerations which complement the written papers and commentaries. The discussion centered around physico-chemical properties, definition, analysis, energy value and labelling of dietary fibre. In conclusion, large bowel diseases and some general difficulties related to investigation of connections between diet and disease are discussed.

Kritchevsky: May I suggest we start this discussion with a few questions relating to the background chapters of Thibault, Morris and Read. What does the measurement of physico-chemical properties of concentrated fibre sources teach us about their effect in the gut? What are the physico-chemical properties of the food bolus and chyme in the intestine and how can these be measured? Is there any way to visualise the idea of the intact cell wall not just being cell wall material? And how can we distinguish between soluble and insoluble dietary fibre? A lot of this is related to food labelling. These questions are certainly of interest for the host organisation, and the answer should have a firm scientific basis and be relevant for labelling. Do you have any comments, Dr. Asp?

Asp: Yes, I think it would be a good start to talk a little bit more about physico-chemical measurements. Is it possible at all to measure, for instance, viscosity in food as eaten with lumps, or should we go for measurement on intestinal aspirations, or could we simulate digestion by treatment with pepsin and pancreatin before making measurements?

Kritchevsky: And what does all this tell us? Will it be useful to us once we know how to do it?

Asp: Of course, provided we agree that the physico-chemical properties in the stomach and gut matter for physiological response.

Read: I think we have generally agreed that the physico-chemical properties may be very important for acute responses. Whether this is at all important for any chronic effects is a different question.

Kritchevsky: Dr. Morris, do you have a contribution to this?

Morris: A central problem, both conceptually and technically, is how to characterise the rheological properties of something that is grossly heterogeneous. At its simplest, how do you describe the viscosity behaviour of a pot of vegetable soup? It would be fairly easy to measure the properties of an individual pea or an individual cube of carrot, and trivial to measure the viscosity of the liquid surrounding them, but these are not representative of the behaviour of the whole system. What is really needed is a measurement that would describe the resistance to the spoon going round in the whole pot. So, for characterisation of digesta, one important consideration would be to make sure that the measuring system is large in comparison with the size of any solid lumps. A practical problem, that is not at all trivial, is coping with the lumps settling out during the measurement, or preventing it happening.

Kritchevsky: I guess one other very important aspect that has not been enough addressed here is still the question of how to define and name dietary fibre.

Mauron: To an outsider of the field represented in this workshop, it appears that the main stumbling block for translating the present scientific knowledge on dietary fibre into practical recommendations for the consumer, the industry and the legislator, is still a matter of semantics. In contrast to the classic nutrients, which are well defined chemical entities independent from their food source, dietary fibre is essentially a concept comprised of four elements: chemical nature, physical structure, food origin and physiological behaviour. In this broad sense, dietary fibre is defined as "non-carbohydrate and carbohydrate material, present as skeletal remains of the cell walls of plant origin, that are not digested by the endogenous secretions of the human digestive tract".

Although this historic definition has been largely abandoned because it is not suitable for testing scientific hypotheses, it still constitutes a sort of ideological basis used to improve the nutritional behaviour of the consumer and to evaluate the proposed, newer and simpler definitions. In order to arrive at a more concise definition of dietary fibre, many modifications of the original concept have been proposed involving three of the four elements of the concept. As regards chemical entity, only lignin has been retained as non-carbohydrate compound and carbohydrate specified as polysaccharides or, by some, as non-starch polysaccharides. The structural feature, the cell wall architecture has been dropped since it is ill-defined and its physiological function not yet established. The plant origin is, generally, not stated but often implied. The last element, the physiological behaviour in the gastro-intestinal tract has been maintained integrally and is not controversial, namely the non-digestibility by endogenous enzymes leading to non-availability in the small intestine. This is the common denominator of all dietary fibre concepts and should therefore be the backbone of a pragmatic definition and analysis of a dietary fibre.

In view of the fact that it is presently not possible to reach a complete consensus on the definition and analysis of dietary fibre, the only way out is to establish a convention about a pragmatic and simple definition to be used for food labelling and everyday life leaving to the care of the scientists the definition of the dietary fibre employed in a particular investigation.

I propose, therefore, for daily use in industry and legislation the term "conventional dietary fibre", defined as follows:

Conventional Dietary Fibre = lignin + polysaccharides unavailable in the small intestine

This definition is based on physiological behaviour, i.e. unavailability for small intestinal absorption, for which there is a consensus, and retains lignin, a typical plant cell wall material never found in animal tissues. It includes, logically, resistant starch, since the latter is unavailable for small intestinal absorption and fermented in the colon like the other types of dietary fibres. Conventional dietary fibre is presently best analysed by the AOAC method, but other methods could be adapted to measure it also.

This proposed new definition is certainly not perfect but represents in my opinion a valid compromise to end a deadlock that has already lasted too long and hampered the practical implementation of the dietary fibre concept in industry and legislation. The term "conventional" clearly shows that it is based in a convention for practical, immediate use that does leave the field open for scientific investigation and further evolution of the concept.

Truswell: I would think this is a very promising proposal and I hope we hear more about it.

Kritchevsky: Yes, I agree. But what about oligosaccharides like stachyose and raffinose? They do not seem to be classified. They are not resistant starch. Are they cell wall polysaccharides?

Truswell: No. They are certainly not available in the small intestine.

Mauron: But they are not completely unavailable: they are fermented in the colon.

Southgate: I think it is better to think of the carbohydrates in food as falling into three principal categories: sugars, which I would probably include up to the disaccharides, then the oligosaccharides, which according to the IUPAC rules include three to ten units but which could go to some higher values, if you are assuming that a polysaccharide should exhibit a tertiary structure. In practice, the amounts of these oligosaccharides present in the diet are quite small, except in specific foods like glucose syrups and some of the fructan-rich vegetables. So I think you would probably find intakes of possibly two or three grams a day in a "normal" Western-style diet. I personally think the IUPAC definition of polysaccharides, as containing ten or more monosaccharide units is probably a bit low in relation to tertiary structures and also in a pragmatic context, because practically everybody who is analysing these materials is using 80% alcohol to precipitate the polysaccharides. Some polysaccharides with 10 to 15 units will not be precipitated in 80% alcohol, particularly if they happen to be branched. A realistic definition of a polysaccharide from a nutritional point of view would be at least 20 units. But that is an arbitrary definition as well.

Asp: This points to the need to consider and discuss more than in the past the very arbitrary cut-off obtained by 80% alcohol solubility. But I would like to come back to the need of a pragmatic or realistic definition and that this must be related to a method. At the "FIBRE 90" meeting in Norwich, Dr. Hans Englyst suggested that the colorimetric variant of the Englyst method might be used optional to the AOAC method as a pragmatic method and fibre definition. I think that was a very good suggestion, which is even more well founded when we see now the almost final evaluation of the MAFF IV study [see Chap. 4 for a detailed explanation] showing rather good agreement with these two methods in most foods.

Englyst: Even so they do differ and we still have a major problem with the resistant starch. How do you think it should be defined and measured?

Asp: The analytically resistant starch present in the AOAC method and the Uppsala method [see Chap. 4] is a reasonably well-defined fraction of the total amount of starch not absorbed in the small intestine. In most foods, it gives a small contribution compared with the analytical errors and the variation between various laboratories. I agree that there may be problems with some special food ingredients or processing techniques, for example with repeatedly autoclaved starch.

Englyst: Could you comment on the preliminary results from the part of the Euresta [EURESTA (European Resistant Starch) designates a European Flair Project which includes analytical studies of resistant starch. The June 1991 meeting of EURESTA defined resistant starch as "any starch which escapes digestion in the small intestine of man".] trial aiming to measure retrograded amylose (the fraction of resistant starch which the Prosky/Asp/Schweizer and Theander procedures include as dietary fibre)? It does not seem to be easy to measure nor to reproduce any measurements of these types of starch. It depends on the enzymes and conditions you use.

Schweizer: There appears to be a difference in attitude with regard to resistant starch vs. the lower molecular weight polysaccharides and oligosaccharides. People tend to agree on a pragmatic stand in saying that 80% ethanol is fine to define the cut-off, well knowing that this does not correspond to a precise degree of polymerisation. There seems to be much less desire to have a pragmatic standpoint regarding the discrimination between the starchy materials which do or do not escape small intestinal digestion. However, the food industry and legislation need a pragmatic solution. As for all food constituents, it is really the method which defines the component which is measured.

Morris: Dr. Englyst knows what I am going to suggest because we had a long discussion on this last night. Acceptable values for routine analysis might be the overall estimate from the AOAC procedure or the sum of the individual values for NSP and retrograded amylose from the Englyst colorimetric assay.

The effective equivalence of these two values should be tested by analysis of representative food products, using best working practice for both methods. If the agreed criterion of acceptable equivalence is met, both methods should be recommended for legislative and labelling purposes. For food tables and analysis of unprocessed foods, individual values for NSP and for "resistant" and "available" starch fractions, should be reported separately.

Turning now to oligosaccharides, I am not sure that precipitation in 80% ethanol is quite as arbitrary as it sounds. In terms of physical properties, the number of sugars in carbohydrate chains is less important than whether or not they are long enough to stick together to form solid lumps or hydrated networks. This will obviously affect their behaviour in the gut and, for exactly the same reasons, affect their precipitation. Thus, although the 80% alcohol "cut-off" can occur at different chainlengths for different carbohydrates, it may not be a bad guide to their physiological action as dietary fibre.

Schweizer: From the discussions I have had with several observers in this room, I presume that this could be a good option to which I would like to add a time schedule. During a five-year period, for instance, we would have the AOAC procedure, with which many are familiar. In parallel and with equal right an "NSP + resistant starch" procedure which gives similar values could be used. Then, during these five years, we could make progress, further clarify the resistant starch issue and others, without having continually to discuss regulatory issues.

Kritchevsky: Any other comment? Well, what we are talking about is satisfying the need for labelling and I thought that Dr. Morris's and Dr. Schweizer's suggestions might be helpful. You have to have a basis from which to start drawing conclusions or doing more work, and regulatory agencies are not interested in scientific arguments.

Southgate: In the introduction to the analytical paper [Chap. 4], it is stated that a different approach is needed from a research point of view and for the regulators. I agree that for routine quality control some sort of simple, pragmatic and rough method, provided it is reproducible, is the obvious answer because of the context in which the analyses have to be carried out. The real issue is the problem of translating that definition into other areas. One of the areas that does concern me is in relation to the dietary advice that has been given to populations. There, you have to consider that the original dietary fibre hypothesis refers to the protective effects of a type of diet which is characterised by the foods that contain plant cell wall materials.

Now, the problem is to know whether regulatory analyses properly reflect that nutritional advice to populations. I am offering this as a point for debate: the real issue is that people are advised to increase their dietary fibre intakes and then may see foods labelled with dietary fibre contents, which actually bear no relationship to the origin of the nutritional guidance that they have been given, because there are many materials that would analyse as dietary fibre which exert no beneficial physiological effects at all. There are lots of plant residue materials that you could use to create dietary fibre-rich foods. The consumer will consume them in the belief that he was eating a high-fibre diet. Therefore, I can see a need to make sure that a regulatory analysis actually is translatable properly to the consumer, and I am not sure whether that can be done adequately in the ingredient descriptions. I am not sure whether consumers read the list of ingredients in a proper way or whether they are just looking at the number.

Kritchevsky: The regulator should be able to regulate what goes into the food and make sure that it is not mixtures that can be put together to resemble fibre and really are not.

Southgate: But the real point is if you then define dietary fibre in terms of a method, then there is no way that the regulator can stop those constituents going into foods.

Schweizer: I think there is a way, because the regulator not only regulates on methods, but also on ingredients. And if there are certain ingredients which the legislator has reasons not to allow in foods, he can regulate on the ingredients.

Mauron: We have a certain analogy with protein measured as N × 6.25, because some people can cheat and have a higher protein content just by putting in urea, e.g. for animal feed. So, here again, the legislator must of course not only insist on a method like Kjeldahl, but also on the ingredients. I think that should not stop us from having a relatively simple method. The legislator has not introduced amino acid analysis instead of Kjeldahl: that was too complicated. Of course, that is just an analogy, the fibre issue is more complicated.

Heaton: I am not happy with that analogy. Fibre, as David Southgate and I conceive it, is not a substance, or even a group of substances: it is a concept. It reflects the cellular structural integrity of food. Could you devise some sort of score for structural integrity which can be put onto your label? Probably not, but I think that we are dealing with something more subtle, difficult and complicated than anything else in nutrition, and to pretend that we can reduce it to a single number which gives useful information about the metabolic and gastro-intestinal effects of that food on your body is to deceive ourselves and the consumer.

Schweizer: Maybe, but this limitation is by no means unique to dietary fibre. The numbers on food labels refer to what a food contains rather than to what it does in the body.

Truswell: If you look at present dietary guidelines around the world, this group of foods will have one of these headings: they will say either "eat more" or "eat plenty of starchy foods", or they will say "eat plenty of foods containing dietary fibre" or "eat plenty of vegetables, cereals, fruit and legumes". And, whatever the heading, the next sentence will say "eat plenty of wholegrain cereals, vegetables, fruit and legumes, preferably without added fat, sugar and salt". People who are framing dietary guidelines have managed to deal with this in an admittedly simple way, but it can be dealt with. The practice of adding dietary fibre to foods, as a sort of food additive to make it more attractive, could be dealt with in the same way as adding vitamins to foods, i.e. with some recommendation: there is no need to add extra fibre to our foods. Maybe I am wrong, maybe there is a need.

Southgate: Defining dietary fibre as endogenous material would in fact protect. I am not one of those people who believe that the food industry manipulates the diets. I believe that most companies are honest and reliable, but dietary fibre does lend itself to being manipulated, particularly in the advertising of foods. You only have to look at all the claims that are being made for cereal products enriched with oats.

Schweizer: No method will resolve this particular problem, because what you call endogenous and exogenous materials are most often indistinguishable in complex foods.

Truswell: With fibre, the position may be the same as, for example, with vitamin C and polyunsaturated fat or linoleic acid. Some manufacturers will wish to guarantee their margarine to contain a certain amount of linoleic acid. If the source of linoleic acid, sunflower or safflower, has a lower analysis in a particular batch, the manufacturer has to do something to get it back. The same situation can occur with fruit juices, guaranteeing at least 50 mg of vitamin C per 100 ml. Now, considering the variability of the composition of oat bran, the manufacturer of a breakfast cereal guaranteed to contain a certain amount of beta-glucans may have to adjust certain batches so as to maintain his claim. That is not adding some useless extra fibre; that is maintaining the quality for something which the public considers important. And I think we have to bear that usage in mind as well.

Fondu: I would like to address the problem from another point of view. The European Community has decided on a Directive on Nutritional Labelling where the indication of quantities of fibres in foods will be mandatory in certain cases. There is no definition as yet within the EC of fibres nor of the method of analysis. If the scientists do not accept their responsibility now, the civil servants of the governments will discuss and establish definition and methods without experts.

Southgate: Unfortunately, with due respect to all the people who have developed the methods, none of these methods can be regarded as analytically accurate and they are certainly not precise, especially when compared with the other methods that are used for measuring macronutrients. So, I think we must recognise them as practical but at the present stage, quite rough methods. Therefore, we should be thinking about the levels of accuracy and precision we are going to imply by the numbers that we put on the labels. If the legislation was such that all dietary fibre sources should be labelled to the nearest whole percentage point, which is the limit that the methods will allow at the present time, then in fact we could have a system whereby we can accept any method that gets comparable results within that limit. That would resolve a lot of the problems over which method should be used.

Truswell: It sounds to me as a total outsider on this that there are two methods that are both very strongly defended and which are very near to true, whatever that means. One is the AOAC method and the other the Englyst-UK method. Now, why would it not be possible for the EC to state that dietary fibre must be declared, that there are two methods permitted and that the method has to be stated in brackets. So, you say on the product, dietary fibre (AOAC), or (A), if you like, and dietary fibre (UK-Englyst) or (E).

Schweizer: These two methods in the methods comparison gave more or less indistinguishable results. Thus, the bracket could be omitted which would correspond to the suggestion which Prof. Morris made earlier in this discussion.

Truswell: I would still like to have a bracket.

Cummings: Three things: one on definition, one on labelling and one on starch. We have sat around many tables over the years, discussing the definitions of dietary fibre and I do not think we are any further forward now than we were in 1970, when we first started talking about it. I do not expect we will get any further forward, largely because, as Ken Heaton says, dietary fibre is a concept. The nearest thing in words we can come to is, I think, that dietary fibre is plant cell wall material. This encompasses the sort of physical and chemical concept without leading one into too many difficulties in terms of physiology. If you start putting a physiological rider to your definition, you run into all sorts of problems, because you have got to say which physiological effects you are talking about, for example is it suppression of appetite, changes in gastric emptying, effects on cholesterol or steroid metabolism or glucose absorption or large bowel function. So, it is very difficult to get agreement for a form of words, but the simplest is that dietary fibre is plant cell wall material. We ought maybe just to say that to the EC. We do have problems, as agreed when we talked about this on the first day, e.g. what do we do about the non-plant cell wall, but very similar polysaccharides? Well, we have to accept that. When it comes to research and labelling they can easily be incorporated, because we are then talking about analysis. If we go back to the original concept, it is the plant cell wall which is central.

When we come to labelling one needs compromises and one needs to be pragmatic. We have got a problem in that we have to put a single number on a packet that means something to the consumer in terms of this concept. No single number is going to be of much use to the consumer, but we have to keep faith with the consumer and I think that the labelling method should principally reflect cell wall material. Therefore, if we have a method, it should reflect the cell wall. It should also give results which are very similar to those from detailed methods, such as in food tables. I think it would be very dangerous to have a labelling method which gave results which are significantly different from what you might find in food tables. Finally, if we have a range of methods, and I do not object to having a range of methods, they should give similar results, if possible. The main problem at the moment in the current two methods is the inclusion of some resistant starch in the Prosky procedure.

The third thing I want to say is that I do not believe that starch has any place in this whole discussion. I doubt if it was ever intended to be part of the cell wall concept and I think it complicates matters enormously to have some starch in one of the methods. It is only there by chance, because the gravimetric method was originally designed to measure cell wall material, but happened to include some starch in it. So, we have to find some good reasons for keeping it there. But as far as I can see, it can be quite easy to get rid of it by adding DMSO to the method.

If that was done, the gravimetric method would presumably become quite a good reflection of the cell wall material. People who say that resistant starch and cell wall material are physiologically similar are making a very brave statement which could be countered so easily and in so many ways. In summary, I would like to see fibre defined as plant cell wall material. Different labelling methods may co-exist but should give equivalent results to more detailed methods and should give similar results to each other. Finally I think that if we get rid of resistant starch, we probably could get rid of most of our problems.

Kritchevsky: Thank you very much. That is a good summary. And I think it is now time to go on to discuss in detail what we heard about the physiological effects of fibre.

Schweizer: Just to clarify two points: first, to my knowledge, the resistance to small intestinal digestion is the only physiological "rider" ever put to the definition and, second, DMSO does not seem to be selective enough a solvent to discriminate between starch and non-starch polysaccharides, as mentioned also in Chapter 4.

Kritchevsky: I would like to continue the discussion by bringing up the subjects of protein and carbohydrate and mineral absorption: what are, for instance, the practical consequences of bringing digestion and absorption to the more distal parts of the gastro-intestinal tract?

Truswell: David Jenkins has nice diagrams, in which he has the rapidly digested carbohydrates going into the top of the small intestine, and the "lente" carbohydrates, slowly digested, going down a longer length of the small intestine. So, that is the image of it, but whether that is a good thing or a bad thing, apart from the effect on the blood glucose, I would not know.

Heaton: We do not know whether it is a bad thing for the gut if digestion takes place rapidly high up, rather than more slowly throughout the gut, but I think it is reasonable to speculate that the commonness of disease at the lower end of the gut, rather than the upper end is connected with the general fact that when an organ is underused or not exercised it usually suffers and, maybe, becomes diseased. I know that this is a crude concept, but I think it is generally true that the more an organ is exercised and used, the healthier it is. It is certainly true for the teeth, for example, and it might be true for the ileum, which I think is a pretty superfluous organ for people on a Western diet, except that you need it to reabsorb bile acids.

Read: I think it is a misconception that the ileum is underused. It is actually quite important. Food going down the gut gets to the ileum very quickly. Then something happens in the ileum to help to control its passage. The other thing is that fat in particular is digested and absorbed rather slowly, and quite a lot of fat gets to the ileum. Patients who have had a resection of the ileum do not just suffer from problems with bile acids and Vitamin B_{12}, they can have quite gross steatorrhoea and diarrhoea.

Heaton: I am of course aware of these other problems associated with ilectomy but I would point out that nearly everybody who gets an ilectomy loses the ileocaecal valve.

Johnson: One of the things that needs to be borne in mind about the small intestine are these regulatory peptides, presumed hormones that, I am sure, play a much bigger role in the control of gut function and probably of other aspects of metabolism than is really understood at the moment. There is good evidence from animal work and some human work that the release of these hormones is modified by fibre, probably because of delayed nutrient absorption. There is a very wide area for further research.

Asp: I would like to bring up again the question of whether there is a place for added fibre in food production. One aspect that we have not addressed is that some fibres can be used at rather low concentrations as water binders which could, in some cases, help to make low fat food, thereby exerting an indirect effect. There are many different kinds of such supplements, and I think brans are one group with some unique features in that nutrients are carried with the fibres, because the aleuron layer is attached to the fibre-rich outer layers. So, when you add bran, you also add nutrients – but also phytic acid, which is the other side of the coin. Then we have another category which is represented, for instance, by sugar beet fibre or soy cotyledon fibre which are preparations that still carry some structure. One can regard them as cell walls of empty cells. Finally there are the really isolated fibres such as pure cellulose or gums. Is there any reason to distinguish these types? Can you gain anything nutritionally from some remaining, more or less intact cell wall structures?

Kritchevsky: Are they additives or not?

Asp: That differs, I think, between countries. In Sweden these "upgraded waste" products are regarded as ingredients and not as additives, whereas pectins for example are additives.

Truswell: I would like to support the triple division which Nils Asp has just suggested. The first group, that is the brans, consists of total cells on the outside of the endosperm and contains nutrients as well as fibre. The second and third groups would not as a rule have any additional vitamins or minerals. I think that it is very helpful to have that subdivision into three potential types of fibre which can be added to foods from the nutritional point of view.

Kritchevsky: Well, does this refer to just using it, or labelling it or . . . ?

Asp: No, not labelling it. Of course, it will appear in the ingredient list, but not in any figures, because we can't characterise these properties in analytical terms. It is also questionable whether you can restore any cell wall effects. My personal view is that one cannot restore much, if any, of these effects, because the cell walls as a package around the nutrients within the cells cannot be restored. Concerning the brans, some intact aleuron cells are retained, but not the structure of the grain, of course.

Kritchevsky: When including purified polysaccharides in the measurement of fibre, even if they have originated from plant cell, the result is no longer an index of cell wall material. That could be a reason to separate them.

Let us now turn to the caloric value of fibre. Dr. Southgate said that it was a maximum of 3 kcal/g and a minimum of zero – you cannot get below that, can you?

Southgate: Some of the polysaccharides do apparently have a negative energy value. But that is probably because there is an effect on fat absorption.

Asp: I would like to ask if you feel that the caloric value of 2 kcal/g that we discussed yesterday is better founded than the zero value which is approved in the United States and in many other countries? The loss of starch, fat and protein on a high-fibre diet could balance some of the caloric content of fibres.

Also, I think that high-fibre foods generally have a lower protein digestibility than low-fibre foods and we usually do not correct for that. So, my feeling is that the zero value can so far be defended as well as any other value between zero and four.

Southgate: It is very important to recognize that the way we calculate metabolisable energy of foods is a convention, just as is using a factor of 6.25 to calculate protein from nitrogen. Strictly speaking, all our values in food composition tables should have inverted commas around the protein. Very few food composition tables have actually measured protein. They should indicate crude protein, but we tend to forget the "crude". Bearing in mind the errors in measuring food intake, in measuring differences in the efficiency of digestion of nutrients between individuals and in a whole host of things, I think that for practical dietetic purposes, a value of zero is perfectly acceptable. However, in connection with the labelling of a food containing a significant proportion of a sugar alcohol, or a non-starch polysaccharide, the manufacturer wants to express a reasonably reliable metabolisable energy value. I would have thought that 2 kcal/g was a reasonable value. What is actually needed are specific values for specific ingredients. ILSI has a research programme specifically to look at methods for measuring these and when their methods are agreed, we will be able to get more specific values.

Kritchevsky: Dr. Cummings, do you have a comment on the energy of fibre?

Cummings: Of NSP! It clearly does have an energy value, otherwise half of the animal kingdom would be dead. I am prepared to accept a value of 2 kcal/g.

Mauron: I suggest we look again at a practical aspect of mineral absorption. If industry adds bran or increases fibre content, especially from cereals, and thereby increases phytic acid content must the consumer be warned that it can have an effect on mineral absorption? I understand that there is an effect, at least on iron and zinc, but some people say that one adapts and that the favourable effects of fibre overrule these possible negative effects on mineral absorption.

Kritchevsky: Is there a discussion on that point?

Sandström: Well, as we write in our paper, it will be important for the consumer to have information about phytate content for products making up a substantial part of his or her fibre and mineral intake, while for products only eaten occasionally, it might not be necessary. On the other hand, it is relatively easy to reduce the phytate content and keep the fibre and the minerals in the product. So, I would recommend that the food industry do it.

Truswell: One of the most important conclusions of this meeting, is that it seems now very well established and accepted that it is the phytate and not the fibre which affects mineral absorption. I have been confused about this, but your work and what you have reviewed seems now very clear.

That being so, we need to draw the attention of the food industry to the importance of phytate, looking at the phytate content of the raw material and looking at technological methods to reduce it.

Heaton: Regarding bran and its possible dangers, it is possible to obtain a wheat fibre concentrate which contains no phytate.

Asp: When discussing brans, we must also remember the amount of minerals, because such a product is not only free from phytate but also free from minerals. So, the overall absorption in mg of minerals must be considered. Whenever one can reduce the phytic acid, it is probably good when this can be achieved without reducing the mineral content – but I also think that we still lack long-term studies to demonstrate the importance of consuming phytic acid, at least in a Western diet.

Sandberg: Yes, I agree with that. But still, we have quite a lot of evidence that we can increase the availability of iron and zinc. So, it would be worthwhile doing it, even if increasing bran intake does not mean that lots of people become mineral deficient. In fact, fibre-rich cereals with a low phytate content can become a good source of iron and zinc in the diet. I think it is also important, to reduce the phytate content in formula diets for children.

Kritchevsky: Now, the third section of this workshop was on disease and there were four different presentations: Dr. Heaton went through the list of all the things that fibre was originally supposed to affect, and he was able to show us that several of these were not really important, but irritable bowel syndrome, gallstones, diverticular disease and cancer still are important. We then had a talk on obesity and in conclusion we heard about diabetes and lipids. Dr. Heaton, do you know, is there a clinical trial started on fibre and colon cancer? Are you going to do a study with feeding fibre and looking at colon cancer outcome or feeding fibre to old people and looking just at a general health outcome?

Truswell: There must be several trials in progress looking at people who have adenomatous polyps.

Heaton: Yes, that is my understanding, too. Obviously, there is a possibility that bran, or some fibre-associated material might affect the carcinoma sequence at some level, other than the production of the adenomas. It may affect the malignant change of adenomas. The trouble is that it would be very difficult, ethically, to take a group of people with adenomas and put one half on some possibly protective agents and the others not and wait to see how many of them get cancers.

Nagengast: Actually, in Europe, there is one multicentre study going on, the European cancer prevention study, in which people with adenomas are put on a normal diet, on psyllium husk as a fibre additive and on calcium. One of the objectives of the study was not only to look at a recurrent trend of adenomas, because – as you pointed out – that may not be a good endpoint and have nothing to do with diet, but to look at tiny polyps, which quite often remain after removal of larger adenomas. After three years this polyp is then removed and examined. There are more studies going on with calcium, I think, than with fibre at the moment.

Cummings: I am surprised to hear about the design of that trial, because I would have thought that it is not particularly appropriate to use calcium. I thought that the calcium story was dying. Grégoire et al. 1989, [Gut 30:376–382] showed that calcium supplements increased faecal deoxycholate concentrations and faecal pH in man.

Nagengast: This may be too strong a conclusion at the present time and I would like to wait for the results of studies presently underway. There has also been some evidence that calcium may not lower proliferative activity but rather enhance it. However, this may differ amongst individuals.

Heaton: Could I go back to constipation, which of course is central to a lot of possible effects of fibre. The statement was made that the more you deviate from the norm, the more response you will get to the treatment, with respect to hypercholesterolaemia at least. With constipation, the opposite seems to be true, i.e. the more somebody needs fibre, the less it helps them. I wonder whether anybody would like to comment on this.

Read: If you regard constipation as – I hesitate to say disorder – a change in colonic motility, then the observations, which are quite right, could be explained. If the change in colonic motility is mild, and can be stimulated by bran, then constipation is going to get better. However, the severely constipated patients are resistant to laxatives, they are resistant to bran, they are resistant to everything. I think it is a question of the severity of the disorder. I do not believe that constipation should be regarded as a deficiency of fibre, a fibre-deficiency disease. I think it is a motility change, which can be helped by fibre, if it is reasonably mild.

Heaton: The only thing which bothers me is the implication that there are two kinds of constipation: a mild kind, which is fibre-responsive and a severe kind, which is a motility disease.

Read: Oh no, you could postulate it being a continuum.

Heaton: Yes, I believe it is a continuum. And that of course makes it difficult to know where to draw the line.

Read: You draw the line according to the response of your patient: some patients respond and others do not.

Heaton: I used to baulk at the concept of constipation which you have put forward but I am beginning to think perhaps it is right, in view of the epidemiological findings that I presented. And yet if you compare communities with different fibre intakes there seems to be a good relationship between the mean fibre intake of the community and its mean faecal weight.

Read: The point is that a lot of people passing very little stool are not constipated at all. Constipation, as I see it, is something patients come to me and complain about. And therefore, it cannot be acquainted on the population basis necessarily.

Heaton: That is a very true statement.

Read: Constipated patients could be divided into those who basically get the faeces to the rectum and can't defecate and those that do not even get the faeces to the rectum. But I find now more and more, that most patients have got both. They have got a disorder of colonic transit as well as a disorder of defecation.

Cummings: Just to go back to the question of magnitude of response. It has been said that people with severe slow transit constipation are less likely to respond than those with slight problems. But actually the response is always the same in a group of people, if you look at it as a proportion. In other words, the percentage increase in stool weight – and another example is the percentage fall in cholesterol – is consistent to a given stimulus. But the absolute values do of course vary enormously. So, if you start with a stool weight of 40 g a day and you have a 50% increase, you go to 60 g a day; you start with 200 g, you go to 300. That is the mathematical explanation. Now, the worst affected ones have the slowest transit time. And this is very important, because it allows time for greater degradation of cell wall material in the colon, which ultimately loses its effect completely. Also, long transit times mean less efficient bacterial growth. So, there are two mechanisms which are impaired in people with very slow transit and this explains why the slow-transit people do not respond so well.

Read: But didn't you also show that constipated people require much more bran or fibre to achieve a similar increase in stool weight? In other words, they are relatively resistant to the action of fibre.

Cummings: Their response is dependent on where you start in the scale. It is a proportional thing.

Read: So, again, one can view this as a kind of continuum. Some constipated patients are relatively resistant to the action of fibre and some are completely resistant.

Cummings: No, you will always be able to show a change. But the more constipated you are, the less dramatic that change will be in absolute terms.

Read: I think I can give you some patients where you just cannot show a change at all, you know.

Truswell: As with everything else in medicine, isn't it also a matter of the chronicity of the condition? If somebody has had constipation for 18 years, or somebody has had it for one year, you would expect a different response, actually in defecation frequency, which is different from stool weight.

Heaton: One of the problems here is the dissociation between physiological variables which we can measure and symptoms, which we cannot. Nevertheless, what the patient complains of is what he wants relief from. We may be able to increase the stool weight of our constipated patients, but if they have come to see us because they feel bloated, they may not thank us for giving them bran. They might actually feel more bloated. It is frustrating if you know that the bran is doing something which ought to help them, but they are complaining more.

Read: I agree, it depends really whether you are treating the patient or treating yourself. It does not help those patients to know that their transit time is increased. Their problem is that they find defecation uncomfortable and difficult.

Rowland: I wanted to make a point about these intervention trials with fibre on patients with adenomas, essentially testing the hypothesis that fibre is affecting promotion of the tumours. A lot of the theories about how fibre is acting in colon cancer are based on it interfering with initiation events. I do not know how to study that. But I think it is important not to throw away the hypothesis that fibre may be important in colon cancer, if these intervention trials on these people do not turn out to show an effect.

Kritchevsky: In rats, different fibres have different effects, when comparing initiation and promotion.

Truswell: If you are looking at both development of new adenomas and conversion of existing adenomas to carcinomas, you are looking at both initiation and promotion.

Johnson: I think there is evidence to show that patients with adenomas have a relatively high rate of mitosis throughout the mucosa of the colon. If that is the case it could be that the appropriate endpoint to look at is not the adenoma, but just look with biopsies at an index of mitosis per crypt.

Heaton: Can we turn to diverticular disease for a moment and discuss the question of whether diverticular disease is a disease of fibre deficiency or a disease of ageing or a bit of both? Martin Eastwood's view is that it is primarily a disease of ageing, and he has done ingenious experiments to support this. He has taken operative specimens of human colon and distended them until they burst and shown that differences in bursting tendency relate to age. I am not sure if these experiments tell us a lot about the natural disease, which develops more subtly, quietly and slowly. In addition, elderly Africans do not seem to have diverticular disease.

Truswell: Are you talking about disease or post-mortem appearance in people of 90?

Heaton: I am talking about the pathology. Symptoms of colonic dysfunction (so-called symptomatic diverticular disease) and the pathology have very little to do with each other. If it is correct that the elderly African has not been getting diverticular disease and if it is also true, as Denis Burkitt has published, that black Americans do get diverticular disease as much as the whites, then I think that does throw some doubt on the idea that ageing *per se* is the main cause.

Edwards: I think some of the animal studies done in Edinburgh recently suggest that fibre is acting to delay the ageing process in the colon. Therefore, may be if you just wait long enough in the Africans . . .

Read: It does depend how many rural Africans of 80 to 90 one is able to study, because you are really talking about the rural African, not necessarily the urban African.

Heaton: Yes, but most urban Africans were rural Africans for most of their lives, weren't they?

Cummings: I guess that is true for the older ones. I was in Soweto where there are two million people and there are a lot of first and second generation indigenous Sowetans now. But there are populations that did move in from the homelands originally and they were elderly.

The other interesting thing about the Africans in South Africa is that their intake of cell wall material is very little different from ours, but they have enormously high starch intakes.

Heaton: So, you do believe then that starch does things to the colon.

Cummings: I think there is increasing evidence that is does, yes. But it may not be quite the same as the cell wall effects.

Truswell: It would not take long to write letters to experienced pathologists in different countries in Africa and ask this question: how many Africans eating rural diets come to post-mortem examination with and without diverticulae.

Mauron: Is there something known about diverticular disease in traditional Inuits who eat a very low carbohydrate diet with much fat and protein?

Heaton: I do not think that anything has been written about it. But not many traditional Inuits live into their seventies and eighties, because of the rather harsh life they have to lead.

Kritchevsky: If there are no other burning comments or questions, I would like to conclude this discussion and, in fact, the whole workshop. At this stage it does not seem necessary to draw other conclusions than those contained in the individual chapters which we have already discussed thoroughly and commented on. Let me therefore just thank everybody for their active participation in this workshop.

Subject Index

Absorption
  of nutrients, *see* Carbohydrates, Lipids,
    Minerals
  of SCFA 138
Absorptive site in presence of viscous
    polysaccharides 106–7
Acetate metabolism 141–2, 145
Acetic acid 124, 203
Acetyl-CoA 142, 146, 150
Acid detergent fibre (ADF) 9, 67, 155
Adenomas 344, 347
Adenomatous polyps 344
Adsorption of organic molecules 32–3
Amino acids, catabolism 124–5
Amylolytic enzymes 63
Amylopectin 60, 284
Amylose 44, 284
Amylose-lipid complexes 34
Analysis 8–9, 57–100
  AOAC method 69–73, 89, 92, 100, 335–7,
    339
  choice of method for carbohydrates in
    foods 64
  collaborative studies 85–93
  comparison of methods 72
  requirements of research and regulation 65,
    336–7
  criteria for choice of method 65
  Englyst method 76–82, 90–1, 339
  individual components of dietary
    fibre 75–84
  inter-method comparisons 91–3
  main features of strategies 63–4
  performance criteria 85
  Uppsala method 76–9, 336
  see also under specific methods
Antinutrients 285
AOAC method 69–70, 72, 73, 89, 92, 100,
    335–7, 339
Appendicitis 10, 11, 252–3
Appetite 270
Ascorbic acid 203
Asp et al. method 69, 72
Atherosclerosis 9

Bacteroides fragilis 122
Bacteroides thetaiotaomicron 120, 123
Bacteroides spp. 123
Ballastoffe 9
Beans 320
Bifidobacterium bifidum 122
Bile acids 11, 32, 33, 113, 171, 180, 217–18,
    303, 341
  biliary 220–3
  binding 111–12, 171
  binding capacity 33
  faecal 223–8, 316
  metabolism 12, 217–31
    relation with other dietary factors 223
  output and faecal concentration 219
  studies on effect of dietary fibre 220–7
  synthesis and degradation 218
Blood pressure 274
Bran 24, 171, 199, 200, 220, 311, 324, 342, 344
  see also under specific cereals
Bran particles, laxative action 113–14
Bread 12
Butyrate 124, 131, 259
Butyrate metabolism 144–5

Cabbage 159
Calcium 344–5
Caloric value, *see* Energy content
Cancer 344
  colonic, *see* Colonic cancer
  colorectal, *see* Colorectal cancer
  large bowel 257–9
  prevention study 344
Carbamoylphosphate synthase (CPS) 143–4
Carbohydrates
  apparently digestible 62
  available 5, 6, 60, 62
  categories 335
  classification of 57–62
  complex 58
    see also polysaccharides
  developments in chemistry and analysis of 4

digestion and absorption   181–96
  acute effects of dietary fibre on factors
      affecting   182
  chronic effects of dietary fibre on factors
      affecting   190–2
  direct measurement of   6
  lente   190
  low molecular weight   122
  malabsorption   189–90
  nomenclature for   61
  nutritional studies   5–7
  physiological role   3
  proximate system for   6
  role in foods   16
  slow absorption   189–90
  unavailable   5, 6, 8, 10, 11, 13, 15, 73–5
Cardiovascular disease   11
Cation-exchange capacity (CEC)
  determination of   23
  values of   23–5
Celery fibres   29
Cellulose   7–9, 44, 121, 156, 171, 174, 198,
      316–17
Cellulose fibrils   43
Cell wall, see Plant cell wall
Cereal-based diets   204
Cereal brans   24
Cereal fibres   23, 25
Cereal foods   9, 12
Cereals   199, 201, 239
Chemical treatments   33–4
Chenodeoxycholic acid (CDCA)   217–18
Chitosan   171
Cholate   251
Cholesterol   14, 180, 295–8, 303, 309, 316–19,
      322–4, 346
  synthesis inhibition by propionate   150
  see also HDL cholesterol, LDL cholesterol
Cholesterol saturation index (CSI)   220
Cholic acid (CA)   217–18, 220
Chyme   51
Citric acid   203
Cocoa   199
Colon   112–15
  adaptation to fibre   115
  human models   125–7
  proximal   126
  transit time   113
  transverse   126
Colonic bacteria   115, 119–20, 123–5, 235, 237,
      303
Colonic cancer   218–19, 258, 344, 347
  protective effect   219
  resistant starch in   219
Colonic contents   161
  in vivo dialysis   126
Colonic dysfunction   347
Colonic fermentation   54, 119–132
Colonic function   127, 234, 235
Colonic microflora   119
Colonic motility   125, 345

Colonic propulsion   113
Colonic SCFA   127
Colonic secretion   113
Colonocytes   138
Colorectal cancer   10, 11, 12
  dietary factors   218
Colorimetric analytical procedures   7, 73,
      78–79
Colostomy   127
Constipation   6, 11, 115, 250, 253–5, 259,
      345–6
Conventional dietary fibre   334–5
Coronary heart disease (CHD)   9, 10, 13, 295
Crohn's disease   252
Crude fibre   4, 8
  analysis of   66–7
Curdlan   44
Cyamopsis tetragonoloba   303

Degree of polymerisation (DP)   71
Deoxycholate   251
Deoxycholic acid (DCA)   217–18, 220, 222,
      223, 228
Detergent fibre methods   8–9, 67
Dextran   44
D-galactose   186
Diabetes mellitus   5, 10–12, 274, 292–3, 344
  high-carbohydrate high-fibre diet   282, 283
  insoluble fibres   281–2
  metabolic effects of fibre   280–3
  prevention and treatment   279–93
  soluble fibres   281
  studies including fibre and effect of
      processing   286–7
Diet
  and incidence of chronic disease   3
  fibre as protective component   9–10
  supplementation with non-starch
      polysaccharides   107–8
  supplementation with viscous
      polysaccharides   109
Dietary fibre
  as energy source   14–15
  as protective component of diet   9–10
  conventional   334–5
  definition   13, 19, 62, 334–5
  effects on eating behaviour   270
  increased intakes of   15
  intake benefits of   21
  mode of action in weight control   269, 271–3
  purified sources   157
  use of term   14
Dietary fibre hypothesis   3–19
  critique of   12
  historical perspective   3–19
  major themes in initial development
      of   13–16
  status of   16
Diffusion rates   186–8

Digestible energy (DE) 236
  estimation of 237–9
Digestion
  of dietary fibre, *see* Fermentation
  of nutrients, *see* Carbohydrates, Lipids,
      Protein
Dimeric egg-box structures 44
Dimethylsulphoxide (DMSO) 77, 80, 340, 341
Directive on Nutritional Labelling 339
Disaccharides 335
Diverticular disease 10, 11, 256–7, 344, 347,
    348
Duodenal ulcer 250, 263

Eating behaviour 270
Electrostatic binding 53
Embden–Meyerhof pathway 123
Energy content 237, 342
Energy conversion factors 8
Energy intake 269–70
Energy metabolism 15
Energy source, dietary fibre as 14–15
Energy values 4–5, 146–7, 236–43, 246, 342–3
  of carbohydrates 8
  of SCFA 146
Englyst methods 76–82, 90–1, 339
Enzymatic-gravimetric methods 68, 70–2
  correction for minerals 72
  protein degradation 71
  resistant starch 70–1
Enzymatic methods 67–9
Enzyme inhibitors 285
Enzyme-substrate interaction, reduction
      of 185–6
Enzymes
  involved in polysaccharide degradation 123
  polysaccharide susceptibility to 54
European Community 339
Extrusion cooking 34, 35, 207

Faecal analysis 127
Faecal bulking 7, 15–16, 233–6
  effect of particle size 234
  effect of physico-chemical properties 234–5
  mechanisms of action 235–6
  personality factors in 235
Faecal energy losses 239
Faecal output 6, 254
Faecal weight 234, 259
Fat content in diet 219
Fat intake 13
Fatty acids 113, 303
  volatile, *see* Short chain fatty acids (SCFA)
Fermentation 111, 114, 115, 119, 137–50, 208,
    236, 237, 303
  animal models 127–8
  by gut bacteria 120–3
  continuous and semi-continuous culture
      systems 130–1

gaseous products of 125
  measurement in vitro 128–32
  measurement in vivo 125–8
  products 123–5
  static in vitro systems 129–30
  studies of 131–2
Fibre, *see* Dietary fibre
Flatulence 6, 114
Food industry 323
Food preparation effects 110–11
Food processing 200, 207–8
  in diabetes mellitus 286–7
Forages, indigestible fraction in 9
Fruits and fruit fibres 6, 23–4, 205, 239, 255,
    322, 323

Galacturonic acid 22, 318
Gallstones 12, 250–1, 344
Gas-liquid chromatography (GLC) 7, 64, 73,
    75, 77, 79, 82, 90–2
Gas production 114, 125, 129, 130, 137
Gaseous products 236
  fermentation 125
Gastric emptying 104–5, 182–90
Gastric filling 183
Gastro-intestinal contents, viscosity of 103–7
Gastro-intestinal disease 12
Gastro-intestinal disorders
  prevention and treatment of 249–63
Gastro-intestinal physiology and function 103–
    17
Gastro-intestinal tract 153, 182, 341
  viscosity in 107–8
Gastro-oesophageal reflux 249
Gelatinisation 63
Gluconeogenesis 143
Glucose 6, 182, 187, 188
  absorption 139
  metabolism 283
Glucuronic acid 22–3
Glycaemia 281
Glycaemic index 110, 280
Glycaemic responses 279–80, 284
Gravimetric methods 9, 63–5, 89–90, 340
Grinding 33
Guar gum 14, 52, 53, 121, 124, 156, 171, 173,
    184, 186, 189, 281, 292, 303–9
Gum acacia 317
Gum arabic 124, 317

Haemorrhoids 11
HDL cholesterol 298, 303, 309, 316, 323–4
Heat treatment 34, 207
Helicobacter pylori 250
Hemicelluloses 7, 120, 155
Hexoses 235
Hiatus hernia 11, 249–50
High-carbohydrate high-fibre diet 282, 283

High-performance liquid chromatography
    (HPLC)   64, 82–4
HMG-CoA reductase   146, 150
    inhibitors of   323
Hunger   270
Hydration properties   26–32
    determination of   27–9
    polysaccharides   26–7
Hydration value
    examples   31
    variations associated with method used   29–
        30
Hydrogen   114, 125–7, 129, 136
Hydrolysis products   200
Hyperlipidaemias   33
    prevention and treatment of   295–332
Hypertension and obesity   273–4

Ilectomy   341
Ileostomy   107, 127, 180, 303
Insoluble components   79
Insoluble fibres   80, 91, 281
Insulin   182, 279, 282
Intestinal absorption rates   186–8
Intestinal mixing, reduction of   105–6
Intestinal motility   188–9
Intestinal transit   106–7
Intrinsic viscosity   47
Ion-binding to fibres   24
Ion-exchange chromatography   7
Ion-exchange properties   21–5
Ionic moieties of fibres   22
Iron
    absorption   201, 202, 205–6, 210–11
    bio-availability   204
    solubility   209
Irritable bowel syndrome (IBS)   255–6, 344
Ispaghula   115, 121, 124, 318

Karaya gum   124, 317
Klason lignin   33, 64, 78

Labelling   338–40, 342
Lactic acid   111, 203, 208
Lactulose   124, 126
Large bowel cancer   257–9
Large bowel disease   16
Large intestine, methane production in   136
Laxative action   6, 7, 113–114, 255
LDL-cholesterol   298, 303, 309, 316, 323–4
Legumes   205, 318–22
Lignin   6, 8, 9, 16, 62, 78, 84, 156, 171, 198–9,
    210, 317, 332
    see also Klason Lignin, Permanganate Lignin
Limiting viscosity number   47
Linoleic acid   338–9
Lipase activity, inhibition   169–71
Lipid binding capacity   32

Lipid digestion and absorption   167–79
    adaptation to prolonged fibre intake   174–6
    binding effects of fibre   171–2
    cellular phase   174–6
    inhibitory effects of dietary fibre   169–71
    intraluminal lipid transport   172–4
    mechanisms of   167–8
Lipid metabolism   145–6
Lipid transport, intraluminal   172–4
Lipids   344
Lipolytic activity, inhibition,   169–71
Lithocholic acid (LCA)   217–18, 222, 228
Locust bean gum   317
Luminal contents   53
Luminal mixing   187

MAFF   90–1, 99–100
Malabsorption   189–90
Malic acid   203
Malting   208
Mark–Houwink relationship   47
Metabolic effects   280–3
Metabolisable energy (ME)   236–7, 246
    calculation of   241–3
    estimation of   237–9
    fibre-rich diets   241–3
Methane production   114, 125, 129
    in large intestine   136
4-O-methyl glucuronic acid   22, 23
α-methyl-D-glucoside   186
Micelles, formation and composition   171–2
Mineral absorption and utilisation   197–215,
    343
    effects of fibre and fibre-associated
        compounds in humans   198–207
    fibre-rich diets   204–5
    implementation of present knowledge by food
        industry and legislative bodies   211
    influence of food processing   207–8
    influence of phytate   343–4
    interactions between dietary
        components   205–6
    methodological considerations in studies in
        humans   197–8
    prediction using animal models   210
    prediction using in vitro studies   208–9
Monosarccharides   5, 7, 42, 64
Motility
    small intestinal   188–9
    colonic   125, 345
Mucilages   121
Mucins   122
Mucopolysaccharides   123
Mucosa   137
Mucus production   175–6

Neutral Detergent Fibre (NDF)   9, 67, 160
Newtonian behaviour   48
Nitrogen digestibility   153–4

Normal Acid Fibre method   9
Nuclear magnetic resonance (NMR)   7
Nutrient absorption   175
  degree of   107
  in small bowel   127
  in small intestine   103–12
  reduction by non-starch
        polysaccharides   109–12
Nutrient displacement   109–10
Nutrient transport and release   53–4
Nutritional Labelling, Directive on   339

Oat bran   171, 311, 324
Oat fibre   309–16
Oat meal   311
Obesity   10, 11, 251, 276–7, 344
  an hypertension   273–4
  fibre trial design problems   265–7
  indicators of treatment success   267–8
  modes of action of dietary fibre   268
  prevalence of   265
  prevention and treatment of   265–77
Oligosaccharides   74, 122, 335, 336
  polymerisation degree   58
  removal of   63
Organic acids   203, 208
Organic molecules, adsorption of   32–3
Oro-caecal transit time   188
Oxalic acid   203

Partial digestibel energy values   237–9
Particles, direct irritant effect   113–14
Pectic substances   77
Pectins   14, 32, 120, 171, 184–7, 199, 296,
        298–303, 332, 342
Permanganate lignin   64
pH values   27, 53–4
Phenolic acids   84
Phenolic compounds   203, 209
Phosphoenolpyruvate carboxykinase
        (PEPCK)   143
Phospholipids, binding of   171
Physico-chemical properties   333
Phytate   199, 203, 206–7, 209, 343, 344
  as inhibitor of mineral absorption   199–207
  in cereals and legumes   199–203
Phytic acid   23, 200, 342
pK value, determination of   25–6
Placebo preparations   265–7
Plant cell wall   7, 9, 10, 11, 13, 15, 16, 61, 64,
        72, 120, 153, 332, 340
  effect of material processing   33–4
  network structure   21
  physico-chemical properties   21–39
  polysaccharides   62
Plant gums   120
Plantago ovata   14, 318
  see also Ispaghula
Plasma lipids   295, 296
Polyphenols   203, 209

Polysaccharides   3, 5, 7, 8, 16, 19, 20, 36, 55–6,
        334–6, 342
  additives   56
  available   58
  chain structure and shape   41–2
  charged   53
  classification of   57, 58–61
  co-existence of ordered and disordered
        regions   46
  coil dimensions   48
  coil overlap and entanglement, c*   48–50
  constant of proportionality   48, 51
  degradation   123
  experimental studies   14
  extrinsic   59
  hydrated networks   45–6
  hydration properties   26–7
  hydrodynamic volume of disordered
        chains   47–8
  implications for digesta viscosity   51–2
  industrial   56
  inter-residue linkage patterns   43–5
  intrinsic   58
  isolated   14, 15, 101
  molecular size   52
  natural   56, 101
  neutral   82–3
  nomenclature   61
  non-cellulosic   57
  non-digestible   60
  non-starch   61, 79, 90–1, 103–17, 125, 169,
        198–9, 210, 334
  order and disorder   42–5
  physico-chemical properties   41–55
  physiological boundaries   61
  polymerisation degree   58
  random coil   50
  shear-rate dependence of viscosity   50–1
  solubility   43
  soluble   55
  storage   58, 121
  susceptibility to cleavage by enzymes   54
  true gels   47
  viscous   53, 104–7, 109, 188
  weak gels   47, 51
  zero shear value   48
Polyunsaturated fat   338
Propionate   124
  inhibition on cholesterol synthesis   111, 150
  metabolism   142–4
Propionyl-CoA   143–4
Protein
  cell wall bound   155
Protein binding capacity   59–60
Protein catabolism   124–5
Protein digestion and utilisation   153–65
  experiments with humans   159–61
  experiments with pigs   157–9
  experiments with rats   154–7
Pseudopolasticity index   51
Psyllium   318

Quality control   337

Radio telemetric pills   126
Radioisotope techniques   210
Raffinose   335
Random coil behaviour   42
Regulatory analyses   337–8
Rheological properties of whole foods
      108–9
Roughage   5, 6
Ruminococcus   122
Rye flour   207

Safflower   339
Satiation   270
Satiety   270
Seaman method   64
Sequestration effects   110, 113
Shear-thinning   50
Short chain fatty acids (SCFA)   123–4, 126,
      127, 129–31, 137–50
   and glucose absorption   139
   and lipid metabolism   145–6
   energy contribution   146
   hepatic metabolism   139–45
   metabolism by digestive tract   137–8
   plasma concentrations   139
   uptake by liver cells   140
Sliding hiatus hernia   250
Small bowel, nutrient absorption in, 127
Small intestine
   digestion and absorption   105–107, 185–90
   nutrient absorption in   103–12
   transit and motor activity   188–9
   transit time   106, 188, 235–6
Soaking   207
Solubility   36
Soluble fibres   91, 145, 155, 281
Southgate method   73–5
   limitations   75
   performance   74
   principles   74
Soya beans   319
Specific viscosity   50
Stachyose   335
Starch(es)   6, 8, 348
   available   336
   characteristics   284–5
   effects of mechanical processing   285
   effects of thermal processing   284–5
   granules   43
   nature of   284
   nomenclature   61
   resistant   122, 124, 219, 336
   unabsorbed   190
Steroids adsorption   33

Stool output   112, 234
Stool production, psychological factors in   235
Stool weight   233, 258, 346
   variations in   235
Succinylsulphathiazole   303
Sugar alcohols   16
Sugar beet fibres   30, 34
Sugars   6, 8, 58, 74
   removal of   63
Sulphate reducing bacteria (SRB)   136
Sunflower   339
Swelling   27, 29, 30

Tartaric acid   203
Termamyl-enzyme incubation   77
Total dietary fibre (TDF)   89–90
   AOAC method for   69–70
Triglycerides   316, 324
True protein digestibility (TD)   154–5

Uppsala method   76–9, 336
Ureogenesis   143
Uronic acids   22, 25, 64, 77, 78, 80, 83–4, 235

Vegetables and vegetable fibres   6, 23, 205,
      239, 255, 322, 323
Villous atrophy   111
Villous height   175
Viscosity of gastro-intestinal contents   103–7
Vitamin B$_{12}$ 143, 341
Vitamin C   338, 339
Vitamin D   199

Water, *see* Hydration properties
Water-binding capacity (WBC)   27–9, 35, 235
Water-holding capacity (WHC)   29
Water-soluble components   79
Weende crude fibre procedure   66–7
Weight loss   271–3, 282
Weight reduction   292
Wheat bran   35, 156, 171, 207, 255
   see also Bran
Wheat fibre   296–8
Wheat flours   9
Whole foods   322–3
Whole wheat flour   207
Wholemeal rye bread   280

Xanthan gum   54, 115, 317
Xylose   189

Zinc absorption   204–6, 210–11